*To Stephanie,
Hoping this will help you & happy for many years extra.
Arnold V. Page   20 Feb 2015.*

Twenty-First Century Nutrition and Family Health

How to raise a healthy family in spite of everything!

Arnold V. Page

Published by New Generation Publishing in 2015

Copyright © Arnold V. Page 2014

First Edition

The author asserts the moral right under the Copyright, Designs and Patents Act 1988 to be identified as the author of this work.

All Rights reserved. No part of this publication may be reproduced, stored in a retrieval system or transmitted, in any form or by any means without the prior consent of the author, nor be otherwise circulated in any form of binding or cover other than that which it is published and without a similar condition being imposed on the subsequent purchaser.

ISBN 978-1-78507-177-5

www.newgeneration-publishing.com

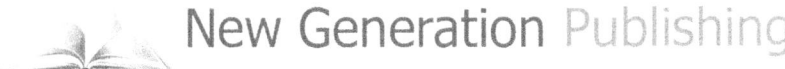

Dedicated to Dr. Mary G. Enig PhD

**who died aged 83 on September 8th 2014,
the week this book was completed.**

A Master of the American College of Nutrition, an editor of the Journal of the American College of Nutrition, and the co-founder of the Weston A. Price Foundation, Dr. Enig was a tireless, courageous and influential campaigner for the truth about healthy and unhealthy food.

CONTENTS

INTRODUCTION	1
CHAPTER 1: WHAT WE USED TO EAT	4
CHAPTER 2: FAT UNDER FIRE	7
CHAPTER 3: THE TRUTH ABOUT SATURATED FAT	23
CHAPTER 4: THE CAUSES OF HEART DISEASE	27
CHAPTER 5: A SICK NATION	34
CHAPTER 6: FATS – THE GOOD, THE BAD AND THE UGLY	48
CHAPTER 7: BATTLE OF THE OMEGAS	57
CHAPTER 8: SUGAR – THE SWEET ASSASSIN	79
CHAPTER 9: CARBOHYDRATES – A WOMAN'S WORST FRIEND	93
CHAPTER 10: CHOLESTEROL – NOT THE BIG BAD WOLF	99
CHAPTER 11: VITAMINS – CAN'T LIVE WITHOUT THEM	110
CHAPTER 12: MINERALS IN MELTDOWN	118
CHAPTER 13: DIETARY DEFICIENCIES	126
CHAPTER 14: ALLERGIES, INTOLERANCES, COELIAC DISEASE AND IBS	140
CHAPTER 15: ARE ORGANIC FOODS BETTER?	150
CHAPTER 18: INFERTILITY – ITS CAUSES AND CURE	179
CHAPTER 19: HOW TO LOSE WEIGHT AND KEEP IT OFF	193
CHAPTER 20: EXERCISE – IT'S WHAT WE WERE MADE FOR	201
CHAPTER 21: REST – NATURE'S MEDICINE	225
CHAPTER 23: A FAMILY HEALTH MANUAL	242
CHAPTER 24: THE COST OF GOOD HEALTH	258

Annexe 1: 3-day menu based on protein:fat:carbohydrate calorie percentages of 25:45:30 ... 262
Annexe 2: Recipes for the 3-day menu 267
Annexe 3: Nutrients, functions and sources 277
Annexe 4: Glycaemic loads produced by typical servings of common carbohydrate foods . 282
Annexe 5: Omega-3 content of marine foods 289
Annexe 6: Derivation of recommended fish oil consumption 295
Annexe 7: Microwaved food – noxious or nutritious? 298

Index 305

Figures

Figure 1: Deaths from coronary heart disease in the U.S.A., 1900-1968 8
Figure 2: Correlation of heart disease and fat consumption, Ancel Keys, six countries 9
Figure 3: Correlation of heart disease and fat consumption, Ancel Keys, all 22 countries ... 11
Figure 4: Margarine consumption and deaths from coronary heart disease in the U.S.A., 1900-2000 11
Figure 5: Annual per capita consumption of butter in the U.S.A. 12
Figure 6: Relationship between stress and disease 30
Figure 7: Trends in adult obesity, U.S.A. and England, 1962-2012 36
Figure 8: Trends in childhood obesity, U.S.A. and England, 1962-2012 37
Figure 9: Coronary heart disease death rates in England & Wales and the U.S.A., 1900-2011 39
Figure 10: Heart disease prevalence, and deaths from ischaemic heart disease, among adults aged 18 and over: U.S.A. 1997-2012 40
Figure 11: Patient admissions for coronary heart disease in England & Wales and number of prescriptions for coronary vascular disease in England: 1960-2010 41
Figure 12: Percentage of population in England and the U.S.A. with diagnosed diabetes, 1958-2010 42
Figure 13: Prevalence of liver cancer in Great Britain, 1975-2010 43
Figure 14: Prevalence of bowel cancer in Great Britain, 1975-2010 43
Figure 15: Fats as a percentage of total fat in some common foodstuffs 49
Figure 16: Association between percentage of omega-6 in highly unsaturated fatty acids and coronary heart disease death rates 61
Figure 17: Ratios of omega-6 to omega-3 for some common sources of fat 73
Figure 18: Ratios of omega-6 to omega-3 for potatoes and some common cereals 74
Figure 19: Relationships between percentage of national population with high cholesterol levels and death rates from coronary heart disease 109
Figure 20: Rates of renal cancer by latitude, 2002 112

Tables

Table 1: Minutes of exercise required to burn 500 kilocalories   5
Table 2: Recommended mixed oily and non-oily fish consumption necessary for cardiac and other health on a Western diet   65
Table 3: Percentage increase in base level of EPA, DHA and DPA in the blood after 12 weeks of omega-3 supplementation among four experimental groups of men   68
Table 4: Methods of obtaining a week's minimum recommended intake of 3,150mg EPA + DHA from fish or the equivalent benefit from oil, and some representative costs in the U.K.   69

Table 5:	Water contaminants and treatment methods	169
Table 6:	Some low energy-dense foods	197
Table 7:	Exercises for children under 5	211
Table 8:	Exercises for children from 5 to 18	212
Table 9:	Exercises for adults	214
Table 10:	Upper body exercises	216
Table 11:	Lower body exercises	217
Table 12:	Abdominal muscle (ABS) exercises	218
Table 13:	Strength-training programme	219
Table 14:	Estimated maximum heart rates by age	221
Table 15:	Recommended daily calorie intakes for children of different ages	246
Table 16:	Body Mass Index ranges for children	247
Table 17:	Guide to waist-to-hip ratios for adults	248
Table 18:	Guide to maximum healthy waist circumferences for children	249
Table A.1:	3-day, 1,823 calorie per day menu for one person based on protein:fat:carbohydrate calorie percentages of 25:45:30	262
Table A.2:	Recipes for the 3-day menu in Annexe 1	267
Table A.3:	The nature, functions, sources and effects of nutrients	282
Table A.4:	Glycaemic loads produced by typical servings of common carbohydrate foods	282
Table A.5.1:	Omega-3 content of marine foods, best sources, in mg per 140gm serving	290
Table A.5.2:	Omega-3 content of marine foods, excellent sources, in mg per 140gm serving	292
Table A.5.3:	Omega-3 content of marine foods, good sources, in mg per 140gm serving	294
Table A.6:	Derivation of recommended fish oil consumptions	295

INTRODUCTION

'*Of the tree of the knowledge of good and evil you shall not eat, for in the day that you eat of it you shall die.*'[1]

An apple itself probably never killed anyone, but much of the food that we consume today certainly is killing us. We've allowed ourselves to be persuaded that it's better to buy and eat foods that men have manufactured or produced artificially than the more natural foods on which people have lived throughout most of human history. Like Adam in the Garden of Eden, we think we know better than God. The result is that the nation's health is suffering and many people are dying prematurely. We die precisely because we do *not* know the difference between good and evil, between good food and bad food, and even when we do, we don't believe it matters enough to change our diet for the better.

Belief is a powerful ingredient in the recipe of life. Believing my daughter to be inside our burning house back in 1981 I went inside to find her without thought of personal safety. When my wife believed that our youngest son had swallowed some poisonous berries she immediately took him to an accident and emergency centre. What we believe determines what we do. The year that we all contracted food poisoning from some infected ice cream, did we continue to feed that same ice cream to our children? Of course we didn't. And if you believed that a certain food or drink would harm your children's health and might even kill them prematurely, would you continue to feed them with it? Of course you wouldn't, not if you really, really believed that it would harm them.

Perhaps your children are not among the one in three children who will be obese by the time they leave primary school and who, by definition, will suffer health problems as a result. Perhaps none of your family will contract the type 2 diabetes, which some children as young as eleven are getting, endangering their sight, heart and kidneys. Perhaps you are fully aware that much of dietary advice given by successive governments during the last 50 to 100 years has actually caused many of the public health problems that have arisen during the same period, and perhaps instead of following that advice you are feeding your children only things that people ate and drank in earlier generations when obesity, type 2 diabetes, coronary heart disease,

---

1 *The Holy Bible*. Genesis chapter 2, verse 17. Revised Standard Version, Collins, 1971.

many forms of cancer and even tooth decay were virtually non-existent.

Or maybe, just maybe, you have to stop believing the diet of falsehoods on which we have all been fed and you need to change dramatically what your family eats and drinks. If so, then somehow I have to make you believe this. For if you don't really believe it then you won't change anything.

Unfortunately it is very hard to change what anyone believes. I know how hard I have resisted changing my own beliefs about a number of major issues in life! It is especially difficult to do this in the areas of food and health, where multimillion dollar food producers and retailers and pharmaceutical companies are daily telling our government and us how their products are good for us, especially the products that make them the biggest profits. So how can I, one small voice, imagine that I can convince you that what they say isn't always the truth? Well, I managed to make the switch in my own thinking, so I'm going to do my best to help you to do the same, if you are willing to read on. I will do it by means of facts, explanations and some earnest prayers. I'll spare you the earnest prayers, but I'll back up every fact with sound supporting evidence, and I'll make my explanations as clear as I possibly can. I'll conclude by telling you how to feed your family in a way that will provide them with the healthiest possible start in life. Then you'll be able to give them a huge reason for being glad that they had you for a parent.

Nutritional science can be horrendously complex. As I was drafting this introduction I came across a research paper entitled, *Isolation of NF-E2-related factor 2 (Nrf2), a NF-E2-like basic leucine zipper transcriptional activator that binds to the tandem NF-E2/AP1 repeat of the beta-globin locus control region*. I'm not going to quote from that particular paper, because I haven't a clue what it was about either. I need you to understand what I am telling you, so if there is something that I feel I can't explain reasonably simply then I'll have to omit it.

By profession I am not a nutritionist but an engineering research scientist. Yet perhaps as an outsider to the subject of nutrition I have not been brainwashed into believing conventional wisdom, but can study the facts with scientific detachment and draw some more reliable conclusions from them. Having authored technical books, manuals and information sheets, and conducted nationwide seminars that consistently received 5-star feedback ratings, I can fairly claim that I am a professional at acquiring knowledge and presenting it in a useful form for the benefit of others. You can make your own judgement on that if you keep reading!

The prophet Daniel wrote that in the final days of this age knowledge would increase. That has certainly happened in our generation with the unbelievable explosion of information freely available on the Internet. What Daniel didn't say was that wisdom would also increase, and that certainly hasn't happened. Governments in the Western world have all been unwise in much of the dietary advice they have given, and most of us have been equally unwise in following that advice and in the way we have lived. It's my prayer that in these pages you will find the knowledge you need to provide yourself and your family with a truly healthy diet and lifestyle, and that you'll have the wisdom to put that knowledge into practice.

In preparing this material I owe a debt of gratitude to the many researchers and scientific institutions who have been willing to allow public access to their findings by publishing them on the Internet, in many cases without charge. That doesn't mean that everything one reads on the Internet is true: far from it. It must all be taken with a pinch of salt, but only a small one, because we are told we should all cut down on our salt intake…

CHAPTER 1: WHAT WE USED TO EAT

Much of the advice about healthy diets that the government and other bodies have been giving us has been wrong. When I was in primary school in the 1940s and 50s we fried our food in pork lard, ate beef dripping sandwiches, put butter on our bread and drank full-cream milk. Nowadays those are all foods that the government tells us to avoid; yet almost nobody was overweight, and we are the generation that is now living so long that pension funds have run out of money.

It is true that people used to take more exercise. Children were generally more active than today's kids are with their Xboxes and PlayStations and car lifts to school. Men worked as dustmen and coalmen and navvies, and women did housework without the benefit of washing machines and other gadgets. But even then not every adult was engaged in manual labour. Even in the 1950s most people who went to work spent their day in factories, shops, banks or offices, or they drove buses, trains or delivery vehicles. People spent most of their working day standing or sitting, as they do now, yet they were not fat.

Yet exercise doesn't have as big an effect on weight as one might suppose. When you exercise a lot you feel hungry, so unless you are very self-controlled you can end up eating more to compensate and thus don't lose any weight at all. When I was training with a team to climb the Welsh 3,000s some of us actually put on weight. No doubt it was extra muscle, but the fact is that we didn't all lose weight in spite of regular, strenuous exercise.

Even if you could lose weight by taking exercise it would take up a lot of time. A 'Big Mac', a deep-pan pizza or a helping of syrup sponge pudding and custard each contain about 500 calories. Table 1 shows that a British adult of 76kg average weight would have to walk up and down stairs for 66 minutes to burn off that amount of energy rather than store it as fat. For most adults 66 minutes of exercise would be an awful lot to fit into the day for every such treat they ate. Even a plain digestive biscuit provides enough fuel to climb up and down stairs for 10 minutes. That's how efficient our bodies are!

Of course exercise is important, which is why I still go jogging three times a week in my seventies. But I don't believe that people used to be slimmer just because they took more exercise than we do nowadays.

Table 1:   Minutes of exercise required to burn 500 kilocalories

Exercise	Your weight in kg				Your weight in lb			
	60kg	80kg	100kg	120kg	150lb	200lb	250lb	300lb
Basketball	62	46	37	32	55	41	33	28
Cycling	62	46	37	32	55	41	33	28
Dancing	83	62	50	42	73	55	44	37
Cross trainer	54	41	33	27	48	36	29	24
Gardening	100	75	60	50	88	66	53	44
Jogging	71	54	43	36	63	48	38	32
Running at 6 mph	50	39	31	25	44	34	27	22
Stairs	83	62	50	42	73	55	44	37
Swimming	63	48	39	32	56	42	34	28
Walking at 3 mph	143	108	86	71	126	95	76	63

So is the reason so many people are overweight now simply that they eat more than they used to? In Britain, and probably in other Western countries too, I think most people do eat more than their forebears did 50 or 100 years ago. In our own family half a pint of custard was enough for six people when I was a child: now it seems to serve only four or five. When our children were growing up a home-made meat loaf served six of us: now, for some reason, it is enough for only five servings. I think supermarkets bear most of the blame for this. They systematically encourage overeating and overdrinking by offering ever larger sizes of sausages, buns, chocolate bars and bottles of fruit juice; ever thicker slices of bread; and ever bigger pre-priced packs of cheese, potatoes, onions, tomatoes and grapes. Multibuy offers such as three for the price of two add to the pressure to buy more rather than less food than we really want or need. The extraordinarily low prices on alcoholic drinks, which all add to our weight, are major incentives to drink more than is good for us.

In spite of all that, I don't believe that we eat very much more than people used to eat, or that eating more is the principal reason for the population's increasing weight. Nowadays a health-conscious individual might have a cup of coffee, a glass of fruit juice and a low-fat yogurt for breakfast. More typically an individual might have a bowl of cereal and a slice of toast with marmalade or something savoury on it. But when my sisters and I went to school we always had for breakfast a bowl of porridge, followed by a boiled egg or scrambled egg or fried sausages or fried bacon and tomatoes, usually with fried bread. That wasn't less than a modern breakfast.

On schooldays we had a cooked school meal, which would always include meat or fish with two veg, followed by a dessert such as semolina and red jam that we called 'murder on the Alps', baked apple with currants where the core had been ('rabbits' lavatory'), tapioca ('frogspawn'), steamed pudding and custard, or perhaps apple crumble and custard. In the evening we'd have tea, which was mostly bread and butter, not bread and margarine, and not bread made by the Chorleywood process, which involves preservatives and other artificial materials. We'd also have home-made cakes of some kind (my mother's rock buns lived up to their name), and these were cooked, as most home-made and bakery cakes were cooked, with a mixture of butter and lard, at least until the end of the war. Once we started to go to secondary school we had a bowl of cereal and milk for supper. Oh! And a third of a pint of full-cream milk on schooldays, and a milky drink at supper time.

I can't remember what we ate for Saturday lunches (I probably never got up in time to find out) but on Sundays there was always a full roast dinner, usually with batter pudding, followed by a proper pudding such as plum duff (a pudding made with suet, which is made from beef fat, and from flour, breadcrumbs, currants and raisins), a rhubarb and apple crumble, a syrup pudding, a steamed fruit pudding, or something like that. The puddings were always with custard, which was generally green, pink or blue, since making the Sunday custard was my job. Even as a boy I believed that variety was the spice of life.

It's true that in our family we used to eat thin sliced bread. The thick sliced bread that most people buy nowadays we'd have called doorsteps, the kind that only road menders and boy scouts would have cut for themselves. But maybe because our bread was sliced thinly we ate more slices of it, especially at teatime, and that meant relatively more layers of butter and fish paste, Marmite or jam.

So I really don't believe that we ate much less than people eat nowadays. The main difference was that that we ate a different kind of food. We certainly didn't try to keep to a low-fat diet as bodies like the NHS and health charities keep telling us we should. So why do they tell us to do that? The answer is in Chapter 2.

CHAPTER 2: FAT UNDER FIRE

There are at least eight reasons why the government and other official bodies advise a low-fat diet or other unhealthy food choices, and none of them has a proper scientific basis.

Ancel Keys and saturated fat

The first reason goes back to a research paper published by an American scientist called Dr. Ancel Keys in 1953. Actually it goes back further than that to an experiment carried out in 1913 by a Russian scientist named Dr. Nikolai Anitschkow. He fed rabbits massive amounts of cholesterol, and the rabbits died of heart disease. This was, of course, a ridiculous experiment, because a rabbit's digestion system isn't designed to ingest cholesterol, any more than ours is designed to ingest grass. How long would we live if we ate nothing but grass?

By the early 1950s it was realized that a lot of people in the U.S.A. and similar countries were dying from coronary heart disease, or CHD. It's hard to believe this now, but before about 1930 in the U.S.A. and 1940 in the U.K. deaths from CHD were almost non-existent. There were other types of heart failure, but not the kind that happens as are result of artery-blocking blood clots. It was only in the middle of the last century that CHD deaths started to appear in any significant way in Western countries. If you have a look at Figure 1 you'll get the picture, in the U.S.A. at least.

CHD deaths in the U.K. followed a similar pattern to the U.S.A., but perhaps 10 years later. After 1968 the numbers of deaths in both countries started to diminish, but this was because diagnosis and treatment improved, not because heart disease itself became less common. In fact the number of people actually suffering from heart disease has remained more or less constant since then.

Figure 1: Deaths from coronary heart disease in the U.S.A., 1900-1968[2]

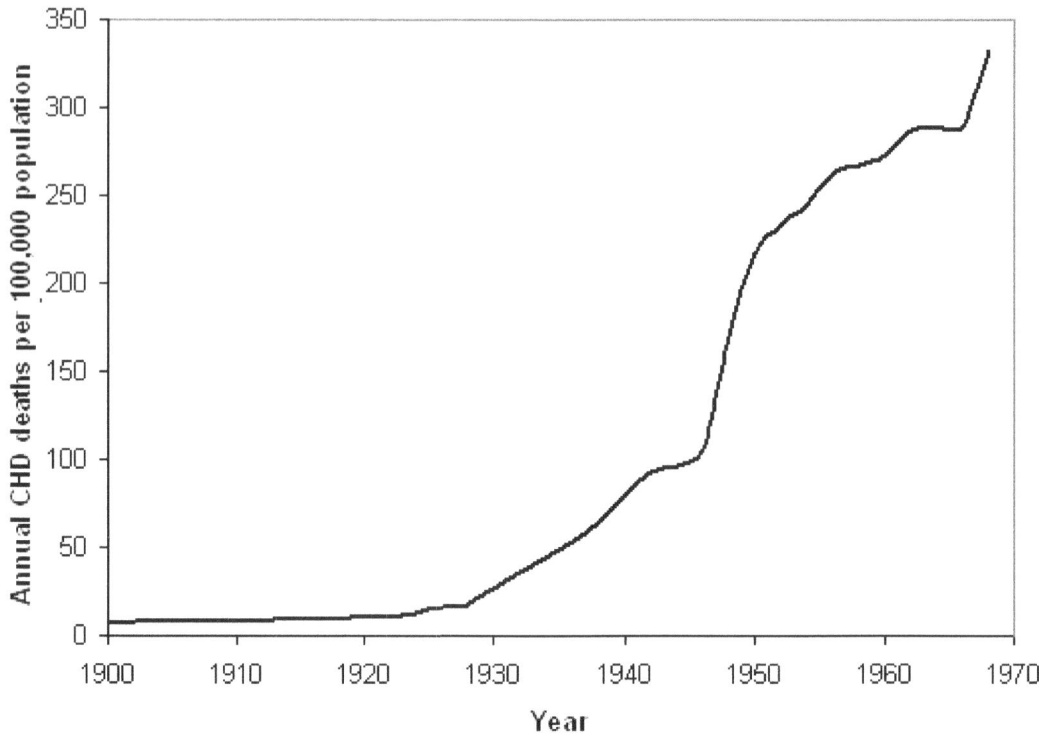

Dr. Keys was naturally concerned about what was causing so many people to die from heart disease, so he travelled to various countries where the rates of death from CHD were known and he recorded the kinds of diet that people ate. He was convinced that the epidemic must have something to do with diet, and in that respect he was right. What he discovered was that in six countries with wide differences in their diet there was a direct relationship between the number of people dying from heart disease and the percentage of their total calories that they obtained from fat. Since the U.S.A. topped the list of both fat consumption and heart disease while Japan was at the opposite end of the scale he concluded that eating too much fat was what was causing heart disease. Here in Figure 2 is the original graph that he published in 1953.[3]

---

2   Reproduced from Colpo A. *The Great Cholesterol Con* 2010. Figures were extracted from *Vital Statistics of the United States.* Centers for Disease Control and Prevention, National Center for Health Statistics. Available online at www.cdc.gov/nchs/products/vsus.htm#natab2003.

3   Keys A. *Atherosclerosis: a problem in newer public health. Journal of Mount Sinai Hospital*, 1953; 20:118.

Figure 2: Correlation of heart disease and fat consumption, Ancel Keys, six countries[4]

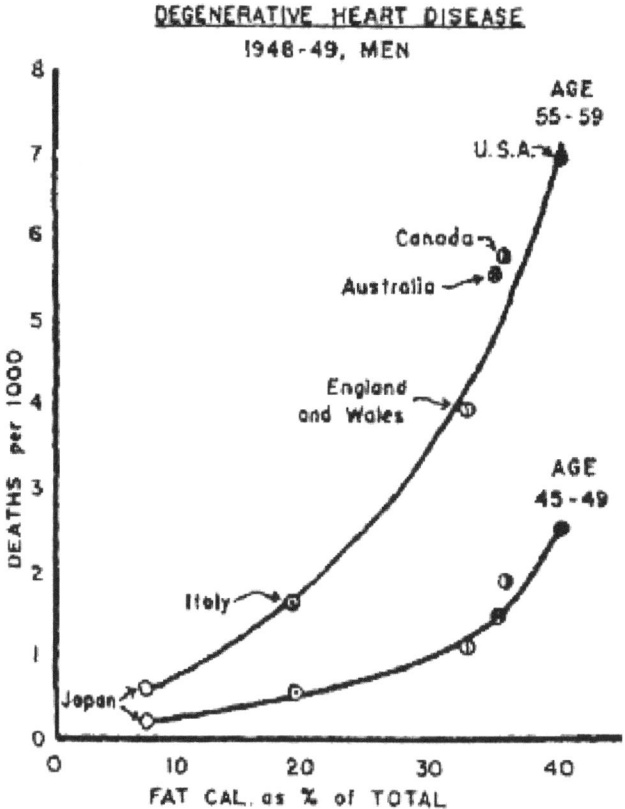

However, Keys's conclusion that eating fat caused heart disease was wrong for three reasons.

First, an association between the two things doesn't prove anything in itself. If he had plotted sugar consumption against heart disease in those same countries he would have obtained a similar graph, and this would have 'proved' that it was sugar that caused heart disease. But if you look carefully you'll see that what the graph actually proves is that speaking English is the cause of CHD. From an American's point of view the further up the slope you go the better English you speak, so it is obvious from the graph that speaking English is what kills people! Clearly, an association can never prove that one thing causes another, unless somehow all other possible causes can be eliminated. However a *lack* of association can *disprove* a causal relationship. For example, if Dr. Keys had found that in China people ate even more fat in their fried food than Americans did, yet had little or no heart disease, this would have proved that eating fat does *not*

---

[4] Reproduced by Yerushalmy J & Hilleboe H E in *Fat in the diet and mortality from heart disease: a methodologic note*. New York State Journal of Medicine, July 15, 1957; 57(14):2343-54.

cause heart disease (or, to be precise, that it doesn't if you are an average Chinaman living in China on a typical Chinese diet).

And that is the second reason that Keys's conclusion was wrong. For there were, and are, at least half a dozen countries where a lack of association between diet and heart disease disproves his conclusion. In the early 1960s, Professor George Mann of Vanderbilt University visited the Masai tribe of Kenya in the hope of confirming Keys's theory. He went there because the diet of this tribe consisted entirely of milk and meat. They ate no vegetables whatsoever and consumed excessive amounts of saturated fat. But in direct contradiction to Keys's theory, they had no incidence of heart disease and their cholesterol levels were 50% lower than those of Americans![5] This couldn't have happened if eating animal fat caused heart disease. Again, people in northern India consume seventeen times more animal fat than people in southern India but they have an incidence of CHD seven times lower.[6] And in Europe, French people eat more dairy fat per head than in any other industrialized nation, yet until recently France had the second lowest rate of CHD in the industrialized world, behind Japan.

Thirdly, and perhaps most damning of all, Keys didn't report all the evidence he found, such as the data from France. When you look at all 22 countries that Keys studied, the association between deaths from heart disease and diet is far less obvious. Figure 3 shows a plot of all his original data points.

As you can see, it's now impossible to draw a neat curve through all the points. Basically Keys was reporting only the evidence that supported his theory.

His chicanery did not pass unnoticed. Jacob Yerushalmy and Herman Hilleboe, two other researchers, published all his data 4 years later, but by then it was too late to undo the damage. Keys had got a picture of himself on the cover of '*Time*' magazine and the margarine and cooking oil manufacturers were publicizing his findings as fast as they could, to persuade consumers that fat made from vegetable sources was healthier than animal fats, which were the kinds most commonly eaten by the people Keys had studied.

The truth is that eating saturated fat, the kind of fat found mostly in meat and dairy products, doesn't cause heart disease, as demonstrated by populations in Africa, India and France. However, there are other kinds of fat that might be a cause. Unsaturated fats are the kinds that come mostly from plant seed oils such as sunflowers, maize ('corn' in North America), oilseed rape (or 'canola') and soya (or 'soy'). And trans fats, sometimes called hydrogenated fats, are plant oils that have been artificially thickened to make them spreadable like margarine and to last longer before going rancid. Too much unsaturated fat and trans fat are almost certainly a cause of heart disease. Margarine is made mainly from seed oils and for many years it contained trans fats. Here's a graph showing the consumption of margarine and deaths from coronary heart disease in the U.S.A.

---

5   Mann G V et al. *Atherosclerosis in the Masai*. American Journal of Epidemiology, 1972; 95:26-37.

6   Malhotra S L. *Epidemiology of ischaemic heart disease in India with special reference to causation*. British Heart Journal, 1967; 29: 895-905.

Figure 3: Correlation of heart disease and fat consumption, Ancel Keys, all 22 countries[7]

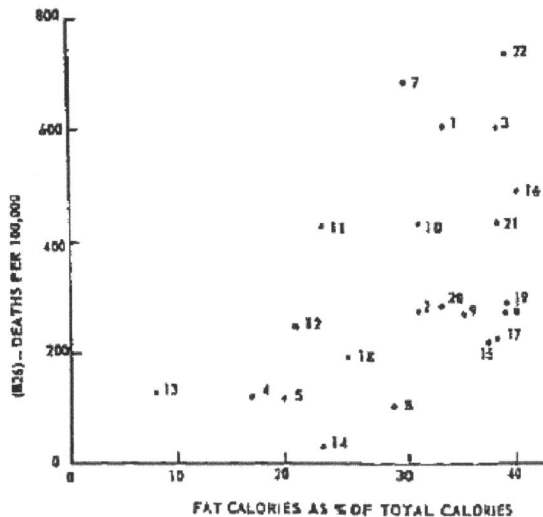

Figure 4: Margarine consumption and deaths from coronary heart disease in the U.S.A., 1900-2000[8]

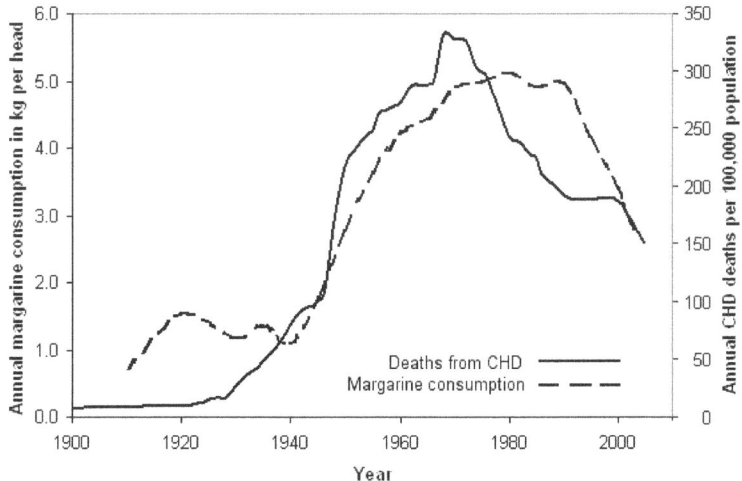

---

7   Reproduced by J Yerushalmy and H E Hilleboe in *Fat in the diet and mortality from heart disease: a methodologic note*. New York State Journal of Medicine, July 15, 1957; 57(14): 2343-54. (Also cited previously.)

8   CHD deaths extracted from *Vital Statistics of the United States*, Centers for Disease Control and Prevention, National Center for Health Statistics. Margarine consumption from USDA Economic Research Service 2004.

The two curves look remarkably similar, don't they? They certainly made me question the idea that margarine is healthier than butter. All right, I know I said that an association, even a remarkably close one like this, doesn't prove a cause. But if one thing does cause another then there will be an association, so Figure 4 certainly suggests that eating margarine might be a cause of CHD. More importantly, as I said just now, a lack of association can *disprove* a causal link. So what the next figure, Figure 5, proves is that eating butter, which is mostly saturated fat, *does not cause heart disease*.

Figure 5: Annual per capita consumption of butter in the U.S.A.[9]

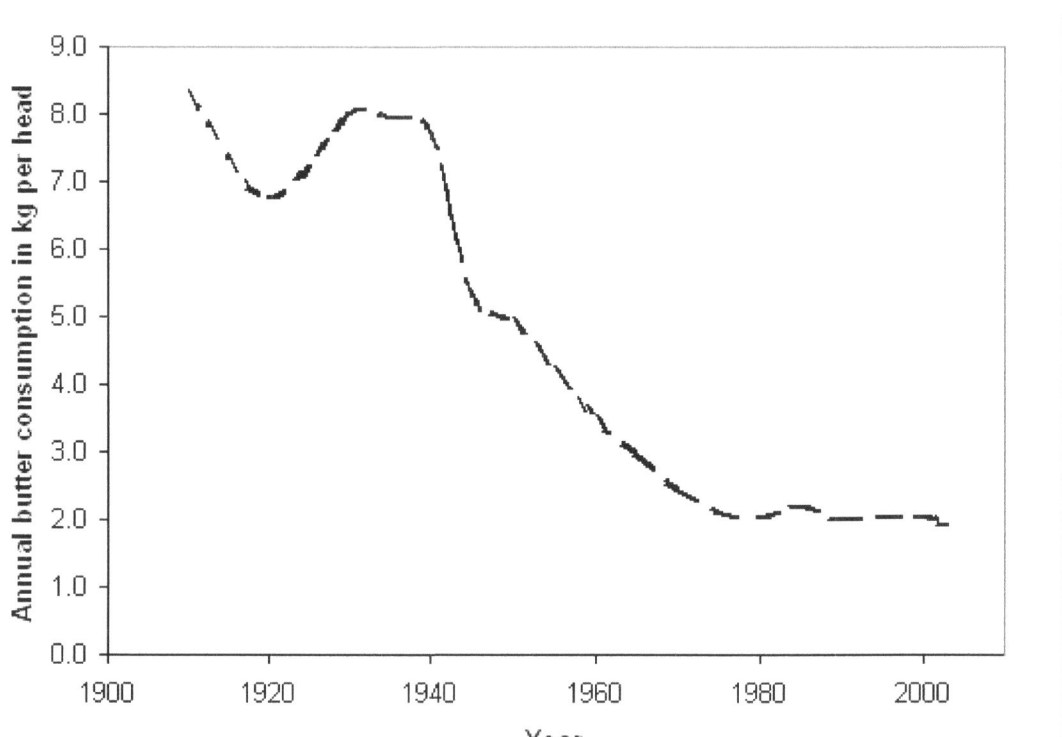

There was almost no heart disease when people were eating an average of 8kg of butter a year, yet when butter consumption fell by 75% coronary heart disease rose dramatically over exactly the same period. If eating butter were the cause of heart disease then the rate of heart disease would have fallen as butter consumption fell. But the opposite happened. So don't blame butter if you get a heart attack!

In support of this, a U.K. Medical Research Council survey in 1991 showed that men eating butter ran half the risk of developing heart disease as those using margarine.[10]

---

9   USDA Economic Research Service, 2004.

10 Nutrition Week, March 22, 1991; 21:12:2-3.

I wish that butter producers would have the courage to label their products as 'heart health*ier*' with *two* heart symbols on them!

Bad advice comes from bad advisors

Once again this raises the question, why are we still told that we should avoid eating butter and other saturated fats? As I said earlier, there are at least eight reasons. The first, as I have already explained, was Ancel Keys's false theory and all the publicity he generated for it.

A second reason is that most government ministers aren't experts on whatever they are ministers of, especially scientific matters, so they turn to advisory bodies for advice. And unfortunately many of the bodies that give advice on diet and health issues rely on food or drug manufacturers to fund them, so their advice isn't always impartial. For example, the website of the British Nutrition Foundation, which was founded in 1967 to '*deliver authoritative, evidence-based information on food and nutrition in the context of health and lifestyle*', currently lists twelve 'sustaining members' including Coca-Cola, Sainsbury's, Nestlé, PepsiCo, Tate & Lyle and Unilever. It is hard to imagine Nestlé advising the government that eating chocolate is bad for the teeth, or Tate & Lyle endorsing a report stating that adding sugar to food is a principal cause of type 2 diabetes.

In 2009 the U.K. Food Standards Agency produced a 40-second film designed to convince people that eating butter, fatty meat and other sources of saturated fat was unhealthy.[11] The film bore no relation to any scientific facts, the Agency itself described it as an 'advertisement', and it openly informed us that it was supported (which probably means 'funded') by 'major supermarkets, manufacturers and some caterers', bodies who make a large slice of their profits from food manufactured with unsaturated fats.

The situation is similar in the U.S.A. The influential U.S. International Food Information Council claims to give impartial and scientifically-based advice on nutrition, but it is financially supported by some twenty food industry companies including Coca-Cola, Del Monte, Heinz, Kellogg's, Kraft, Mars, Nestlé, PepsiCo, Sara Lee, Tate & Lyle and Unilever.

The website of the American Heart Association openly tells us that it is sponsored by CanolaInfo. CanolaInfo is a company that supports the manufacturers of Canadian rapeseed oil, so it is hardly surprising that the website advocates the consumption of unsaturated fats – the main kind you get in temperate vegetable oils such as rapeseed oil.

Hence much of the information fed to governments comes from sources which are not free from vested interests.

---

11 www.food.gov.uk/news/pressreleases/2009/feb/launchsatfatcampaign

Food retailers

The third reason that the government and other influential bodies keep playing the same old record is, I think, to do with the economic power and influence of the big food retailers, who are among Britain's biggest employers. A huge slice of their income comes from selling low-fat spreads and yogurts, cooking oils, diet foods, and cakes and pastries baked with unsaturated fats. No government would dare tell them to put a health warning on them all. Right-wing governments in particular are more concerned with helping big business to make profits for its shareholders than protecting citizens from its activities. Any suggestion that there should be some effective intervention to stop people buying unhealthy food would be lambasted as setting up a 'nanny state' and an attack on personal freedom.

Food manufacturers

Fourthly the food manufacturers naturally have a vested interest in convincing us and the government that their products will keep us healthy. At the time of writing, for instance, the Flora pro.activ® website states that using its products will lower one's cholesterol level, which is true, but it goes on to say that '*too much cholesterol in the blood can build up in the walls of the arteries causing them to narrow*'. That is mostly untrue, according to a medical paper published in a prestigious international medical journal, '*The Lancet*', in 1994.[12] The plaque that builds up in the walls of our arteries contains very little cholesterol. It is mostly polyunsaturated fat, one of the main groups of fats that vegetable oil spreads are made of! The authors concluded, '*These findings imply a direct influence of dietary polyunsaturated fatty acids on aortic plaque formation and suggest that current trends favouring the increased intake of polyunsaturated fatty acids should be reconsidered*'. If the ministers at the Department of Health read that then they might think twice about telling people that cooking oils and spreads made from vegetable oils are healthier than lard and butter. You may still be able to read a summary of the report itself. At the time of writing it's available on the Internet at www.ncbi.nlm.nih.gov/pubmed/7934543.

The U.K. National Institute for Health and Clinical Excellence, otherwise known as NICE, advises the medical profession on the appropriate use of drugs. It recommends that patients should *not* routinely be advised to take plant sterols and stanols for the primary prevention of cardiovascular disease. It says this is because although they reduce cholesterol levels '*there have been no controlled trials to determine whether this*

---

[12] Felton C V et al. *Dietary polyunsaturated fatty acids and composition of human aortic plaques.* Wynn Institute for Metabolic Research, London, U.K. Lancet, October 29, 1994; 344(8931):1195-6.

has any effect on cardiovascular health'.[13]

In spite of that, cholesterol-lowering spreads containing these chemicals are still sold at premium prices, their manufacturers relying on the popular myth that lowering cholesterol is good for one's health.

Actually the opposite may be true. There are responsible warnings on such spreads that '*pregnant and breastfeeding women and children should not use this product*', as well as the recommendation not to exceed three 20g servings a day. The warnings are there because the plant sterols and stanols, which are added to these spreads to reduce cholesterol levels, behave like sex hormones. They have been shown to provoke the growth of breast cancer cells and alter sex hormone levels in animals. A Swedish review of the effects of plant sterols concluded that '*further studies are required of their phyto-oestrogenic and endocrine effects, and their effects on growing children, particularly regarding subsequent fertility in boys*'.[14]

The website Patient.co.uk, which generally takes a rather positive stance on the benefits of such products, nevertheless states that plant sterols and stanols impair the absorption of fat-soluble vitamins. It says they are not recommended for pregnant or lactating women or for children aged under five because they reduce the level of carotenoids including vitamin A, which is closely associated with foetal development,[15] and because the developing brain needs cholesterol. The nerve synapses in our brains are made almost entirely from cholesterol.

Apart from all those warnings, there is sound evidence, which I will address later, that men over 70 years old and women of all ages are more likely to have a heart attack if they have a *low* cholesterol level than a high one. So if cholesterol-lowering spreads are unsuitable for children, women, and men over seventy, the only people who might benefit from eating them are middle-aged men! And even for them there is an alternative: eating more fruit and vegetables would be just as effective for many people in lowering their cholesterol levels, without the potential downsides. Curiously, no manufacturer seems to have funded any research to compare the effectiveness of eating its spreads with eating more fruit and vegetables, even though one of them has an annual turnover of £75 million a year in the U.K. on its cholesterol-lowering range. I wonder why that is?

---

13   *Lipid modification - cardiovascular risk assessment and the modification of blood lipids for the primary and secondary prevention of cardiovascular disease.* NICE Clinical Guideline (May 2008, amended May 2010)

14   Wikström A C. *Is the Finnish 'healthy margarine' food or medicine? Addition of plant sterols can lower cholesterol levels.* [Article in Swedish] Lakartidningen, November 11, 1998; 95(46):5146-8.

15   *Vitamin A: a multifunctional tool for development.* Seminars in Cell and Developmental Biology, August 2011; 22(6):603-10. Epub June 13, 2011.

Food growers

In 2012 there was a fantastic illustration of the lengths to which food growers will go to ensure that people will buy their products, whether or not they are healthy. In California a man called James Wheaton proposed a new state statute that all food containing genetically modified material should state this on the food label.[16] This was not unreasonable: it is a legal requirement in over 40 other countries. So in accordance with federal procedure arrangements were made for the population to be balloted on whether the new law should be enacted. Wheaton's 'Right to Know' campaign was financially supported by individuals and small businesses to the tune of 3.9 million dollars. A lot of money, you might think. But opposing the new law were the companies who own patents to genetic modifications, federations representing big farmers and the major food manufacturers, a total of over 43 companies and organizations. Between them they poured no fewer than 32.5 million dollars into the 'No' campaign to keep Californian residents in the dark about what they were eating![17] Needless to say, the law was not passed. That is the power that food manufacturers have over the rest of us.

In some cases governments act as little more than marketing organizations for their major food growers. The independent charity Food and Water Watch examined cables from the U.S. State department sent between 2005 and 2009. It concluded, *'The United States has aggressively pursued foreign policies in food and agriculture that benefit their largest seed companies. The U.S. State department has launched a concerted strategy to promote agricultural biotechnology, often over the opposition of the public and government, to the near exclusion of other more sustainable, more appropriate agricultural policy alternatives. The U.S. State department has also lobbied foreign governments to adopt pro-agricultural biotechnology politics and laws, operated a rigorous public relations campaign to improve the image of biotechnology and has challenged common sense biotechnology safeguards and rules – even including opposing laws requiring the labeling of genetically engineered (GE) foods'*.[18]

---

16 *California Proposition 37, Mandatory Labeling of Genetically Engineered Food (2012).*

17 According to ballotpedia.org some companies well known in the U.K. who financed the 'No' vote to prevent consumers knowing if they were eating genetically modified food were Monsanto (US$8 million), E.I. du Pont de Nemours & Co., PepsiCo Inc., Kraft Foods Group, Coca-Cola North America, Nestlé USA, Kellogg Company, Del Monte Foods, Campbell Soup Company, Heinz, Ocean Spray, Mars Chocolate North America, and Sara Lee Corporation. http://ballotpedia.org/California_Proposition_37,_Mandatory_Labeling_of_Genetically_Engineered_Food_%282012%29, accessed October 2014.

18 http://www.foodandwaterwatch.org/reports/biotech-ambassadors. Accessed August 2014.

Pharmaceutical companies

Sixthly, I can say with some confidence that the pharmaceutical manufacturers don't want people to be healthy without the use of drugs, for if they found a way to stop people getting ill without their help then nobody would need to buy their products and they would go out of business. According to one source statins earn their US manufacturers US$26.2 billion a year. It's obvious that statin manufacturers will do everything possible to maintain the myth that cholesterol causes heart attacks and that artificially lowering the cholesterol level in the blood will reduce the risk of having one. So how do they maintain such myths?

Pharmaceutical manufacturers fund most medical research, and the main reason do so is to prove that their drugs are effective and safe. That kind of research is very different from impartial research to discover whether or not a drug is effective and safe. Since universities and other bodies know that they won't receive further funding if they keep turning up results that their sponsors don't want this can affect the impartiality of their experimental methods or conclusions or both. A few years ago two doctors looked at all the research projects that were reported at the annual meeting of a medical professional society. They kept the society's name anonymous to protect its reputation, but they discovered and reported that every paper presented at the conference on research funded by a pharmaceutical manufacturer ended up by recommending the use of the product tested. And this was not so in the case of the relatively few papers on research which had been funded independently.[19] Another researcher concluded that much of the '*pharmaceutical company-sponsored research in medical journals, and its presentation at conferences and meetings*' is '*designed to look like traditional academic work, but performed largely to market products*'.[20]

Early in 2014 the U.K. government expressed concern that while pharmaceutical companies are obliged to report the principal results of their researches, they do not have to report all the results, making it possible for them to conceal any negative results to present their products in a better light.

Even the advice provided by apparently independent bodies that have no direct link to pharmaceutical companies might be influenced by them. For example the British Medical Association and the British Dietetic Association are combinations of a trade union and a professional body to cater for the needs of health professionals and dieticians respectively and to regulate their work. They are not scientific bodies, and so far as I know they don't conduct any research, yet they do make recommendations to the government. In practice these are only the recommendations of their more influential

---

19   Finucane T & Boult C. *Commercial support and bias in pharmaceutical research.* American Journal of Medicine, Volume 117, December 1, 2004.

20   Sismondo S. *Ghosts in the Machine: Publication Planning in the Medical Sciences.* Social Studies of Science, April 2009; 39:171-198.

members, and many overworked health professionals don't have time to keep abreast of the latest medical knowledge by reading scientific research papers. My own doctor seemed to be totally unaware of research papers reporting that older people are less likely to die of a heart attack if their cholesterol level is on the high side, even one that had been published in the '*British Medical Journal*'.[21]

Health professionals in the U.K. generally specify medication in accordance with the current recommendations from NICE, the National Institute for Clinical Excellence, but if these offer alternatives then their choice may well be influenced by advertising literature sent to them by pharmaceutical companies advertising the superior benefits of their own particular products. Furthermore, NICE itself may not be immune from external influence. In 2014 a letter signed by the President of the Royal College of Physicians and another eight authoritative figures asked NICE to reconsider its reasons for advising the wider use of statins. After listing extensive medical evidence opposing its advice, the writers pointed out that eight members of NICE's panel of twelve experts for its latest guidance had direct financial ties to the pharmaceutical companies that manufacture statins.[22]

The media

Newspapers and other popular media don't seem to mind distorting the truth if they can grab an eye-catching headline as a result. A typical example was the BBC website headline in August 2014: '*Low vitamin D boosts dementia risk*'. The article itself, beneath the selfsame headline, said, '*A study like this can't tell us whether being deficient in vitamin D can cause dementia*'.

In May 2011 The Independent newspaper ran a story under the headline, '*Scientists confirm direct link between bowel cancer and red meat consumption*'. The story began with the alarming words, '*A new report described as "the most authoritative ever" to confirm the link between red meat and the risk of developing bowel cancer has experts around the world sounding the alarm on keeping meat consumption to a minimum*'. Those were eye-catching headlines! And numerous websites purporting to give dietary advice reproduced this story, so it appeared all over the Internet.

However, readers who took the trouble to read the report for themselves were bemused

---

[21] Ravnskov U. *Diet-heart disease hypothesis is wishful thinking.* British Medical Journal, 2002; 324:238.

[22] The letter was dated 10th June, 2014. It was addressed to Professor David Haslam, Chairman, National Institute for Health and Care Excellence, and copied to The Right Honourable Jeremy Hunt, MP, Secretary of State for Health.

by what it actually said.[23] 'The U.K. Dietary Cohort Consortium has recently reported *no evidence of association* between red meat consumption and colectoral cancer risk in a pooled analysis of food diary data from seven prospective studies...Preliminary results in an abstract from pooling 14 prospective studies and 7743 colectoral cancer cases *did not support* a positive association between red meat intake and colectoral cancer risk...' It is true that the report said some researchers had found a statistical association between red meat and cancer for people who eat very large quantities of red meat and few vegetables, but even those researchers found that eating less than half a kilogram of red meat a day was found to create little or no increased risk of contracting cancer. So The Independent's story was a clear distortion of the fact that eating red meat in any normal quantities does not increase one's risk of bowel cancer.

One can guess what happened to the sales of red meat after this article was published. Evidently the editor of this newspaper, or at least his so-called science reporter, preferred printing an eye-catching scare headline to keeping honest meat-producing farmers in business, regardless of the truth.

Health charities

This brings me on to the eighth reason that I believe there is so much bad information around. Surprisingly, it is connected with some of the health charities. The British Heart Foundation and similar charities do fund lots of research into heart disease, but nearly all of it is to do with finding better ways to treat people who already have heart trouble. They spend relatively little money looking for a way to stop people getting heart disease in the first place.

I do wonder if some health charities, particularly some of the big American ones, actually don't want to stop people getting heart disease or diabetes or what have you, because if they did then they wouldn't be needed. The American Heart Association has assets of US$1 billion, and according to Alan Watson of dietheartnews.com the CEO earns over US$500,000 annually, giving him a very comfortable lifestyle in return for telling people to eat a low-fat diet which, I believe, is actually a principal cause of the problem. The city of Dallas even built the 1,000-bed 4-star Dallas Convention Center Hotel to help accommodate 22,000 people who were expected to attend the AHA's grand annual conference in November 2013, after the AHA threatened to go elsewhere if they

---

23 The report to which the story referred was the World Cancer Research Fund/American Institute for Cancer Research report *Continuous Update Project Report Summary: The Association between Food, Nutrition and Physical Activity and the Risk of Colectoral Cancer.* May 2011.

didn't.[24,25] So you can understand my scepticism about the true goals of some health charities.

Health charities are fundraising organizations: they are not scientific institutions. So the only 'facts' one will learn from them are statements that support their primary raison d'être, to persuade people to donate money to them. Of course they will use much of this money to fund health education and research, but it is no good looking to them for independent information and advice on healthy eating.

Heart U.K., for example, describes itself as 'The Cholesterol Charity', so one can understand why its director has a vested interest in maintaining the myth that cholesterol is what causes heart attacks. On their website in 2012 there was a tab which said 'Evidence base'. When I saw this tab I thought, "Ah, let's find out what is the scientifically factual basis for these claims." And when I clicked on it all I found was a list of similar recommendations from other charities and organizations – no evidence at all!

Most of the health charities seem to follow a similar line. In 2012 the chief executive of Diabetes U.K. told the BBC that thousands of diabetics were putting themselves at risk from heart attacks because they were not lowering their cholesterol levels by statins and other means. I wrote to Diabetes U.K. asking how they knew that cholesterol caused heart attacks. I received a polite personal reply from a representative. He began by quoting another organization which said the same thing, so that wasn't particularly helpful, but he then referred me to a long and impressive scientific report that looked as though it would be helpful. It was called '*European guidelines on cardiovascular disease prevention in clinical practice: executive summary. Fourth Joint Task Force of the European Society of Cardiology and Other Societies on Cardiovascular Disease Prevention in Clinical Practice. (Constituted by representatives of nine societies and by invited experts)*'.[26] Something with a title as impressive as that must be right, I thought! The report said, '*There are strong, consistent and graded relationships between saturated fat intake, blood cholesterol levels, and the mass occurrence of CVD (that's Coronary Vascular Disease or CHD). The relationships are accepted as causal.*' That statement is very clear, and I'm sure that Diabetes U.K. isn't the only organization to have quoted it. Unfortunately both sentences are factually incorrect, for there *are* many inconsistencies and many doctors do *not* accept a causal relationship. Those are undeniable facts, as we've seen already.

Further on under the heading, '*Plasma lipids: scientific background*', the

---

24   www.bizjournals.com/dallas/stories/2008/02/11/story1.html?page=all

25   my.americanheart.org/professional/Sessions/ScientificSessions/Scientific-Sessions_UCM_316900_SubHomePage.jsp

26   *European guidelines on cardiovascular disease prevention in clinical practice: executive summary Fourth Joint Task Force of the European Society of Cardiology and Other Societies on Cardiovascular Disease Prevention in Clinical Practice (Constituted by representatives of nine societies and by invited experts).* European Heart Journal, 2007; 28, 2375–2414.

same report stated, '*The relationship between a raised plasma cholesterol and atherosclerotic vascular disease fulfils all of the criteria for causality*'. That's even clearer, and here at least it did quote another report in support of its claim.[27] So I read this second report. It showed that on average a number of independent tests on the effectiveness of statins had demonstrated that taking statins reduced blood cholesterol *and* that subjects who took statins were less likely to suffer a heart attack. That sounds like good news for statins, but before you rush off to your doctor and demand a prescription, remember that most statin tests are carried out on middle-aged men, so the results may not be applicable to women or older people. And even for middle-aged men there is a major problem in claiming this proves that cholesterol causes heart attacks. Statins not only reduce cholesterol levels: they also reduce the blood's clotting ability. And since in the end it is a blood clot blocking an artery that causes a heart attack, it is quite possible, if not likely, that where statins do reduce the occurrence of heart attacks it is by reducing the blood's coagulability. That is exactly how aspirin and even small quantities of alcohol help to prevent heart attacks in people who are at risk. A friend of mine is on statins, not because her cholesterol is high – it isn't – but to stop her blood clotting and causing a stroke. More than that, statins are powerful anti-inflammatory agents and have antioxidant properties which reduce damage to the arteries.[28]

So if the statins in the trials reduced the incidence of heart attacks either by preventing blood clotting or by protecting the arteries from damage – and both seem exceedingly likely – then the fact that statins also happened to lower the subjects' cholesterol levels is totally irrelevant. In this case the 'proof' that it is cholesterol that causes heart attacks evaporates into the mythical mists of the borogrove swamps. So long as there is a *possibility* that the observed reduction in heart attacks was caused by something other than the reduction in cholesterol, it is *un*true, *un*scientific and *un*professional to conclude that '*the relationship between cholesterol and atherosclerotic vascular disease fulfils all of the criteria for causality*'. One of the criteria for causality must be that there can be no alternative cause.

If the papers cited are the best evidence that Diabetes U.K. can come up with in support of its chief executive's statements to the BBC about cholesterol causing heart disease then I am not impressed. Actually, statins might prevent heart attacks more effectively if they did *not* lower cholesterol levels. Our livers manufacture cholesterol because our bodies need it, and one reason they need it is to repair damaged arteries. So interfering with the cholesterol level might be doing more harm than good.

For some researchers, food and drink growers and manufacturers, retailers,

---

27   Baigent C et al. (Cholesterol Treatment Trialists' (CTT) Collaborators) *Efficacy and safety of cholesterol-lowering treatment: prospective meta-analysis of data from 90,056 participants in 14 randomised trials of statins.* Lancet, 2005; 366:1267–1278.

28   Cortese C et al. *Atherosclerosis in light of the evidence from large statin trials.* Annals of the Italian Medical Institute. 2000; 15(1):103-107.

pharmaceutical companies, news media and even health charities, truth is like a second home: they don't live in it all the time. So where can we find the truth about saturated fat and heart disease? Surely someone somewhere has done some proper research into the matter?

CHAPTER 3: THE TRUTH ABOUT SATURATED FAT

The Prudent Diet

In reality there has been a lot of proper experimental research carried out to discover the truth about saturated fat, even if the Secretary of State for Health has never read any of it. For example, in 1957 a group of 1,113 New York businessmen were put on what was called a 'Prudent Diet'.[29] They were aged from 40 to 59 years old, because men in that age group, especially overweight businessmen, are most at risk of heart attacks. They replaced butter with cooking oil and margarine, eggs with cold cereal and skimmed milk, and beef with chicken and fish. A second group of 467 similar men ate whatever they had been eating before. After 9 years the number of men who had developed some symptom of coronary heart disease was much higher in the second group than those in the first group who had kept to the diet.[30] So it did appear that a low-fat diet was beneficial in preventing *symptoms* of heart disease. However there were nine *deaths* from heart disease among the Prudent Dieters and *no deaths* from heart disease in the control group. I would have preferred to be in the test group of men who ate saturated fat and stayed alive.

The Multiple Risk Factor Intervention Trial

Since the Prudent Diet experiment was inconclusive, a much bigger study was organized in the 1970s. This involved 12,866 middle-aged men. They were all deliberately chosen as men who were thought to be at risk of heart failure because of their weight, blood pressure or cholesterol level. It was called the Multiple Risk Factor Intervention Trial.[31] Over an average period of 7 years half the men were encouraged, through regular visits to a clinic,

---

29   Cristakis G. *Effect of the Anti-Coronary Club Program on Coronary Heart Disease Risk-Factor Status.* Journal of the American Medical Association, 1966; 198: 129-35.

30   69.0% higher for men who were 40 to 49 years old at the start of the trial, and 53.6% higher for men who were 50 to 59 years old when it started.

31   *Multiple Risk Factor Intervention Trial.* Journal of the American Medical Association, 1982; 248:1465-77.

to reduce their saturated fat and cholesterol consumption and increase their consumption of polyunsaturated fats (the fats that come from plants), to give up smoking cigarettes (which many of them did), and, where necessary, to lower their blood pressure by means of prescribed drugs. The other half were left to more conventional medical care.

And what was the result? The researchers wrote, '*The overall results do not show a beneficial effect on coronary heart disease or total mortality from the multifactor intervention.*' In fact in half of the 22 test centres the number of deaths from coronary heart disease was actually greater in the intervention group which had cut their saturated fat consumption, in spite of the fact that a significant number of men in this group also stopped smoking during the trial period.

The Helsinki Study

A similar study started in Helsinki in 1974, involving 1,222 businessmen who were at risk of cardiovascular disease. Half of them went on a strict low-fat diet for 5 years, reduced or cut out smoking, and were treated with drugs for high blood pressure where necessary. But in this experiment they also took more exercise. And guess what? The results were as bad as before for the low-fat diet supporters. After 15 years 65 men in the group who continued life as normal had died, but in the group who had been on a low-fat diet and adopted a healthier lifestyle 95 had died![32]

The Coronary Prevention Study

Again the results of the World Health Organization's European Coronary Prevention Study published in 1983 were called 'depressing' because once more no correlation between fats and heart disease was found. The researchers had cut saturated fats down to only eight per cent of the subjects' calorie intake, yet in the U.K. section there were once again more deaths in the intervention group than in the control group.[33] To be honest the researchers ought to have expected this, knowing that coronary heart disease had become an issue only since people switched from eating things like butter, lard and full-cream milk to margarine, vegetable oil and low-fat diets. One really wonders why they went on spending money trying to prove the opposite.

---

32   Strandberg T E et al. *Mortality in participants and non-participants of a multifactorial prevention study of cardio-vascular diseases: a 28 year follow up of the Helsinki Businessmen Study.* British Heart Journal, 1995; 74: 449-454.

33   World Health Organization. European Collaborative Group. *Multi-factorial trial in the prevention of coronary heart disease: 3. Incidence and mortality results. European Heart Journal*, 1983; 4:141.

The Caerphilly Project

Finally I have another paper,[34] which was published in the British Journal of Nutrition in 1993. It is based on a very comprehensive 18-year study of the health of nearly all the men who were aged 45 to 59 when it first began and who lived in and around Caerphilly in Wales between 1979 and 1997 – around 2,500 of them. I say it was a very comprehensive study because it even recorded how frequently the men shaved and had sexual intercourse. One dependent study actually examined whether these factors might contribute to heart disease! The project was funded by the Medical Research Council and I believe it was managed by my old university at Bristol. Some 200 papers have been published on its findings, a remarkable indication of its value and importance. The authors of my paper were interested in the relationship between diet and IHD. IHD stands for ischaemic heart disease or reduced blood supply to the heart. This is usually caused by coronary heart disease, so the two terms are very similar. After 13 years the authors reported, *'There was some evidence suggesting a positive association between total fat intake and IHD risk, but the trend was not consistent and not statistically significant. There was no association for animal fat.'* So they found *no evidence whatsoever* that eating animal fat caused heart disease, although they did find a slight indication that other kinds of fat might be linked to heart disease. What is especially interesting is that the authors then stated that their findings were consistent with other studies, and they cited a list of them in support of this assertion.[35]

The verdict

All this means it is absolutely certain that eating animal fats is not responsible for the heart disease epidemic which began around the time I was born. It is really extraordinary that the government and so many semi-official organizations continue to this day to ignore all this authoritative research. The saturated fat in butter and meat and lard and dripping and full-cream milk and full-fat cheese will not block your arteries or cause heart failure, whatever the government or the popular press or health charities or the food manufacturers may tell you.

Of course the popular view, as promulgated by the Food Standards Agency in the film I mentioned earlier, is that saturated fats cause a build-up of plaque in the arteries that eventually restricts the flow of blood to the heart causing a heart attack. The truth is that the plaque that causes our arteries to narrow doesn't build up in the arteries themselves,

---

34 Fehily A M et al. *Diet and incident ischaemic heart disease: the Caerphilly Study*. British Journal of Nutrition, 1993; 69:303-314.

35 Fehily A M et al., cited above – *Table 10: Relationship between intake of total fat and of saturated fatty acids (or animal fat) and incidence of ischaemic heart disease in major prospective studies.*

the channels through which the blood flows, but in the actual *wall* of the arteries. It is produced when the endothelium, the thin slippery lining of our arteries, is damaged in some way. As to what happens next, there seem to be two different stories. One is that when the damage is repaired scar tissue is formed, and if this happens repeatedly it narrows the arterial channels until a blood clot comes along and blocks the channel altogether resulting in a heart attack. The other story is that because the damaged endothelium is no longer slippery, small blood clots get stuck in it, where they turn into plaque, which again narrows the channels as before. Whichever it is, or perhaps both, it is the initial damage that produces the blood clots which block our arteries and cut off the supply of blood to the heart. Rather than blame blocked arteries on pork lard or dripping, as the film did, we have to discover what is causing the initial damage to the cell walls.

In any case meat fat doesn't go into the arteries, it goes into the stomach and intestines where it is changed into other things. And even if it did go into the arteries it would remain liquid at body temperature: it wouldn't solidify as it would if you poured it down a waste pipe, which is what the film claimed. And if fat entered our arteries directly as the film implied then so would popcorn and peanuts, and I can't imagine anything that would block our arteries more effectively than popcorn and peanuts would!

Finally, as I said before, the main component of arterial plaque, measured in autopsies of people who have died of coronary heart disease and as reported in the Lancet,[36] is not saturated fat but *polyunsaturated* fat, the very kind of fat that the film told us we *should* be eating.

So it was a silly, ignorant film, but at least it taught us something. It taught us how unscientific and misleading the government's propaganda on healthy eating can be, including that of the Food Standards Agency.

---

[36] Felton C V et al. *Dietary polyunsaturated fatty acids and composition of human aortic plaques.* Wynn Institute for Metabolic Research, London, U.K. Lancet, October 29, 1994; 344(8931):1195-6. (Also cited earlier.)

CHAPTER 4: THE CAUSES OF HEART DISEASE

The major causes of heart disease appear to be:

- smoking
- stress
- diet other than saturated fat and cholesterol

Let's look at these in turn.

Smoking

First smoking. Smoking is estimated to kill 100,000 people a year in the U.K. mainly as a result of heart disease and various cancers.[37] In the U.S.A. smoking kills 443,000 people a year.[38] As well as damaging the endothelium, which results in narrowed arteries in the body and brain, nicotine increases the blood's coagulability, in other words it makes the formation of blood clots more likely. That's why smokers are more likely to get a heart attack (when the blood supply to the heart is blocked), or a stroke (when the blood supply to the brain is blocked). And that's also why a daily dose of aspirin or small amounts of alcohol have been found to reduce the risk of heart attacks and strokes, because they thin the blood. But aspirin and small amounts of alcohol are beneficial only if you have damaged arteries: they don't stop such damage developing in the first place. So if you are fit don't consume aspirin or alcohol for medical reasons (a) because they are of no benefit, and (b) because it's important that your blood *does* clot properly if you have an accident, otherwise you could bleed to death.

Nowadays almost everyone accepts that smoking is a principal cause of lung cancer. It seems incredible that it wasn't until 1949, when I was 7 years old and my father smoked 40 cigarettes a day, that any statistical evidence linking smoking with

---

[37] Cancer Research U.K. quoted 102,000 deaths from smoking-related diseases in 2009.
[38] The National Cancer Institute quoted 443,000 deaths from smoking-related diseases in 2012.

lung cancer was found.[39,40] But 10 years later coronary heart disease was linked to smoking even more strongly than lung cancer was. A mammoth study made by the American Cancer Society showed that *four times as many* smokers died of coronary disease as died of lung cancer.[41] The report of this study attributed one out of every three *coronary* deaths in the U.S.A. to smoking. Thankfully this last figure has fallen now that fewer people smoke, but the main result remains true, that if you smoke you are four times as likely to die of heart disease as lung cancer, so smoking is clearly a major cause of heart disease. Anyone who spends his money on cigarettes needs his head examined as well as his lungs, especially if the result is that he can't afford to buy good quality food.

The good news about smoking cigarettes is that one can stop it. That will probably sound too simplistic to a smoker, because everybody knows that nicotine is a strongly addictive drug. It's also a very deceptive one, because smoking appears to calm one's nerves, whereas the nervous tension one feels after a few hours without a cigarette is actually a withdrawal symptom caused by lack of the drug to which one has become addicted: a non-smoker wouldn't have any nerves to calm! However, I firmly believe that if we really want to do something then we can find a way to force ourselves to do it however troublesome, costly or outrageous the way may be. For example, a smoker who is a married man could cancel all his personal credit cards and bank accounts and have his pay go into his wife's bank account, thereby ensuring that for 3 months, or 12 months if necessary, he has no money of any kind to spend. His wife would have to pay all the bills and he'd have to walk or cycle to work, take sandwiches for lunch, and pass on the church collection bag, but you get the idea. The Queen gets by without carrying any money so it can't be that hard! This solution may sound ridiculous, but what I am saying is that where there's really a will there's a way.

Naturally the first step for most smokers would be to ask their doctor or local pharmacist for advice on quitting. And then they should tell their families and friends what they are doing and ask for their support: that's very important. Furthermore, someone who has a genuine relationship with God as his heavenly father could ask for God's help too. I knew a pipe-smoking church minister in Somerset who prayed to be filled with the Holy Spirit. When his prayer was answered the first unexpected result was that he no longer wanted to smoke, so he just stopped. There were no withdrawal symptoms. He just didn't want to smoke any more, and so far as I know he never touched his pipe again.

---

39 Wynder E L & Graham E A. *Tobacco smoking as a possible etiologic factor in brochiogenic carcinoma - a study of 684 proved cases.* Journal of the American Medical Association, 1950; 143:329-336.

40 Doll R & Hill A. *Smoking and carcinoma of the lung; preliminary report.* British Medical Journal, 1950; 2: pp. 739-48.

41 Hammond E C & Horn D. *Smoking and Death Rates - Report on 44 months of follow-up of 187,783 men.* Journal of the American Medical Association, March 1958.

Stress

Next on the list of the causes of heart trouble is stress. When populations undergo disruption or rapid social change, such as occurred in Eastern Europe following the end of communism, or among Asian emigrants to Western countries, the rate of coronary heart disease rapidly increases. When I first read this I did wonder if the reason was simply that such people exchange their traditional diet for a modern Western diet, but apparently the opposite was true in the case of Japanese people who moved to the U.S.A.[42] Those who continued to eat Japanese food had double the rate of heart disease as those who adopted an American diet, whereas heart disease in Japan itself, at least among those who continue to eat a traditional diet, is comparatively rare. More generally, actuaries calculate that a 40-year-old who experiences two very stressful events in one year will on average live 0.2 years less in consequence.

Stressful employment has been linked directly to the development of coronary heart disease. It was found that 71 coronary patients out of a group of 100 under the age of 40 had been working for more than 60 hours a week for a prolonged period, compared with only 18 out of 100 in a control group of similar people who had no evidence of heart trouble.[43] Some other studies have not shown any such connection between long working hours and heart disease in men, but most women, who tend to have more family responsibilities as well, are more likely to develop heart trouble if they spend more than 50 hours a week in paid employment.[44]

These and other observations suggest that stress may be a major factor in the development of heart disease. Stress can be caused by constant overwork and fatigue, worry, injury, depression, anger, hatred, relationship problems and even conflicting demands on one's time or priorities. Death, divorce, redundancy and moving to another town or country are particular culprits. When our bodies experience stress, adrenaline is injected into our bloodstream to enable us to fight or run away. It makes our heart beat faster, raises our blood pressure, and accelerates our breathing. This is called the fight or flight reaction, and it's rather like what happens in a fire station when the fire alarm sounds. It's fine when it is needed, but if it is happening all the time then it can produce wear and tear on our heart and arteries. Birds have relatively large adrenaline glands because they have to be constantly on the watch for cats and other enemies and be ready to fly at a moment's notice. Most birds live for only 10 to 20 years if they are not killed first. Crocodiles on the other hand laze around without fear of any attack.

---

42 Marmot M G & Syme S L. *Acculturation and coronary heart disease in Japanese-Americans.* American Journal of Epidemiology, 1976; 104: 225-247.

43 Russek H I & Zohman B L. *Relative significance of heredity, diet and occupational stress in coronary heart disease of young adults.* American Journal of Medicine, 1958;325:266-75.

44 Spurgeon A et al. *Health and safety problems associated with long working hours: a review of the current position.* Occupational and Environmental Medicine, 1997; 54:367-375.

They have tiny adrenaline glands and can live to 100. The picture in Figure 6 was published in the New York State Health News back in 1955, but its message remains true today.

Figure 6: Relationship between stress and disease

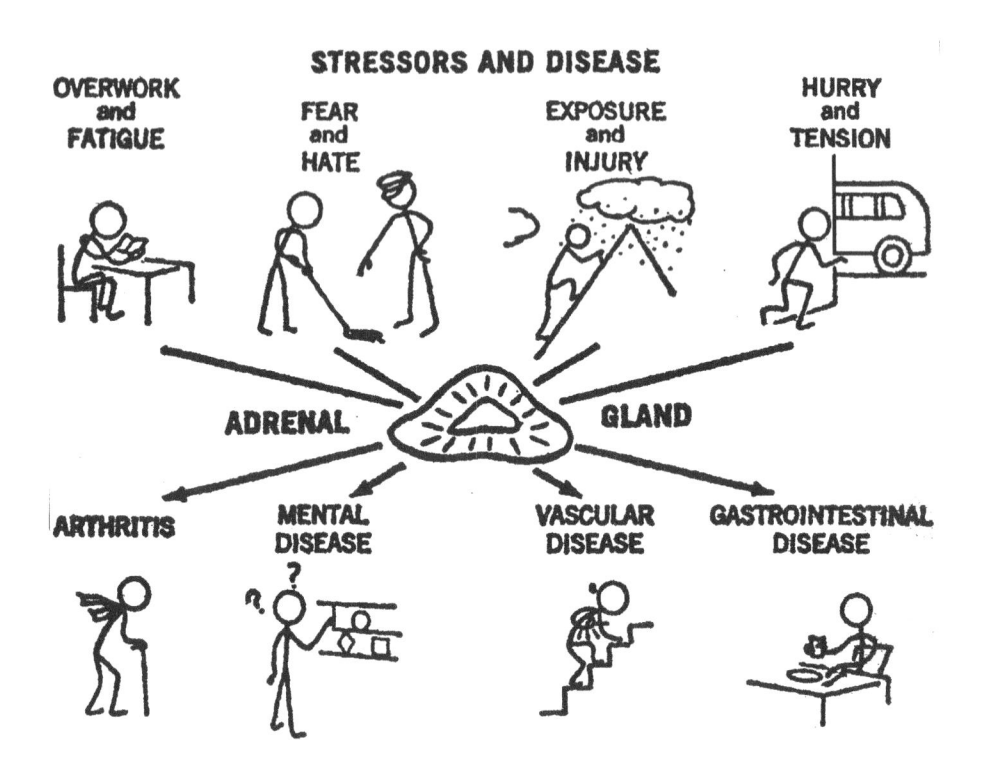

It's true that some people seem to enjoy stress, perhaps because an adrenaline rush does initially feel rather pleasant. Other people find stressful situations very unpleasant indeed. Since work occupies such a large part of our time it is unwise to allow an unpleasantly stressful situation at work to continue for long. Anyone who feels that his job is getting too stressful should first talk to his manager about it. It is better for everyone if you can be happy in your work, for people who feel themselves to be unduly stressed don't work at their best, and if they become ill they can't work at all. A good manager will recognize this and will do his best to find a way to reduce the stress you are experiencing. A bad manager is probably best left by applying for another post, either in the same firm or elsewhere.

We all know that family life can be stressful, particularly if there is a shortage of discipline, order, money or love. I don't need to tell any parent that children can cause a lot of stress. But, with young children at least, the important thing to remember is that our job as parents is to train them, not to be their servants or to act simply as unpaid childminders. With older children friendship is often a key. There are ways to deal with most problems in family life if we are willing to ask for advice and support from more experienced people and to make changes. Some churches, mosques and other organizations provide helpful teaching on marriage and family life. There can be huge benefits in belonging to such a body: once, when I was unemployed, the other members of my church home group surprised me by delivering a huge box of groceries to our house.

One of the most effective ways to reduce the levels of stress hormones is to take regular exercise. It is also the most effective way to reduce insulin resistance for type 2 diabetics or to prevent its onset in the first place. When I was in full-time employment I was one of the few people who went out for a walk every lunchtime, and perhaps that is one reason why so many people still say that I look younger than my years. For many years I cycled to work. Cycling to and from work is excellent exercise because it saves money as well.

Not all exercise is relaxing. A highly competitive game of squash might be a rapid way to get physically fit but I'm not sure that it would be the best way to reduce stress. And I certainly don't recommend a game of croquet or even bowls against anyone who takes such games very seriously. Watching other people exercise can be even worse, especially if you are watching your home team lose. When Los Angeles lost to Pittsburgh in a close, nerve-wracking Super Bowl game in 1980, deaths in the city due to heart and circulatory issues rose by 15% in men and 27% in women during the following 2 weeks!

Dr. Malcolm Kendrick, a member of the BMA's General Practitioners Sub-committee and the author of '*The Great Cholesterol Con*',[45] believes it is particularly important not to eat while under stress. He points out that French people take a long time over their meals and have very little heart disease compared with people in Great Britain. If you eat while under mental or physical stress, he says, your body generates adrenaline, cortisol, glucagon and growth hormones, which produce surges of blood sugar, insulin and triglycerides, all of which are strongly associated with heart disease.

So the advice is:

- don't rush your meals
- don't eat while working
- don't eat standing up
- don't eat while watching a TV programme or film that annoys, frightens or excites you
- don't eat while watching your local football team play, especially if you are the manager

It is perfectly possible to set your alarm clock (or 'opportunity clock' as the American

---

[45] Kendrick M. *The Great Cholesterol Con*. John Blake Publishing Ltd, 2007.

writer Zig Ziglar calls it) to rouse you in time to have a proper breakfast seated round a table, with time for conversation and some encouraging words to one another, before going out to school or work or starting the day's chores. Of course this requires an effort, like most things in family life. It's something that parents have to believe and agree is important, and they then have to plan a routine that will make it happen.

What most commonly puts me under stress is getting behind with things. I dream that I have been left behind, or have run out of time to do something important. While I have not fully mastered the secret of controlling my use of time to my own satisfaction, I do think that some keys to keeping on top of things are:

- an organized daily and weekly timetable
- learning to say, "No"
- delegation (particularly to our children!)
- conquering procrastination
- learning not to waste time on trivialities

When I was 10 years old I was the only child in my class who could spell 'procrastination' and who knew what it meant. Guess why! Procrastination is closely linked to time-wasting, which in turn is linked to a lack of purpose or passion. Anyone who spends hours every week working for an employer in return for, say £10 an hour, must feel that an hour of his time is worth 'selling' for £10 or he wouldn't do it. So why are so many of us willing to give our time away for *nothing* the moment we get home, by watching some mindless entertainment on television or playing an addictive computer game or reading about the latest 'celebrity's' goings on? If your time is worth £10 an hour, isn't spending an hour on some pointless activity equivalent to deliberately stuffing a £10 note down a drain? And who would do that? Well, we all do it to a greater or lesser extent. But if it means that we end up being stressed out because relationships with our spouse and children and wider family members are neglected, or because jobs are piling up in the house or garden, or we are receiving flashing red reminders from HMRC or the water company because we 'haven't had time' to deal with our bills and correspondence, where is the sense in it?

Spend a few moments imagining how good you will feel when you have actually done a job you've been putting off for weeks. Then grab some good feelings by doing it. Once you've done it you'll be able to relax without feeling so stressed.

One amusing way to stop feeling stressed about all the jobs you haven't had time to do is to make a list on Monday evening of the jobs you *have* done that day. Then head it, 'Tuesday's To-Do List'. Pin it up in a prominent place next morning and you'll feel great!

As you have probably noticed, I seem to have wandered off the subject. I was explaining that arteries get blocked when they are damaged, and this is caused either by smoking, stress or diet, so let's make a start now on diet.

Diet

According to Dr. Kendrick, high blood levels of sugar, insulin,[46] triglycerides and an acid called homocysteine all seem to be associated with coronary heart disease. Insulin is a hormone that tells our bodies what to do with sugar in the blood. Triglycerides are packages of three fats in a form that can be carried around the bloodstream to take energy to the brain and muscles or be stored as fat in our fat cells. Homocysteine is an acid that, over time, eats away at the protein in our arteries.

High levels of *all* these substances occur when we consume too much sugar or starchy carbohydrate. Our digestive systems turn both sugars and starchy carbohydrates into glucose, raising the level of *sugar* in our blood. Glucose in turn triggers the release of *insulin*. And the US Medline website says that *triglyceride* levels can become too high if we eat too much sugar, starch or fibre.[47] (It also says triglyceride levels are increased if we eat too *little* protein, which is interesting.)

So a major cause of elevated levels of these four substances appears to be eating too much sugar and starchy carbohydrates. When we do that, of course, we put on weight, which explains why obesity is associated so strongly with heart disease, whether or not it actually causes it. But, as in the case of smoking and stress, this is good news because our diet once more is something we can change if we really want to.

While smoking and stress are factors, my personal opinion is that the main cause of coronary heart disease is our diet. After all, people used to smoke like factory chimneys in the early part of the last century, when CHD was not an issue. Watch an old black and white film and you'll wonder how anyone who didn't smoke could get a job as an actor. As for stress, there must have been an awful lot of it throughout Europe during and after the First World War, when 16 million people died and 20 million were injured, not to mention the Great Depression of the 1930s when up to 25% of the population in the U.S.A. and U.K. were unemployed.

In spite of widespread smoking and the stress caused by unemployment and war, the CHD epidemic didn't really take off in the U.K. until the 1950s, when Prime Minister Harold Macmillan was telling us, "You never had it so good," the war had ended and the use of tobacco was at last starting to fall. So what else happened round about then, the period when the CHD epidemic really got underway? That is when the kinds of food we ate really started to change.

---

46 Actually a high level of insulin is associated with an increased risk of heart disease only in women. However, low insulin *sensitivity*, which can occur as a result of prolonged high levels of insulin, is a strong risk factor for both men and women.

47 www.nlm.nih.gov/medlineplus/ency/article/003493.htm. Accessed November 2013.

CHAPTER 5: A SICK NATION

I will explain what I believe is wrong with our diet, but before I do so I want to convince you how serious the issue of public health has become. I'm now talking about much more than heart disease. The situation is very serious, both for individuals and for the National Health Service. In March 2013 obesity-associated health problems were costing the NHS £5 billion every year.[48] A study by the Royal College of Physicians in the same year said drink-related health problems could account for up to £3 billion of spending in NHS hospitals. The cost to the NHS of coronary vascular disease was estimated at an astonishing £14.4 billion. Diabetes UK estimates the cost of treating diabetes at another £14 billion annually. And these horrendous costs don't allow for the yet greater cost to the U.K. economy in terms of lost production, sickness benefits, road deaths and other related matters.

Such huge costs illustrate how serious the issue of diet-related health problems has become. It's absolutely essential to grasp this, especially if you have children, for only then will you really be motivated to take action to prevent your children from dying young as the result of a pattern of life and diet which you might otherwise be passing on to them.

Obesity

First of all, there's obesity. Obesity is a condition in which someone is so overweight that it either causes health problems or will do unless the person returns to a more normal weight. In the U.K. the term is applied to adults whose body mass index is 30 or more. Men with a waist circumference of 94cm or more and women with a waist circumference of 80cm may also be regarded as obese. In the case of children the term is applied to those whose body mass index is in the top 2% of children of the same age and sex. Does being obese really matter? It certainly does, especially for children.

BUPA lists the following consequences in later life of being obese as a child:

- Obesity increases the risk of heart disease, strokes, type 2 diabetes, liver disease,

---

[48] *Reducing obesity and improving diet*. U.K. Department of Health, 25 March, 2013.

osteoarthritis and some cancers.
- Other associated problems include high blood pressure, orthopaedic problems (joints, bow legs and other abnormalities), asthma and sleep apnoea (when a person stops breathing while asleep).
- Obese children can suffer teasing, name-calling and exclusion. Their appearance can make them unhappy. Such psychological effects that can lead to bulimia, or to comfort eating, which makes matters even worse.
- Young people who develop type 2 diabetes are at an increased risk of developing eye, heart and kidney disease.
- Obese teenagers are fifteen times more likely to become obese adults.

In 2008 the BBC reported that over 25% of children in England were going to suffer health problems because they were so seriously overweight. But only 3 years later in 2011 national newspapers reported that one in three children leaving primary school in the U.K. was clinically obese – the figure had risen to 33% in only 3 years! In June 2011, based on figures released under the Freedom of Information Act, several national newspapers reported that acute hospital trusts in Britain were treating 2 to 3 thousand children every year for clinical obesity. As a consequence, many were suffering diseases that normally appear in later life such as breathing difficulties and diabetes.

It's easy to assume that this is another family's problem, even when your own children are clinically obese, because most parents of overweight children don't recognize or acknowledge their child's condition. Researchers at Derriford Hospital in Plymouth found that only a quarter of the parents of overweight children that they questioned recognized that their children had a problem.[49] Similarly a study at Newcastle University showed that seven out of ten parents of overweight children were in denial about the problem and underestimated the risk.[50] So if you are ever in the slightest doubt about your offspring, whatever their age, please have a word with your doctor while there is still time to put things right.

Obesity is affecting adults too, of course. In 2013, the U.K. Department of Health stated that in England 61.9% of adults and 28% of children aged between 2 and 15 were overweight or obese. The story is similar in Scotland, Wales and Northern Ireland. Figure 7 shows the remarkable rise in obesity in the U.S.A. and England in recent years. Between 1978 and 2012 the number of obese people in England increased from 7.5 in every 100 to 25 in every 100. That's a 230% increase! And many, many more people are overweight, but not so overweight as to be obese. Figure 8 illustrates in graphical form a similar problem among children. Thankfully it appears that rates of childhood obesity

---

49 It is interesting that three years later the Guardian reported that half the *staff* at the same hospital were medically overweight!

50 Jones A R et al. Parental perceptions of weight status in children: the Gateshead Millennium Study. International Journal of Obesity, July 2011; Vol. 35, Issue 7:953-962.

may have stopped increasing, but a study at University College, London, suggests that this is mainly due to improving health in the children of only the better-educated and wealthier families.

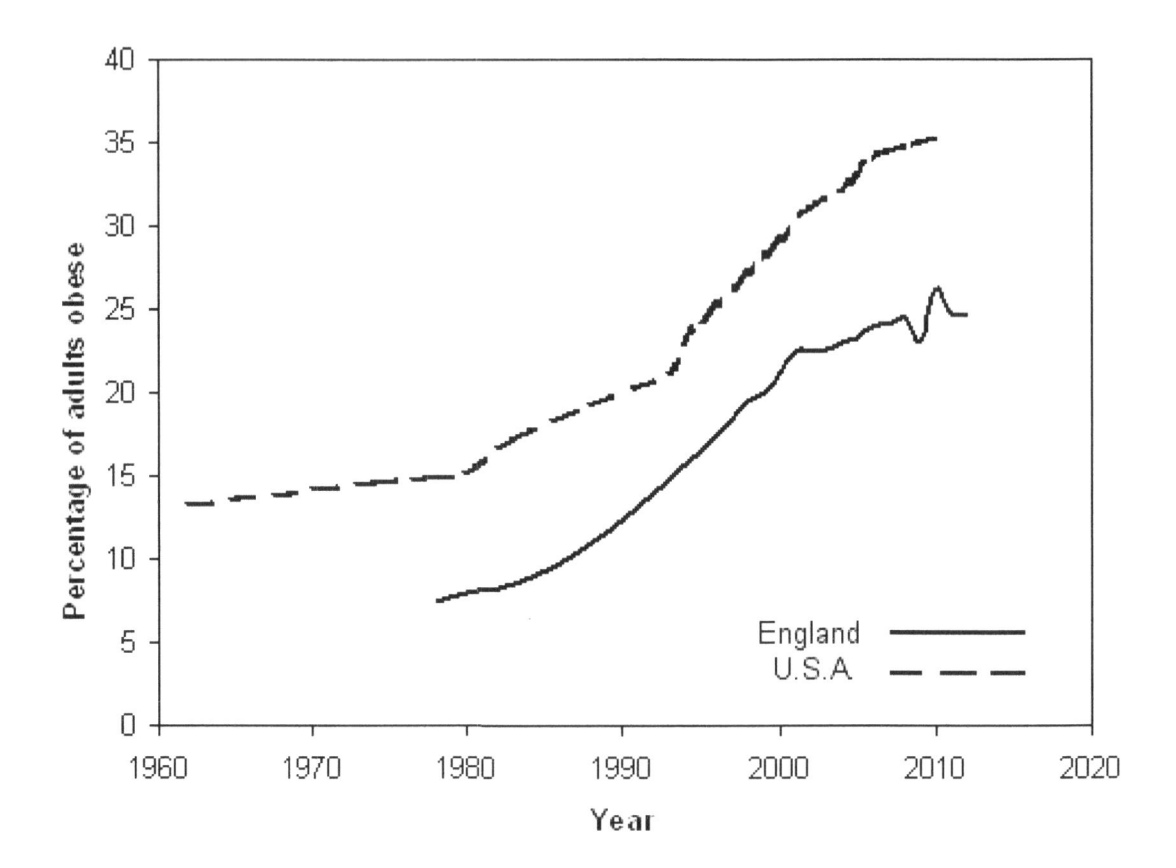

Figure 7: Trends in adult obesity, U.S.A. and England, 1962-2012[51,52,53]

---

51 *Trends in obesity prevalence.* Department of Health: Public Health England. Accessed January 21, 2014.
52 *Health Survey for England - 2012. Trend tables.* Health and Social Care Information Centre, December 2013. (Obesity is defined as having a Body Mass Index of 30kg/m² or more.)
53 *Health, United States, 2012.* Centers for Disease Control and Prevention. U.S. Department of Health and Human Services.

Figure 8: Trends in childhood obesity, U.S.A. and England, 1962-2012[54,55]

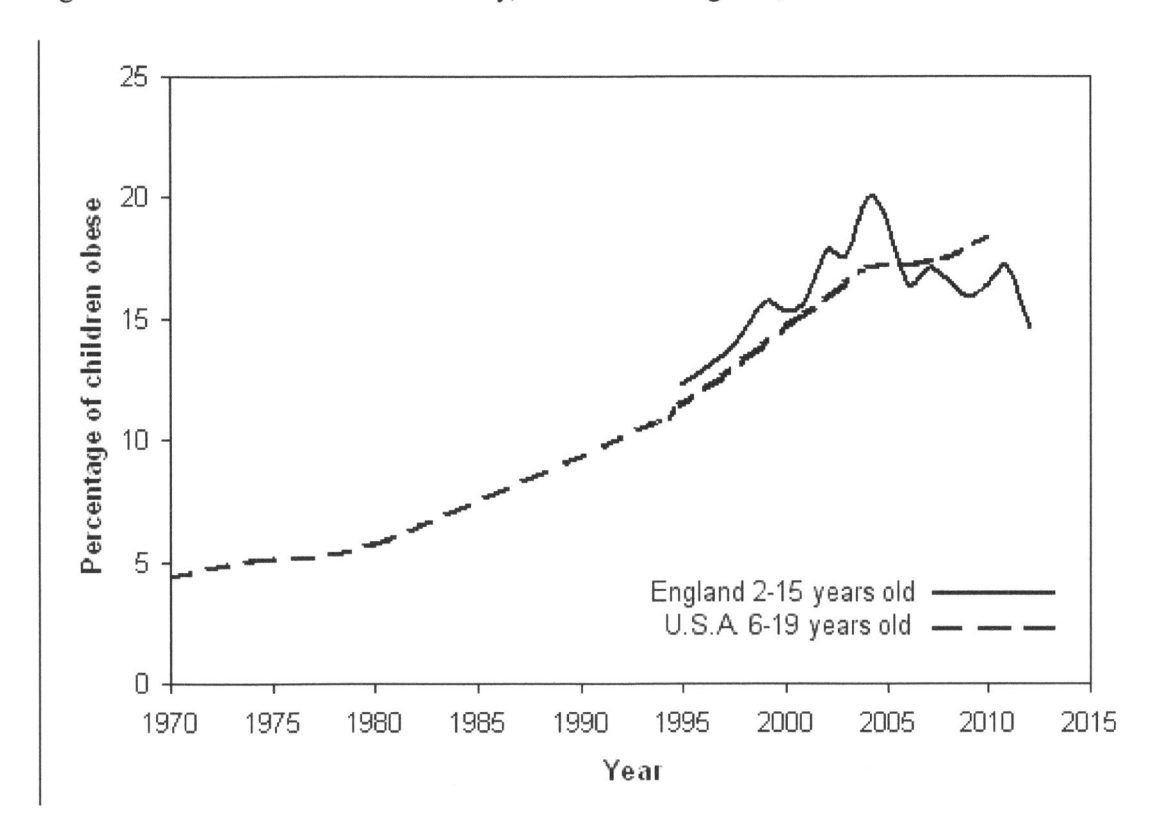

[Graph showing percentage of children obese from 1970 to 2015, with lines for England 2-15 years old and U.S.A. 6-19 years old]

Even being overweight matters. People who are overweight have a higher risk of getting type 2 diabetes, heart disease and certain cancers. They may find it harder to obtain or keep work. Their self-esteem and mental health can be affected. While health problems associated with being overweight or obese currently cost the NHS more than £5 billion every year, the Government Office of Science has forecast that, unless effective actions is taken, the total cost to the nation of people being overweight and obese will rise to £50 billion per annum in England alone by the year 2050.[56]

Heart disease, diabetes, and liver and bowel cancer

But now let's move on from obesity to other health problems. Look at Figures 9 to 12.

---

54 *Health Survey for England - 2012. Trend tables: Children trend tables.* Health and Social Care Information Centre, December 2013.

55 *Health, United States, 2012.* Centers for Disease Control and Prevention, U.S. Department of Health and Human Services.

56 *Mid-Term Review November 2008 – September 2010.* Foresight, Government Office for Science.

These illustrate the growth of various diseases in the U.S.A. and England since the Second World War.

Figure 9 shows that during the last century death from coronary heart disease (CHD) increased from almost zero in 1900 to a maximum in about 1970, when 3 in every 1,000 people in England, Wales and the U.S.A. died of it each year. Since then deaths from heart disease have steadily decreased on both sides of the Atlantic due to improvements in diagnosis and treatment, but as Figure 10 shows the number of people actually suffering from heart disease is not falling at all. Even worse Figure 11 shows that since 1970 the number of people being treated for CHD in England and Wales has increased by 600% and the number of prescriptions issued for heart trouble has risen by 600% since 1980. The cost of treating heart disease is immense and it continues to rise!

In England the number of people with diagnosed diabetes has increased more than threefold since 1990, affecting 3.2 million people or 6% of the population in 2010 and still rising. The condition kills an estimated 24,000 people a year,[57] and accounts for nearly 20% of all the patients in NHS hospitals.[58] In the U.S.A. the problem is even worse, as Figure 12 shows. According to figures published by the U.S. government's Centers for Disease Control and Prevention the true numbers are about 40% greater than the numbers of diagnosed patients shown on the graph, with over 10% of the population actually suffering from type 2 diabetes in 2011. Much of the recorded increase is due to improved diagnosis, but not all of it is, and according to Diabetes U.K. several associated problems such as retinopathy are growing worse.

Figures 13 and 14 show that both liver and bowel cancers have also become increasingly common at least since 1975, with diagnosed liver cancers increasing threefold since that year.

---

57 *National Diabetes Audit Mortality Analysis 2007-2008.* The Health and Social Care Information Centre (NHS), 2011.

58 *State of the Nation. 2012 England.* Diabetes U.K., updated to 2013. From the society's website.

Figure 9: Coronary heart disease death rates in England & Wales and the U.S.A., 1900-2011[59]

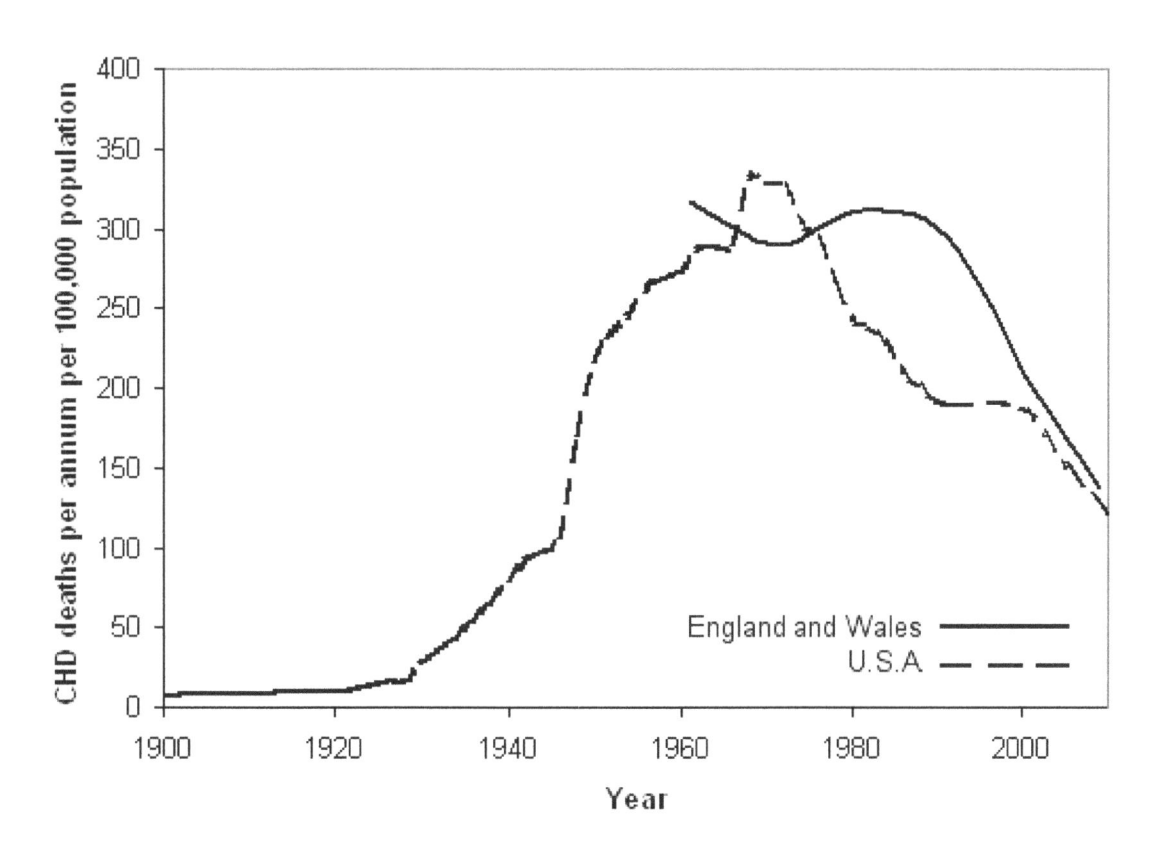

---

[59] *Trends in coronary heart disease, 1961-2011*. British Heart Foundation.
Vital Statistics of the United States: 1900-1960. Centers for Disease Control and Prevention. www.cdc.gov/nchs/products/pubs/pubd/vsus/vsus.htm.
National Vital Statistics Reports, Volumes 47-61. Centers for Disease Control and Prevention. www.cdc.gov/nchs/products/nvsr.htm

Figure 10: Heart disease prevalence, and deaths from ischaemic heart disease, among adults aged 18 and over: U.S.A. 1997-2012[60]

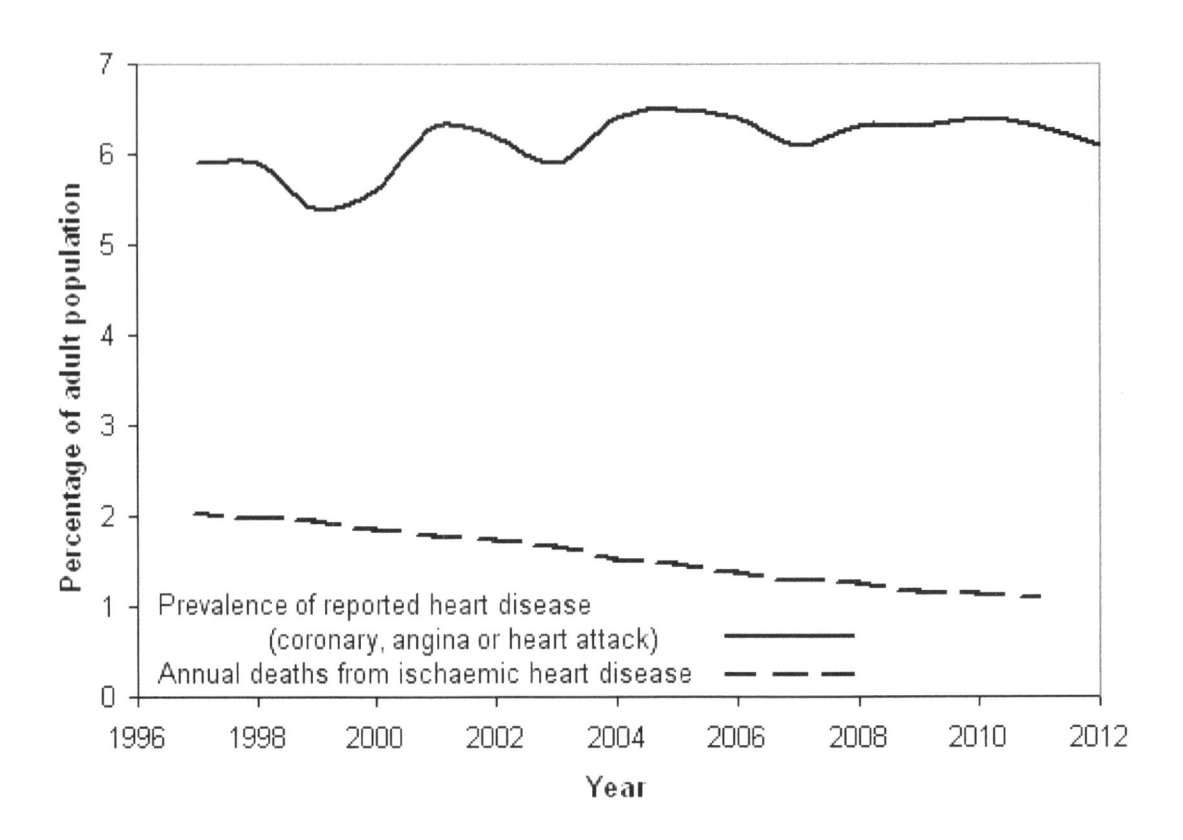

[Graph showing two lines from 1997 to 2012. Y-axis: Percentage of adult population (0 to 7). X-axis: Year. Upper line (solid): Prevalence of reported heart disease (coronary, angina or heart attack), fluctuating between approximately 5.4 and 6.5. Lower line (dashed): Annual deaths from ischaemic heart disease, declining from about 2.0 to 1.1.]

[60] Prevalence data from *Vital and Health Statistics, Series 10: Data from the National Health Interview Survey, Tables 2: Age-adjusted percentages of selected circulatory diseases among adults aged 18 years and over, by selected characteristics: United States.* Centers for Disease Control and Prevention., U.S. Department of Health and Human Services. www.cdc.gov/nchs/products/series/series10.htm
Mortality data from *Health, United States, 2012, Table 20, Age-adjusted death rates for selected causes of death, by sex, race, and Hispanic origin: United States, selected years 1950-2010.* Centers for Disease Control and Prevention, U.S. Department of Health and Human Services. www.cdc.gov/nchs/data/hus/hus12.pdf#listtables

Figure 11: Patient admissions for coronary heart disease in England & Wales and number of prescriptions for coronary vascular disease in England: 1960-2010[61]

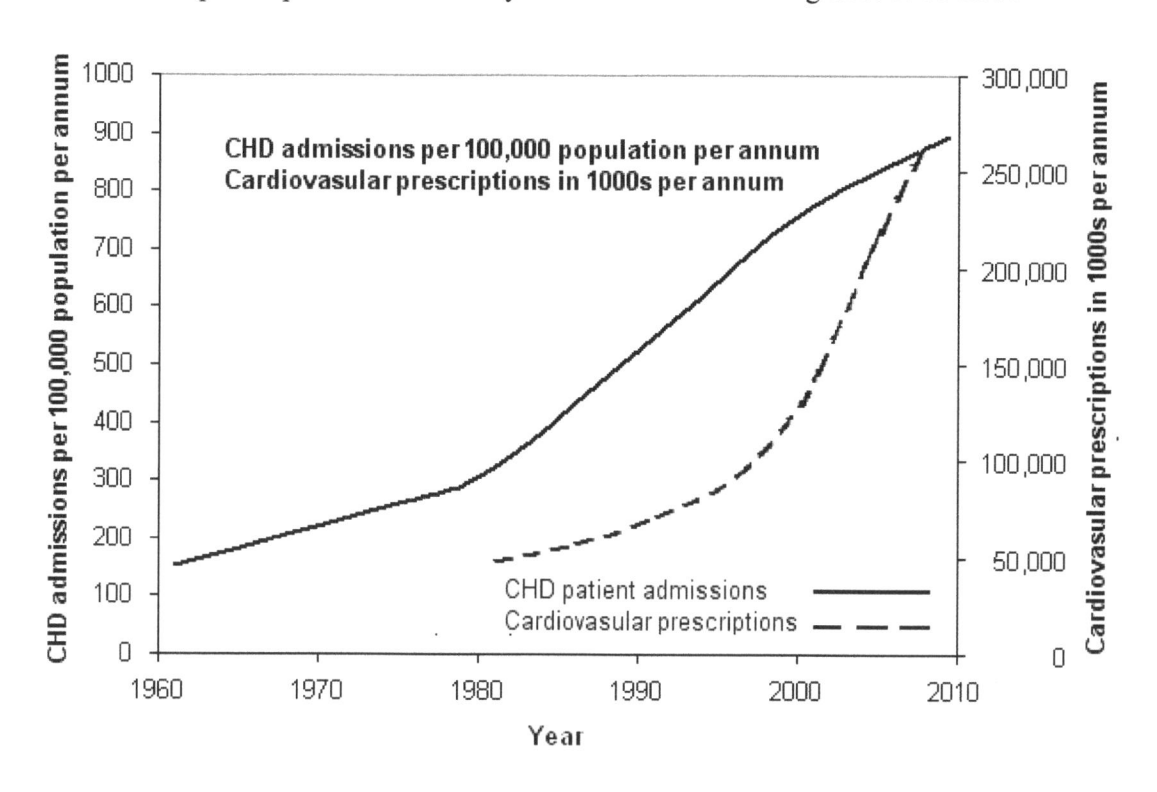

---

[61] British Heart Foundation. *Trends in coronary heart disease, 1961-2011.*

Figure 12: Percentage of population in England and the U.S.A. with diagnosed diabetes, 1958-2010[62]

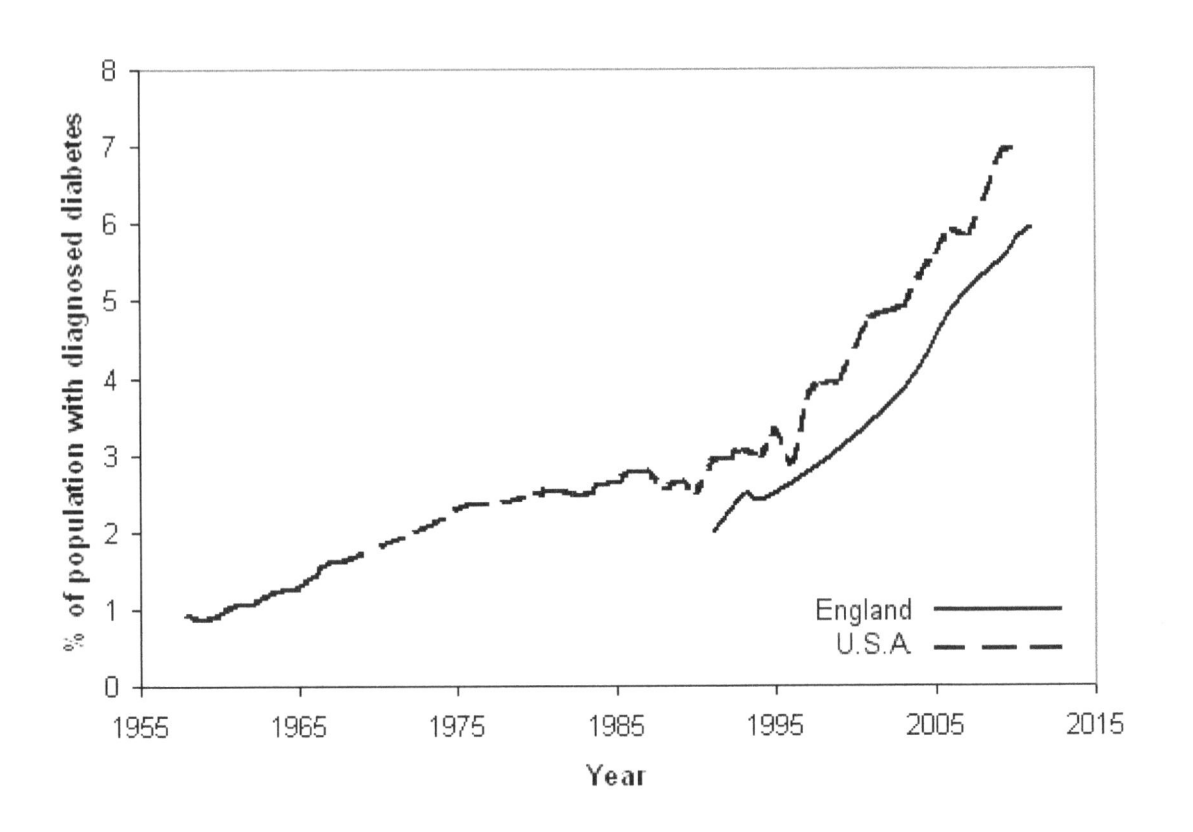

---

[62] England data from *Health Survey for England, 2011. Trend tables. Table 13. Prevalence of diabetes, by survey year, age and sex.* Health and Social Care Information Centre (NHS). December 2012 (and previous editions).
U.S.A. data from *Long-Term Trends in Diagnosed Diabetes.* Centers for Disease Control and Prevention, Division of Diabetes, Translation, October 2011.

Figure 13: Prevalence of liver cancer in Great Britain, 1975-2010[63]

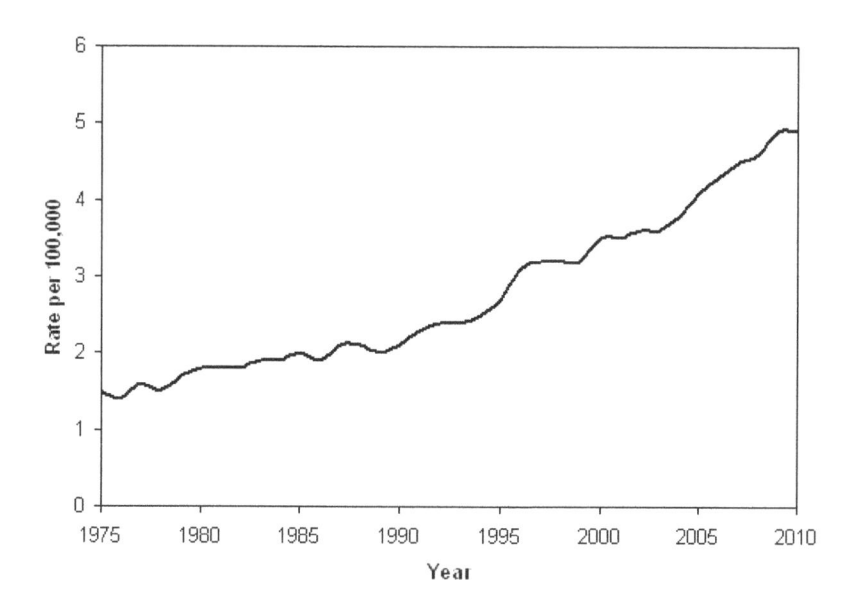

Figure 14: Prevalence of bowel cancer in Great Britain, 1975-2010[64]

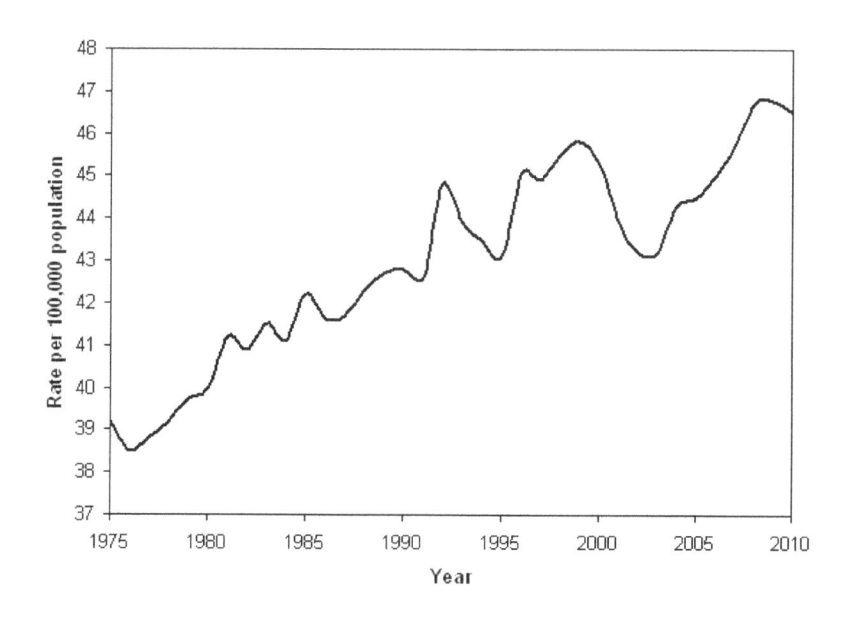

---

[63] *Liver cancer incidence statistics: Trends over time. Figure 1.2.* Cancer Research U.K., 2014. www.cancerresearchuk.org/cancer-info/cancerstats/types/liver/incidence/#trends

[64] *Bowel cancer incidence statistics: Trends over time. Figure 1.2.* Cancer Research U.K., 2014. www.cancerresearchuk.org/cancer-info/cancerstats/types/bowel/incidence/#Trends

With all this evidence of serious, and in most cases worsening, health problems in our nations, many people will shrug their shoulders as if to say, "Illnesses like these are a fact of modern life that we have to put up with. There's nothing much we can do about them." I hope that wasn't your reaction, because there is something you can do about them, something that most probably will keep you and your family completely safe from them. And that something is shown right there in Figures 7 to 12. Can you see what I am talking about?

If you look at the dates you will see that widespread obesity, coronary heart disease and type 2 diabetes are relatively new diseases. They hardly existed before 1930 in the U.S.A. or before 1940 in Great Britain. And there was very little cancer of the liver or bowels, two parts of our body most closely involved with digesting food. Something caused these diseases to appear, for you don't get an effect without a cause. Something new began to affect the populations of Britain and America as well as many other Western countries. That something new was almost certainly a widespread, major change in our diet. And we can do something about our diet!

Dietary changes in the mid twentieth century

In the 1940s our diet in the U.K. was based on advice published by the government back in 1938. According to the Social Issues Research Centre in Oxford:[65]

'The BMA and the government, based on the research in the 1920s and 1930s by Sir John Boyd Orr and others, recommend that the British people should drink eighty percent more milk, eat fifty-five percent more eggs, forty percent more butter and thirty percent more meat.'

In keeping with these recommendations, in 1944 the government introduced free, full-cream milk for all school children up to the age of 18, in the 1950s we were all encouraged to 'Drinka Pinta Milka Day', and in 1957 the Egg Marketing Board encouraged us all to 'go to work on an egg'. And what happened? Did everyone put on weight and suffer heart attacks? No. After the war, child deaths from diphtheria, measles, scarlet fever and whooping cough fell dramatically. Rickets and other vitamin deficiency diseases were relegated to the past. Obesity wasn't a problem. In my last primary school class in 1952 there was only one slightly plump child. At secondary school, as late as 1960, I remember only one fat boy and maybe two or three boys who were on the plump side, one of whom was the school's champion pole-vaulter. I and the other children whose parents followed those recommendations are now the very people who are living so long that pension funds are short of money.

So how did our diet change after this time? Between about 1935 and 1975 in the U.K. people started to replace butter, made by cows, with margarine made from plant

---

65   www.sirc.org/timeline/1938.shtml

oils and all kinds of chemicals. Lard, made by pigs, was replaced by Trex, Cookeen, Crisco, Spry and similar products that were also made from plant oils. These substitute products were used more and more in homes for frying and baking and spreading on bread. Commercial fryers such as fish and chip shops and later fast-food outlets like McDonald's also replaced lard by plant-based oils. In most cases these oils contained trans fats as well as much higher levels of polyunsaturated fat.

Trans fats are polyunsaturated fats which have hydrogen forced into them at high temperature to make them more solid and to stop them going rancid, and it is almost certain that they have been responsible for much of the increase in coronary heart disease. A study of over 85,000 female nurses who were initially healthy in 1980 showed that the likelihood of their contracting heart disease or dying from a heart attack during the following 8 years was directly proportional to the amount of trans fats they consumed.[66]

Other significant dietary changes in this period were that people gradually consumed more sugar, and food manufacturers began to use more chemical additives to improve appearance, taste and shelf life. And what happened to public health? By 1975 it was clear that a major epidemic of heart disease had begun in Western countries, and it was getting worse. Not only that: type 2 diabetes was starting to become an issue.

Various national and international bodies correctly decided that the appearance of these major health epidemics must be due to diet, but instead of recommending a return to the diet which people had lived on earlier in the century, when there was little or no heart disease, they recommended almost the exact opposite: that we should consume even less animal fat, and obtain most of our calories instead from carbohydrates! Throughout the 1980s various reports were published by bodies like the World Health Organization (WHO), the American Heart Association, the U.K. National Advisory Committee for Nutrition Education, and the Scottish Home and Health Department, and these all recommended that we obtain more and more of our calories from starchy carbohydrates and plant-based oils, and less and less from saturated fat in the form of fatty meat and full-cream dairy products. The final 1990 WHO report recommended obtaining only 15% to 30% of our calories from fat, with as nearly as possible zero per cent from saturated fat and free sugar, and from 50% to 70% (nearly all) of our calories from starchy carbohydrates. A supporting publication called 'Eat Well... Live Well!' produced by the U.K. Guild of Food Writers and endorsed in 1991 by the Secretary of State for Health, actually said, '*Eat bread, cereals and potatoes and other starchy goods with every meal, and snack on sandwiches and other breads.*' That was terrible advice, as you'll see shortly.

At least these various reports recommended eating less sugar and more fresh fruit and vegetables, so their recommendations were not all bad. Some also advocated an increase in fibre, which may or may not be a good thing, and some a reduction in alcohol

---

66 Willet W C et al. *Intake of trans fatty acids and risk of coronary heart disease among women.* Lancet, March 6, 1993.

consumption, which certainly would be.

So what exactly happened once people started to adopt these changes? Figures 7 to 14 give the answer. There was an explosion of obesity, particularly among children; bowel cancers doubled and liver cancers tripled. The incidence of heart disease stubbornly remained at the same high level, while type 2 diabetes continued to rise without a halt. Not exactly a good result really, was it? And, if you look at Figure 4 again, you'll see a strong hint that the only reason the incidence of heart disease stopped rising was that people started to eat *less* margarine.

When the low-fat fad was first introduced it wasn't universally supported. In 1986 the American Academy of Pediatrics objected to the idea that even children over 2 years old should eat a low-fat diet.[67] '*Meat and dairy products, which would be restricted, form an important source of protein,*' they declared. '*Dairy products provide 60 per cent of dietary calcium; and meat is the best source of available iron. Current dietary trends in the United States - decreased consumption of saturated fats, cholesterol and salt, and an increased intake of polyunsaturated fats - should be followed with moderation. The optimal fat intake cannot be determined, but 30% to 40% of calories seems sensible for adequate growth and development.*' However these apparently rational objections were soon drowned under the onrushing tide of vegetable oil and skimmed milk. At the time of writing it is recommended in the U.K. that low-fat milk and other foods should start to be introduced from the age of 2. They are still doing it!

The current U.K. dietary recommendations published by the Food Standards Agency and the National Health Service are based on the 1990 WHO report, even though it is nearly 25 years old. We are advised to eat:

- as many vegetables and fresh fruits as we like, but at least five portions a day
- plenty of starchy foods such as rice, bread, pasta, potatoes and cereal foods with every meal
- moderate amounts of protein-rich foods such as lean meat, fish, eggs, nuts and pulses
- moderate amounts of reduced fat milk and dairy products or small amounts of full-fat versions
- as little fat, sugar and salt as possible

Thus, in an attempt to halt heart disease, the experts who wrote the 1990 WHO report decided to encourage people to eat as much starchy carbohydrate as they like, apparently oblivious of the fact that one of the first things our digestive system does is to turn starch into glucose and then, if it isn't needed for immediate energy requirements, to store it as fat. No wonder there has been an explosion of obesity, as well as a continuing increase in type 2 diabetes resulting from excessive glucose levels in the blood. Any first-year

---

[67] *Prudent Life-style for Children: Dietary Fat and Cholesterol.* Pediatrics, 1986; 78:521.

medical student could have predicted such an outcome, at least until he was brainwashed into believing the exact opposite!

One of the more reliable predictors of heart disease is the level of triglycerides in the bloodstream.[68,69] E. J. Parks[70] described research in which 34 patients with coronary heart disease changed from a diet high in carbohydrates and low in fat (59% of energy from carbohydrates: 21% from fat) to a diet *very* high in carbohydrates and *very* low in fat (76% of energy from carbohydrates: 8% from fat). As a result, the triglyceride level increased by 30% in those with a body mass index of 28kg/m^2 or more (very overweight or obese), but it remained the same in those with a lower BMI. Although this research did not measure the long-term effects of such a diet on triglyceride levels it does suggest that people who are very overweight will increase their risk of a heart attack if a very high proportion of their calories come from carbohydrates and only a small proportion from fats.

In conclusion, bingeing on bagels, buns, baps and bread increases blood sugar and insulin levels and bolsters the triglyceride levels of very overweight people. Since high levels of all three substances in the blood seem to be associated with arterial damage, let's find out now why this is. Why exactly is our food is killing us?

---

68 Austin M A et al. *Hypertriglyceridemia as a cardiovascular risk factor.* American Journal of Cardiology, 1998; 81:7B–12B.

69 Sarwar N et al. *Triglycerides and the risk of coronary heart disease: 10,158 incident cases among 262,525 participants in 29 Western prospective studies.* Circulation, 2007; 115:450–458.

70 Parks E. J. *Dietary carbohydrate's effects on lipogenesis and the relationship of lipogenesis to blood insulin and glucose concentrations.* British Journal of Nutrition, Volume 87, 2002; Supplement 2, S247–S253.

CHAPTER 6: FATS – THE GOOD, THE BAD AND THE UGLY

Oscar Wilde was probably right when he said that the truth is rarely pure and never simple. All the same I'll try in this chapter to make it as pure and simple as possible.

Types of fat

Saturated fats are the main kinds of fat found in animals and human beings, and in tropical oils like coconut and palm oil. They are solid at room temperature, but if they are warmed up they melt.

Unsaturated fats are the main kinds of fat found in the seeds of cereals and other plants that grow in temperate countries, and in oils obtained from their seeds, such as sunflower oil. They are also found in oily fish such as tuna and sardines, but not in great quantities. Unsaturated fats are liquid at room temperature. Fish have to have unsaturated fat otherwise they would go stiff in the cold sea and wouldn't be able to swim. 'Unsaturated' means that the chemical molecules are not full: they have room for other atoms or molecules to join them.

Actually, there are two kinds of unsaturated fat, '*monounsaturated*' and '*polyunsaturated*'. A monounsaturated molecule has room for one or two additional atoms or molecular groups, while polyunsaturated ones can accept more. So when the polyunsaturated molecules in sunflower oil, for example, are exposed to the air, they partner up with multiple oxygen atoms in the air. This is called oxidation, and it means that the oil goes rancid. The resulting bad taste indicates that it is no longer good for us.

Trans fats, as I said, are polyunsaturated fats which have hydrogen forced into them at high temperature to make them more solid and to stop them going rancid.

Cholesterol is a special kind of fat that is an essential part of all the cells in our bodies and is used to make a number of equally essential hormones or messenger cells. Some foods such as eggs contain small quantities of cholesterol, but most of it is generated internally by our liver.

Figure 15 shows the relative amounts of each kind of fat in some common food sources. You'll see that round about half the fat in meat and dairy products is saturated, but in most cooking oils and nuts it is mostly unsaturated fat that will go rancid after a period of exposure to the air.

Figure 15: Fats as a percentage of total fat in some common foodstuffs[71]

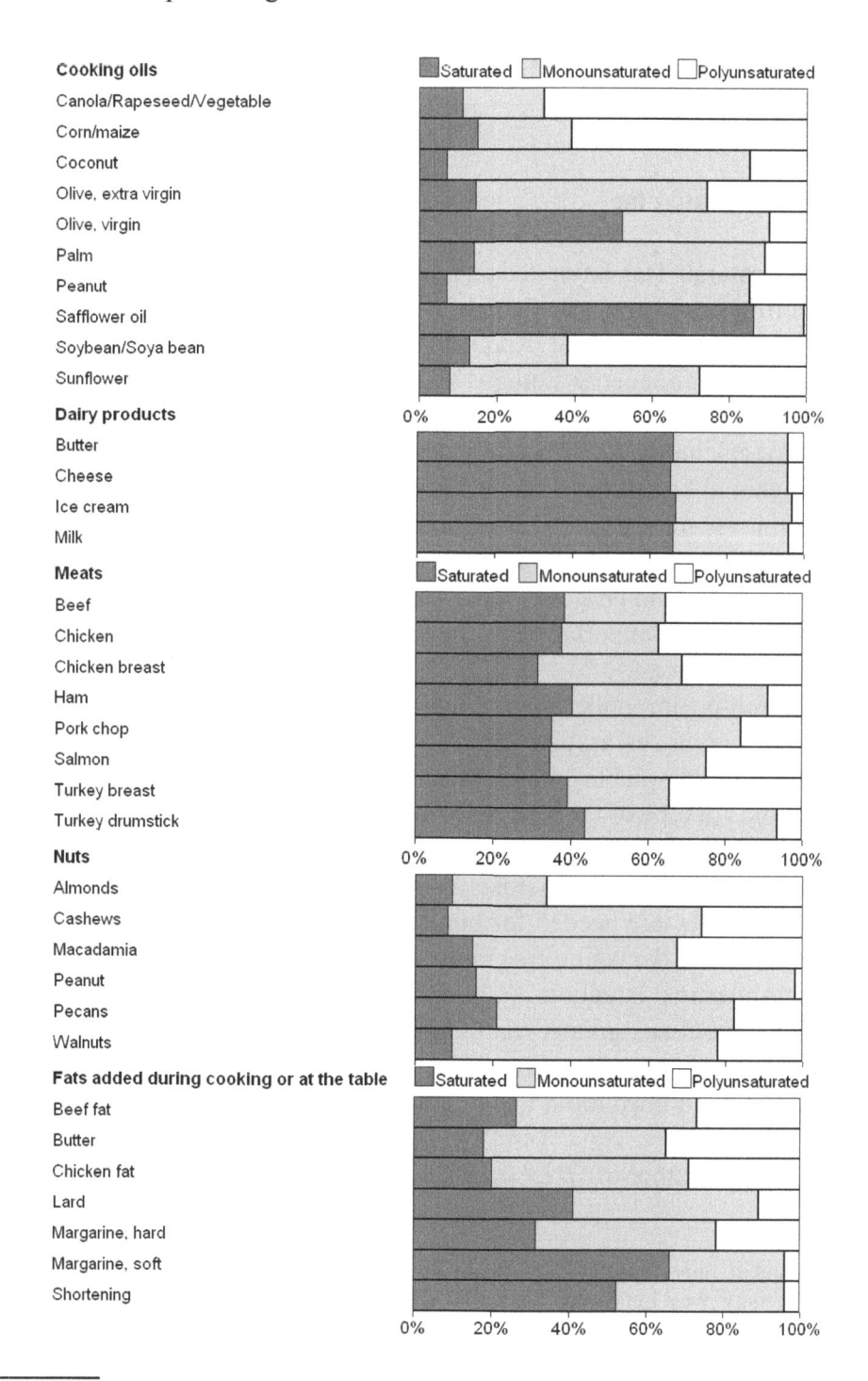

---

71 Sources: Best consensus of information from Wikipedia: Cooking oil; Wikipedia: Monounsaturated fats; About.com: Culinary arts.

Now I can explain what's wrong with the fats in our current diet and why they are killing us. I just hope that some intelligent person in the government will read this and will do something about it. Basically, there are three things wrong with the fats in our typical Western diet.

1. Not enough saturated fat

Our bodies need saturated fat. Saturated fats constitute at least 40% of our cell membranes, giving them stiffness and strength. 50% of our brain consists of saturated fat. 100% of our lung surfactant is saturated fat. And saturated fat is the main kind of fat our bodies use for insulation and for energy storage.

Saturated fat is essential for our lungs to work properly and to avoid asthma and emphysema. For calcium to be incorporated properly into our bones, at least 50% of the fat in our diet should be saturated fat.[72] Our white blood cells need it to recognize and destroy foreign invaders such as viruses, bacteria, and fungi. The liver needs saturated fat to make cholesterol, which is used to make critical hormones such as cortisol, testosterone, oestrogen and progesterone, as well as vitamin D and bile.

So saturated fat is as important as water and air. When we don't eat enough of it things go drastically wrong.

Butter and full-cream milk are particularly important sources of saturated fat, for saturated fat comprises around 40% of the fat in full-cream milk. Furthermore, cream contains the fat-soluble vitamins A, D, E and K_2, lecithin, iodine, selenium, glycosphingolipids (a type of fat needed by the brain) and (if the cows are fed on grass) conjugated linoleic acid. Between them these various substances provide a degree of protection against cancer, heart disease, calcification of the joints, osteoporosis, and thyroid problems. They are needed for human fertility and normal reproduction. They neutralize the effects of damaging free radicals and help our bodies to fight infection, in particular gastrointestinal infections. (Children who drink skimmed milk have diarrhoea at rates three to five times greater than children who drink whole milk.[73]) And these important substances are not found, or else are found in much smaller quantities, in semi-skimmed and skimmed milk, the very kinds of milk we are always being told are healthier for us!

As Barry Groves, author of '*Trick and Treat: How Healthy Eating Is Making Us Ill*', writes:

---

72 Watkins B A et al. *Importance of Vitamin E in Bone Formation and in Chrondrocyte Function.* Purdue University, West Lafayette, Indiana, AOCS Proceedings, 1996;
Watkins B A & Seifert M F. *Food Lipids and Bone Health.* Article in McDonald R E & Min D B (editors). *Food Lipids and Health,* p. 101. Marcel Dekker, Inc, New York, 1996.

73 Koopman J S et al. *Milk fat and gastrointestinal illness.* American Journal of Public Health, 1984, 74:12:1371-1373.

'The fats our bodies store and those that are found in human breast milk are the fats our bodies are designed to use. These contain very little of the polyunsaturated fatty acids found in vegetable oils. Instead, they are made up of a mixture of saturated and monounsaturated fatty acids which are similar to the fatty acid profiles found in the fats of cattle and sheep. Our bodies haven't evolved to do things that harm themselves. As our natural body fat is nearly half saturated, how did we ever come to believe that such fats can be harmful to us? Human breast milk is 54% saturated. Does anyone believe that this is harmful to a human child? How did this ridiculous idea (that saturated fat is harmful) *ever get started?'*

2. Too much unsaturated fat

Unsaturated fats are mainly found in plant oils and in products like margarine and similar spreads made from them, and in nuts. As I explained, unsaturated fats oxidize on exposure to the air and after a while they go rancid. This is a particular problem for soya oil, sunflower oil, corn/maize oil, canola/rapeseed/vegetable oil and even peanut/groundnut oil, which all have a high proportion of polyunsaturated fat. Oxidation occurs even faster when an unsaturated fat is heated, for example in frying, so it's a very bad idea to allow unsaturated cooking oils to get too hot, or indeed to eat food made with such oils if it has been fried or baked. That includes most of the cooked products and fast-food delicacies kindly provided by your local supermarket or the 'U.K. Chinese Halal Pizzeria' round the corner. In 2001 a review of studies in the U.K., the U.S.A. and Spain during the previous 20 years concluded that the prolonged consumption of burnt oils was likely to lead to *'atherosclerosis, the forerunner to cardiovascular disease; inflammatory joint disease, including rheumatoid arthritis; pathogenic conditions of the digestive tract; mutagenicity and genotoxicity, properties that often signal carcinogenesis; and teratogenicity, the property of chemicals that leads to the development of birth defects'*.[74] The scientists who wrote the report also questioned the advice given by most health authorities to consume large amounts of polyunsaturated fats without taking measures to protect them against oxidative degradation. This is because even our body temperature is above the temperatures that temperate plants experience in the open air so, even without frying or baking them, such fats will oxidize once they are inside us.

People used to fry their eggs and bacon for breakfast in lard, which is what fish and chip shops used before they changed to peanut oil. Lard is healthier because it is mostly saturated fat, and saturated fat molecules are positively inhospitable to oxygen or anything else. However one practical problem with cooking with lard is that if any liquefied lard is tipped down the sink it will solidify again and in time may block the

---

74 Grottveld M et al. *Health effects of oxidized heated oils.* Foodservice Research International, Volume 13, Issue 1: 41–55. 2001.

drainpipe. One solution is to wipe the pan out with some kitchen paper before washing it up. A more traditional way is simply to leave any excess fat to solidify in the pan ready for use another time. If you adopt this approach you should clean the fat occasionally by boiling some water in the pan and then allowing it to cool. When the fat solidifies again the water can be poured off with the impurities in it. If you still prefer frying in oil, use extra virgin olive oil (which by definition must be produced by a process that doesn't raise its temperature above 30°C), or coconut oil or palm oil. But don't use palm oil from Borneo and Sumatra where tropical rainforests are being cut down to clear the ground for this profitable crop and where the orang-utan has lost 90% of its habitat in consequence. Red palm oil from some African countries comes from sustainable sources and doesn't cause major environmental problems.

When complicated molecules such as unsaturated fat molecules oxidize, parts of them may become 'free radicals'. A free radical isn't a political agitator who hasn't been arrested yet. It's best defined as an incomplete molecule. A complete molecule of H_2O, for example, consists of two atoms of hydrogen and one of oxygen. The reason that these three atoms stick together is that hydrogen atoms each have one 'hand' and oxygen atoms have two 'hands', so the two-handed oxygen atom can hold hands with two hydrogen atoms. Atoms don't like to find themselves empty-handed, so if the oxygen atom loses one of its hydrogen atoms it looks around for something else to take its place. This incomplete HO molecule is called a 'free radical'.

When unsaturated fats oxidize inside us free radicals are produced. The reason that these can endanger our health is that they so much want to find an atom to replace the one they have lost that they are willing to steal the first one they can find from a complete molecule. When that happens the complete molecule is left empty-handed, turning it into another free radical which goes off looking for a third molecule it can steal from and so on. A chain reaction is started. The serious danger that this poses to the cells in our bodies is that when a molecule steals an atom or even part of a molecule to make itself complete again, the part that it steals may be different from the part it had before, so the molecule itself changes into something different, something abnormal which should never have been in our body at all.

Unsaturated fats, especially the polyunsaturated ones, are very easy to steal atoms from. This is because inside each molecule there are carbon atoms holding on to each other with two hands, like the oxygen atoms do. Monounsaturated fat molecules each have just two carbon atoms holding hands with each other: polyunsaturated fat molecules have several. But carbon atoms are special: they have two hands and two feet, so they can hold on with their feet as well! So, while these carbon atoms are holding on to each other with their hands, they are also hanging on to other parts of the molecule, including hydrogen atoms, with their feet. They are so busy clinging on to each other that they forget to hold on equally tightly to the hydrogen atoms, and as hydrogen atoms have only one hand to hold on with anyway they are easily kidnapped by a marauding free radical, leaving a newly created free radical in the form of a degenerate fat molecule.

Wikipedia's article on 'Lipid peroxidation' clearly states, as I have, that the problem most often affects *polyunsaturated* fatty acids, i.e. the ones that the government and food manufacturers are always telling us are the healthier ones.[75]

Our bodies actually generate some free radicals on purpose. They do this for various purposes, such as killing bacteria, fungi and parasites, or carrying messages around. Normally, if the free radicals in our bodies aren't needed to kill infections or carry messages around, they are arrested by the digestive police in the form of antioxidant enzymes such as vitamins C and E and chemicals called uric acid, glutathione and melatonin. These same antioxidants can also neutralize the free radicals generated by the oxidation of fats and alcohol inside us, but if there are too many free radicals or too few enzyme policemen to cope with them then the free radicals run riot and start to cause damage.

Dr. Hari Sharma, who wrote '*Freedom from Disease: How to Control Free Radicals*', lists the results of such damage: '*In a joint, it ultimately results in arthritis, in lungs we have emphysema and bronchitis, in the blood vessels we have atherosclerosis or heart disease, in the stomach we have peptic ulcer, in the skin, ageing and wrinkling. If free radicals are produced in the DNA, the DNA mutates and will produce cancer, leukaemia or lymphoma. Diabetes, kidney problems, liver problems, almost every disease is related to the damage caused by these free radicals. If we remove the cause of the damage, all these diseases can be prevented.*' I must say that I found this hard to believe until I discovered the very same message in Wikipedia's articles on 'Antioxidants' and 'Oxidative stress', backed up by its mandatory reference list of corroborating scientific papers. The article on oxidative stress, which is what happens when one's body cannot effectively deal with free radicals, says that it is thought to be involved in the development or exacerbation of many diseases, including cancer, Parkinson's disease, Alzheimer's disease, atherosclerosis, heart failure, myocardial infarction, schizophrenia, bipolar disorder, fragile X syndrome, sickle-cell disease, lichen planus, vitiligo, autism, and chronic fatigue syndrome.

So the startling conclusion is that consuming too many unsaturated fats, *especially polyunsaturated fats*, causes cell damage that ultimately leads to most types of human disease. You certainly won't hear this mentioned by the companies that produce cooking oils from maize and sunflowers and soya beans, nor from the manufacturers of the margarines that are made from them. However there is a lot of experimental evidence that directly links the high consumption of polyunsaturated fats to human diseases:

---

75 The first paragraph of Wikipedia's entry on 'Lipid peroxidation' talks about stealing an electron rather than a hydrogen atom. This is not in accordance with the subsequent text nor with Wikipedia's accompanying diagram, so it appears to me to be an error.

- Unsaturated fats suppress our immune systems[76],[77] and kill white blood cells.[78] That means they make it harder for our bodies to fight infections.
- Cancer cells are known to have a high level of unsaturated fats,[79] and breast cancer in rats was found to occur only when there were unsaturated fats in their diet.[80]
- Alcoholic cirrhosis of the liver cannot occur unless there is linoleic acid in the diet.[81] Linoleic acid is a polyunsaturated fatty acid found in safflower, sunflower, and maize oils.
- The consumption of unsaturated fat is believed to have a role in skin ageing.[82]
- Lipid peroxidation (the degradation of fats through oxidation) appears to make the skin more sensitive to damage from ultraviolet light so that skin cancers develop.[83]

One obvious question arises: why is the NHS not telling us this? One reason is that the NHS is not primarily a health service. It's a sickness service, and that's where its focus is. Apparently even weight loss isn't taught in medical schools. In 2014 the Daily Mail featured an article by two doctors – identical twins – who both needed to lose weight. One of them wrote, '*Despite being doctors - I also have a degree in public health - neither of us knew much about losing weight and eating healthily. These topics fall between the cracks at medical school. Yes, we understood biochemistry and food metabolism, and knew a lot about the consequences of being overweight. But which diets work, why we eat too much and why losing weight is so hard don't sit within any medical speciality*'. The NHS does fund research through the National Institute for Health Research and the Medical Research Council, but only a minority of that funding is spent on trying to improve public health. Much of it is spent on improving surgical procedures, developing technology aids for the handicapped, or even looking for ways to run the Health Service more efficiently. The vast majority of NHS expenditure goes into treating the sick, and I

---

76   Mertin J & Hunt R. *Influence of polyunsaturated fatty acids on survival of skin allografts and tumor incidence in mice.* Proceedings of the National Academy of Sciences, U.S.A., March 1976; 73(3): 928–931.

77   Mascioll E A et al. *Medium chain triglycerides and structured lipids as unique nonglucose energy sources in hyperalimentation.* Lipids, 22(6) 421-3, 1987.

78   Meade C J & Martin J. Advances in Lipid Research, 127, 1978.

79   Lankin V Z & Neifakh E A. [*Higher fatty acids in the process of malignant growth*]. (Article in Russian.) Izvestiya Akademii Nauk Kazakhskoj SSR, Ser. Biology, March-April 1968; 2:263-8.

80   Ip C et al. *Requirement of essential fatty acid for mammary tumorigenesis in the rats.* Cancer Research 45, 1985.

81   Nanji A A & French S W. *Dietary linoleic acid is required for development of experimentally induced alcoholic liver-injury. Life Sciences,* 1989; 44:223-301.

82   Widmer R et al. *Protein oxidation and degradation during aging: role in skin aging and neurodegeneration.* Free Radical Research, December 2006; 40(12):1259-68.

83   Black H S et al. *Relation of antioxidants and level of dietary lipids to epidermal lipid peroxidation and ultraviolet carcinogenesis.* Cancer Research 45(12, pt 1), 6254-9, 1985.

would guess that less than 1% goes into preventing sickness in the first place.

Perhaps another reason that the NHS is not telling us the whole truth about unsaturated fats is that it is a government-controlled body, and governments are extremely reluctant to take any action that would cause a major disruption to a nation's industrial, commercial and economics sectors. But maybe, just maybe, the polyunsaturated spread manufacturers are themselves beginning to worry about the problem. In 2012 Flora changed the formulation of its 'original' spread in order '*to enhance its health credentials*' by reducing the percentage of vegetable fat from 59% to 45%.[84] So here's a question: if vegetable fat is so healthy, how does reducing the amount of it make a spread healthier?

3. Trans fats

I once heard a speaker named Ronald Dunn say, "*I may be Dunn but I'm not finished yet.*" So I may be A. Page but I haven't reached the last one yet!

One of the more lethal components of our modern diet has been, and still is to some extent, trans fats. In 2006 it was estimated that eating trans fats was causing up to 100,000 deaths a year.[85] Here at least pretty well everyone is in agreement: man-made trans fats are harmful.

Very small quantities of trans fats occur in natural foods such as meat, but nearly all trans fats are man-made. They are made by adding hydrogen to vegetable oils at high temperature to stop them oxidizing. By filling the vacant spaces in unsaturated fat molecules with hydrogen there are no spaces left for oxygen atoms to come in and turn them rancid. So products cooked in or made with trans fats last longer: they can hang around on the supermarket shelves much longer and can be bought before they have to be labelled, 'Reduced for a quick sale'. The result is of course that food manufacturers and supermarkets reduce their costs. An additional advantage of hydrogenation, as it is called, is that it thickens the oil so that it can be spread on bread more easily. This property makes the process ideal for the manufacture of margarine and similar spreads. Trans fats were used on a wide scale in margarine and commercially fried and baked products as a replacement for saturated fats such as lard. This was in the 1970s and 1980s, when people began to think that heart disease was caused by saturated fat. What people who thought they were buying 'healthy' margarine didn't know was that trans fats, or perhaps the chemicals involved in their manufacture,[86] would cause heart disease

---

84 Ford R & Zuke E. The Grocer, March 2, 2012.

85 Zaloga GP et al. *Trans Fatty Acids and Coronary Heart Disease*. Nutrition in Clinical Practice 21: 505–512, October 2006.

86 Chemicals used in the manufacture of margarine may include petroleum-based solvents like benzene, bleaching agents (illegal in the manufacture of bread in the U.K.), caustic soda, nickel (known to cause cancer) as a catalyst, and antioxidants such as the carcinogenic butylated hydroxyanisole (E320), which are usually petroleum based.

and almost certainly a number of deadly types of cancer.

In 1993 eight scientists studied data on the diet and health of 85,000[87] nurses that had been gathered over 8 years by Harvard University during the 1980s. They discovered that *'Intakes of foods that are major sources of trans isomers (margarine, cookies [biscuits], cakes and white bread) were each significantly associated with higher risks of coronary heart disease'*.[88] Professor Walter Willett was the principal investigator of the original nurses' study and the lead author of the 1993 paper. According to an article in the Guardian newspaper[89] he called hydrogenation *'the biggest food processing disaster in US history'*.

In addition to heart disease, the Wikipedia article on trans fats lists seven other deadly diseases that they either cause or may cause.

Thankfully their use has been largely eliminated during the last few years, but they are not actually illegal and are still be present in some products.[90]

In the 1990s McDonald's were pressurized by the so-called Center for Science in the Public Interest to replace beef dripping with deadly hydrogenated vegetable oils. It wasn't until 2007 that they made the decision to eliminate hydrogenated trans fats completely. However they still use a mixture of rapeseed, maize and soy oils, all high in polyunsaturated fat and subject to oxidation on heating, much as other fast-food companies do.

Another expression for trans fat is 'partially hydrogenated vegetable oil'. Fully hydrogenated vegetable oil does not contain trans fats, but unless a food label specifically says 'fully hydrogenated vegetable oil' some of it may be partially hydrogenated. So if you see the words 'partially hydrogenated vegetable oil' or simply 'hydrogenated vegetable oil' in a product's list of ingredients, don't buy it. Even so, food manufacturers in the U.S.A. don't have to include trans fats in the list of ingredients if they constitute less than a certain small percentage. So any substitute for butter or lard and any commercially cooked product manufactured there could contain very small quantities

of man-made trans fats.

---

87   By the time the study ended in 1999 a total of 91,249 nurses had been included.

88   Willett W C et al. *Intake of trans fatty acids and risk of coronary heart disease among women.* Lancet, March 6 1993; 6;341(8845):581-5.

89   Felicity Lawrence, The Guardian, 23 January 2010.

90   In the U.S.A., the 2009 Food and Drug Administration regulations state that if there is less than 0.5gm of an ingredient per serving the label should say '0g per serving'. So even if a food label states that a spread contains zero trans fat one could be eating up to 0.5gm of it per slice of bread. A serving of margarine is considered to be two teaspoonfuls or 10gm, which means that up to 5.0% of a spread can be hidden trans fat. In the U.K. however the Food Labelling Regulations 1996 permit the words 'trace', 'negligible', 'nil' or '0gm' to be used only if a nutrient constitutes less than 0.1% of the ingredients by weight or volume. This limit is 50 times stricter than the limit in the United States.

CHAPTER 7: BATTLE OF THE OMEGAS

Mega trouble

There are some special kinds of fat that we need in very small quantities. Nearly everyone agrees that eating the wrong amounts of them is causing some very big problems. What is not agreed is how to get the right amounts of them into our diet.

Both omega-3 and omega-6 fatty acids are essential parts of a human's diet, but consuming too much omega-6 and too little omega-3 spells mega trouble. You may have seen an advertisement for a 'healthy' spread telling you that it has 'added omega-3'. The reason that some margarine manufacturers add omega-3 fat to their products is that the seed oils from which the spreads are made contain too much omega-6 fat. Omega-3 has to be added to compensate for this. Butter is naturally healthy and doesn't *need* added omega-3, because it already contains enough and has far less omega-6.

Back in 1982 it was discovered that people who ate plenty of omega-3 fatty acids in their diets generally lived longer. In the same year, three scientists called Bergstrom, Samuelsson and Vane won a Nobel Prize for discovering that too little omega-3 produces a whole range of diseases and the reason for this. Both omega-6 and omega-3 fatty acids make some important things called signalling molecules. Signalling molecules tell our cells how to grow and repair themselves and defend themselves against infection, and they send messages around our nervous system. So you can understand that they are essential for keeping us healthy. But omega-3 and omega-6 make two different kinds of signalling molecules, which each do very different jobs. And the problem is that these two kinds of omega fats compete for the same enzyme 'food' in our bodies, rather like red and grey squirrels used to compete for similar food until the little red ones died out in most parts of Britain. So if we eat too many grey squirrel omega-6 molecules there isn't enough food in us for the little red omega-3 ones, and then they can't do their job properly.

Bergstrom and his colleagues discovered that too much omega-6 and too little omega-3 results in painful and chronic inflammation within our bodies, and it is this which causes many of the diseases people suffer from, particularly in Western nations where our diet contains far more omega-6 than omega-3. Inflammation is a major cause of coronary heart disease, many forms of cancer, asthma,[91] and various autoimmunity and neurodegenerative diseases such as coeliac disease, rheumatoid arthritis, Parkinson's and Alzheimer's diseases.[92] Doctors often treat it with nonsteroidal anti-inflammatory drugs (NSAIDs) such as ibuprofen and naproxen, because these block the production of signalling molecules by omega-6. You've probably seen advertisements for ibuprofen on television. NSAIDs produce substantial profits for their manufacturers, costing from £2.50 to £185 a month per patient.[93] The NHS could save millions of pounds if they simply told sufferers to reduce their intake of omega-6 fatty acids, but of course NSAID manufacturers aren't going to mention that in their advertisements.

Too much omega-6 can also result in blood clots, high blood pressure, irritation of the digestive tract, depressed immune function, sterility, cell proliferation and weight gain.[94] It is especially likely to produce insulin resistance, which is a major cause of type 2 diabetes.[95] Margarine is a huge source of omega-6, and even bread has eight times as much omega-6 as omega-3.

Both omega-6 and omega-3 fats are polyunsaturated fats, for there are at least 40 different ones. So, while earlier research identified polyunsaturated fats in general as the causes of obesity and ill health, in more recent years it has been discovered that it is in these two particular groups of omega polyunsaturated fats where a major problem lies. So when I talk about consuming too much omega-6 I am still talking about eating too much food or oil that comes from seeds and nuts, such as polyunsaturated cooking oils, rice, flour, maize and soya products.

Too little omega-3 brings problems of its own. Omega-3 is essential for the proper development of the eye retina and hence for sight. Children whose mothers ate oily fish (the major source of omega-3) during their pregnancy tend to have better eyesight than

---

91   Okuyama H et al. *Dietary Fatty Acids - The N6/N3 Balance and Chronic Elderly Diseases. Excess Linoleic Acid and Relative N-3 Deficiency Syndrome Seen in Japan.* Progress in Lipid Research, 1997; 35:4:409-457.

92   www.drweil.com/drw/u/QAA400149/balancing-omega-3-and-omega-6.html. Accessed February 2013.

93   US$4 to US$300 a month. Consumer reports.org. www.consumerreports.org/health/resources/pdf/best-buy-drugs/Nsaids2.pdf

94   Horrobin D F. *The regulation of prostaglandin biosynthesis by the manipulation of essential fatty acid metabolism.* Reviews in Pure and Applied Pharmacological Sciences, 1983; 4: 339-383;
Devlin T M, ed. Textbook of Biochemistry, 2nd Edition, 1982, Wiley Medical, 429-430;
Fallon S & Enig M G. *Tripping Lightly Down the Prostaglandin Pathways.* Price-Pottenger Nutrition Foundation Health Journal, 1996; 20:3:5-8.

95   Berry E M. *Are diets high in omega-6 polyunsaturated fatty acids unhealthy?* European Heart Journal Supplements, 2001, 3 (Supplement D); D37–D41.

other children.[96] Omega-3 fats are essential for the proper development and functioning of the brain, so a lack of them can cause mental problems. A lack of omega-3, especially before and after birth, has been associated with learning difficulties.[97] It can result in depression,[98],[99],[100],[101] dyslexia, hyperactivity and even violent and criminal behaviour.[102] In several studies it was found that giving omega-3 supplements to violent young men in prison reduced rule breaking, aggressive behaviour and violent incidents.[103],[104] When the supplements stopped the violent behaviour resumed.[105] Before going to a psychologist, any parent with a depressed, dyslexic, hyperactive or violent child should consider what he is eating. Mega problems may have an o-mega cause.

One other effect of a lack of omega-3, which is especially interesting to me as an oldie and has only recently been discovered, is that people who consume more omega-3 fatty acids do not age so quickly and therefore live longer.[106] Remember you'll be an oldie one day, if you remember your Highway Code and the world doesn't end first!

It is not the amount of omega-3 we consume that matters so much as the relative

---

96 Williams C at al. (Longitudinal Study of Pregnancy and Childhood Study Team.) *Stereoacuity at age 3.5 years in children born full term is associated with prenatal and postnatal dietary factors: a report from a population-based cohort study*. American Journal of Clinical Nutrition, 2001; 73:316-322.

97 Okuyama H et al. *Dietary Fatty Acids - the N-6/N-3 Balance and Chronic Diseases. Excess Linoleic Acid and the Relative N-3 Deficiency Syndrome Seen in Japan*. Progress in Lipid Research, 1997; 35:4:409-457. (Also cited earlier.)

98 Maes M et al. *Fatty acid composition in major depression: decreased omega-3 fractions in cholesteryl esters and increased C20: 4 omega-6/C20:5 omega-3 ratio in cholesteryl esters and phospholipids*. Journal of Affective Disorders, 1996; 38:35–46.

99 Edwards R et al. *Omega-3 polyunsaturated fatty acid levels in the diet and in red blood cell membranes of depressed patients*. Journal of Affective Disorders, 1998; 48:149–55.

100 Peet M et al. *Depletion of omega-3 fatty acid levels in red blood cell membranes of depressive patients*. Biological Psychiatry, 1998; 43:315–9.

101 Maes M et al. *Lowered omega-3 polyunsaturated fatty acids in serum phospholipids and cholesteryl esters of depressed patients*. Psychiatry Research, 1999; 85:275–91.

102 www.drweil.com/drw/u/QAA400149/balancing-omega-3-and-omega-6.html. Accessed February 2013.

103 Gesch CB at al. *Influence of supplementary vitamins, minerals and essential fatty acids on the antisocial behavior of young adult prisoners. Randomised, placebo-controlled trial*. British Journal of Psychiatry 2002; 181;22–28.

104 Hibbeln J R et al. *Omega-3 fatty acid deficiencies in neurodevelopment, aggression and autonomic dysregulation: Opportunities for intervention*. International Review of Psychiatry, April 2006; 18(2): 107–118.

105 Zaalbergl A et al. *Effects of Nutritional Supplements on Aggression, Rule-Breaking, and Psychopathology Among Young Adult Prisoners*. Aggressive Behaviour, Volume 36, pages 117–126, 2010.

106 Farzaneh-Far R et al. *Association of marine omega-3 fatty acid levels with telomeric aging in patients with coronary heart disease*. Journal of American Medical Association, Vol. 303, No. 3, January 20, 2010.

amounts of omega-6 and omega-3, in other words how badly the grey squirrels outnumber the red ones. Let's call the ratio between the two kinds the O-6-3 ratio. In the diet of Greenland Eskimos (more correctly the Inuits) the O-6-3 ratio has been estimated at 1:1, i.e. equal quantities of omega-6 and omega-3. In the traditional Japanese diet it has been estimated at around 4:1, or four times as much omega-6 as omega-3. Typical European diets however provide O-6-3 ratios of between 10:1 and 14:1;[107] in the U.S.A. the ratio is higher, and in Israel, where there is a particularly high prevalence of cardiovascular diseases, hypertension, type 2 diabetes, obesity and cancer, the ratio is as high as 26:1.[108] Contrast these O-6-3 ratios in the Western world with values of between 1:1 and 4:1 on which humans are thought to have evolved,[109] and you can see how much our Western diet has been altered by commercial food manufacturers.

Look at the extraordinary chart below in Figure 16. It shows an almost exact association between the death rates from heart attacks and the percentage of omega-6 fats in the highly unsaturated fatty acids (HUFA[110]) found in the body tissues of various population groups. As the percentage of omega-6 fats in a population group increases, its death rate increases in exactly the same proportion. This is the chart that Ancel Keyes should have shown the world back in 1953. Then we wouldn't have had all the nonsense about saturated fat causing heart attacks.

---

107 *Fats and oils in human nutrition: Report of a Joint Expert Consultation.* FAO Food and Nutrition Paper No. 57, 1994.

108 Berry E M. *Are diets high in omega-6 polyunsaturated fatty acids unhealthy?* European Heart Journal Supplements, 2001, 3 (Supplement D); D37–D41. (Also cited earlier.)

109 Budowski P & Crawford M A. *Alpha linolenic acid as a regulator of the metabolism of arachidonic acid: dietary implications of the ratio, n-6:n-3 fatty acids.* Proceedings of the Nutrition Society, 1985; 44: 221–9.

110 Highly unsaturated fatty acids are polyunsaturated fats that contain several double chemical bonds in each molecule and are therefore easily oxidized.

Figure 16: Association between percentage of omega-6 in highly unsaturated fatty acids and coronary heart disease death rates[111]

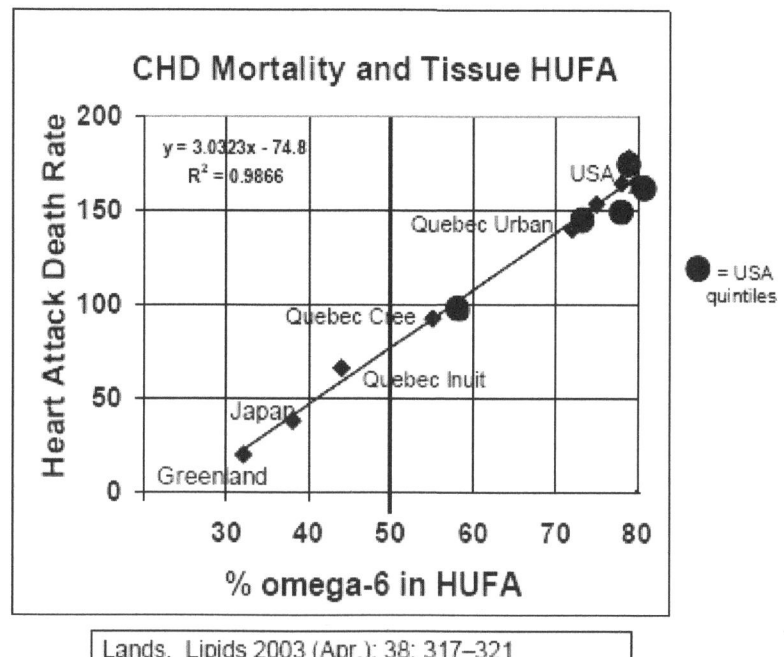

CHD Mortality and Tissue HUFA

$y = 3.0323x - 74.8$
$R^2 = 0.9866$

(Heart Attack Death Rate vs % omega-6 in HUFA; data points labeled Greenland, Japan, Quebec Inuit, Quebec Cree, Quebec Urban, USA; ● = USA quintiles)

Lands, Lipids 2003 (Apr.); 38: 317–321

More recently Dr. Bill Lands, who produced the chart in Figure 16, has shown that the *difference* between the amounts of omega-6 and omega-3 in our diet can give a good estimation of the percentage of omega-6 that will end up in our tissues, and hence a good estimation of the risk of a heart attack.[112] In other words, what matters is both the ratio of omega-6 to omega-3 in a particular food and how much of it we eat. If some food has a bad, high ratio but we eat only a tiny amount of it then our bodies will cope; but if the ratio in a particular food is only moderately high and we virtually live on it, then we probably won't live on it much longer!

"That's all very well," you might say, "but how can one possibly create a family menu that provides an O-6-3 ratio of less than four? It's complicated enough trying to count calories." Certainly most parents wouldn't have the time, inclination or ability to add up the omega contents of food while they are doing their shopping, and even if they wanted to they would find that very few products display the amounts of omega-3 and omega-6 in their nutritional information.

---

111 Lands W E M. *Diets could prevent many diseases*. Lipids, 38:317-21, 2003.

112 Lands B & Lamoreaux E. *Using 3–6 differences in essential fatty acids rather than 3/6 ratios gives useful food balance scores*. Nutrition & Metabolism, 2012; 9:46.

There are three possible ways to correct an imbalance in the omega ratio:

(i) Eat more food that's high in omega-3
(ii) Take omega-3 supplements, e.g. fish oil capsules
(iii) Eat less food that's high in omega-6

Let's look at these three options in turn.

Solution 1: Eat more food that's high in omega-3

It's extraordinary, but the only substantial source of omega-3 fatty acids in the form our body needs them comes from the sea. Some omega-3 can be obtained from grass-fed meat, poultry fed on grass and insects, and eggs from such poultry, and the body can obtain a certain amount in the forms that it needs from plants, but by far the best source of omega-3 is fish, and in particular oily fish. Oily fish also contain vitamins A and D, so it is doubly good for you.

Oily fish are fish that store their fat in their flesh. Some common types are:

- herrings (which include kippers and bloaters)
- sardines and pilchards (pilchards are large sardines)
- mackerel
- salmon
- fresh or frozen tuna
- anchovies
- swordfish
- halibut
- trout
- sprats
- whitebait
- carp

There is a much fuller list of oily fish as well as non-oily fish in Annexe 5. Herrings have the most omega-3 by weight, with the others in approximately descending order. Fish roe, weight for weight, is even better than herrings. Crabs and shellfish are other good sources of omega-3, but the best source of all is caviar. Caviar has three times as much omega-3 as the same weight of herrings, but you'll probably need a much better paid job before you can afford to buy Royal Beluga caviar for your family at £2,570 per kilogram!

In general the omega-3 content of any particular species of fish is similar whether it is fresh, frozen or canned. Fish canned in oil loses some omega-3 because fatty acids dissolve in oil, so when you pour the oil away you pour away some of the omega-3 too.[113] You could drink the oil as well as eat the fish if you wanted to, but whatever you do don't drink it if it is sunflower oil because its omega content is 100% omega-6 so it will completely undo the good of the omega-3 in the fish.[114] Even olive oil has more omega-6 than is really good for you. The healthiest canning mediums for fish are spring water and brine (salt water). Canned tuna however contains very little omega-3 whatever it is canned in, so you can't count canned tuna towards your oily fish consumption.

Non-oily white fish such as cod, haddock and plaice also contains omega-3 and vitamins, but not nearly so much as oily fish does. However cod liver oil is an excellent source of omega-3, because non-oily fish store their fat in their liver. Of course cod liver oil on its own doesn't provide the protein that eating the fish itself does.

So, eating oily fish will increase our omega-3 consumption, but the question is, how much fish do we need to eat before the O-6-3 balance in our diet is at a healthy level? Naturally the answer to that question depends on how much omega-6 we are consuming. Unfortunately all the research into this subject, so far as I know, has been carried out on people who are on a typical Western diet, so the resulting recommendations really apply only to people who are eating high amounts of omega-6, but at least this can give us a start.

The British Food Standards Agency (FSA) says that everyone should eat 'at least' two 140gm portions of fish a week, including one portion of oily fish. However, women who are likely to have a child, and pregnant and nursing women, should eat no more than two portions a week of oily fish, and other people should eat no more than four.[115] The upper limit is set because of concerns about harmful contaminants in sea water such as mercury and dioxins that may get into some fish.

The Scientific Advisory Committee on Nutrition (SACN), which advises the FSA, makes the same recommendations, but adds that everyone should consume a minimum of 450mg per day or 3,150mg per week of 'long-chain omega-3 fatty acids'.[116] For children the International Cod Liver Omega-3 Foundation suggests a minimum intake of 200mg per day or 1,400mg a week.

The two most important long-chain omega-3 fatty acids so far as our diet is concerned

---

113 Tesco states that the omega-3 content of its canned fish is the same whether it is canned in oil or water. I find this hard to understand, especially since Glenryck Ltd states that its pilchards canned in oil contain only half the amount of EPA + DHA that its pilchards in water contain. EPA and DHA are the kinds of omega-3 found in fish which our bodies need. Perhaps the loss of these in Tesco fish canned in oil is made up for by linoleic acid or LA, a kind of omega-3 found in oils such as olive oil and sunflower oil, but which is of far less nutritional value.

114 A 125gm tin of typical mackerel fillets in sunflower oil contains 90gm of mackerel fillets and 35gm of oil. The mackerel contains 2.8 x 90 / 100 = 2.52gm of omega-3. The sunflower oil contains 22.7 x 35 / 100 = 7.95gm of omega-6. The combined O-6-3 ratio is therefore 7.95/2.52 = 3.15:1. This is within the healthy range of 4:1 and 1:1, but it will not help to bring a high dietary O-6-3 ratio down to a healthy level, which eating only the mackerel would do.

115 www.food.gov.uk/multimedia/faq/oilyfishfaq/#.URpmq5Zs9aY June 2004. Accessed March 2013.

116 Scientific Advisory Committee on Nutrition, FICS/04/02, dated 14/04/04. www.sacn.gov.uk/pdfs/fics_sacn_04_02.pdf. Accessed March 2013.

are eicosapentaenoic acid (EPA) and docosahexaenoic acid (DHA), and those are the two main kinds of omega-3 found in fish. A third one, docosapentaenoic acid or DPA, is found in fish in smaller quantities. Another kind of omega-3 is alpha-linolenic acid or ALA. This is found in plants, and the body can convert it to EPA and DHA, so it is an essential source of omega-3 for vegetarians. However, some studies have indicated that ALA is ineffective in reducing the likelihood of a heart attack or the recurrence of one.[117]

In terms of fish, a 140gm portion of the oily fish salmon contains about 2,800mg of EPA and DHA and a similar portion of the non-oily fish plaice contains about 350mg, so a weekly portion of oily fish and one of non-oily fish would provide the 3,150mg weekly ration recommended by SACN for adults. For children two 60gm portions a week would provide the recommended 1,400mg of omega-3.

While at least two portions of fish a week is the official advice given in the U.K., the words 'at least' cover up the fact that for people on a typical Western diet two portions are not nearly enough to keep us healthy, as many other authorities show. Table 2 summarizes the advice from the FSA and other bodies.

---

[117] Wang C at al. *n-3 Fatty acids from fish or fish-oil supplements, but not alpha-linolenic acid, benefit cardiovascular disease outcomes in primary- and secondary-prevention studies: a systematic review.* American Journal of Clinical Nutrition, July 2006; 84(1):5-17.

Table 2: Recommended mixed oily and non-oily fish consumption necessary for cardiac and other health on a Western diet[118]

Source	Recommended number of 140gm portions of mixed fish per week	Comments
UK Food Standards Agency	2 at least	With limitations on maximum consumption for women who may have a child and for pregnant and nursing mothers.
UK Scientific Advisory Committee on Nutrition	2 or 3	To reduce the risk of heart trouble, from various sources.
	4	For people over 65 or those who have survived some form of heart attack.
	6 at least	To significantly reduce the risk of heart trouble.
American Heart Association	2	'Especially oily fish'. With limitations on certain species for pregnant and nursing mothers and young children.
	4 at least	People who have had a heart attack.
	9 to 18	Equivalent in capsule form for people who need to lower their triglyceride level.
Holland & Barrett	Up to 7 portions of fish, or the equivalent in fish oil.	From various cited research sources, for protection from heart trouble, lupus and rheumatoid arthritis.

---

118 See Annexe 6 for detailed references and the derivation of the quoted numbers.

| US National Institutes of Health | 9 or the equivalent in fish oil. | For someone on a 2,000Kcal a day diet, or in proportion. |

It may take from 2 to 6 months for the benefits of increasing one's intake of fish oil to be measurable.

So there you go. Table 2 shows that to be absolutely certain that our diet isn't contributing to a heart attack or other health problems we should be eating six to nine portions of uncontaminated fish a week! This is completely unrealistic, unless one is an Eskimo or a shark. Bearing in mind that on average British people eat only a little over one portion of fish a week, if we all ate only the FSA's minimum recommendation of two portions a week, twice as many fish would have to be taken out of the sea, and it is doubtful if the already depleted fish stocks could survive this. That may be why the government recommends only two portions a week, even though its own Scientific Advisory Committee says we ought to eat at least six portions a week to reduce the risk of heart disease significantly. So let's look at the second solution.

Solution 2: Take omega-3 supplements

Omega-3 supplements come in several forms:

- fish oil and cod liver oil capsules
- krill oil capsules
- flaxseed oil capsules
- omega-3 enriched foods

In general, governments don't recommend the use of such supplements, although the NHS in Britain does provide vouchers for free vitamin drops that contain fish oil for children up to their fourth birthday, if you can manage to get hold of them. While the US Food and Drug Administration (FDA) hasn't published any recommendations for omega-3 supplementation, the American Heart Association (AHA) suggests that people who have been diagnosed as having coronary heart disease should consume 1gm a day of omega-3 (EPA + DHA), either from oily fish or, in consultation with a doctor, from fish oil capsules. The AHA also says that people who need to lower their triglyceride level should take 2gm to 4gm a day of EPA + DHA in fish oil capsules.

There is no apparent reason why governments should not recommend omega-3 supplementation, unless it is that they don't want to admit their existing dietary advice is inadequate, so many people do buy omega-3 supplements in order to keep themselves healthy. However a lot of this is needed in order to provide a significant benefit, as I shall now explain.

(i) Fish oil and cod liver oil capsules

Some Norwegian researchers discovered that over an 8-week period salmon raised the level of EPA + DHA in the blood more than cod liver oil did, even though the amount of cod liver oil they provided contained two and a half times as much EPA + DHA as the salmon did.[119] Another study demonstrated that to obtain the same increase in EPA and DHA in the blood one needs twice as much EPA from fish oil as from salmon, and *nine times as much* DHA.[120] Therefore in this section I am going to assume that to supplement our omega-3 intake from cod liver oil or fish oil we need to consume about three times as much EPA + DHA as we would if we obtained it from fish.

(ii) Krill oil

Other researchers in Norway found that krill oil was more beneficial than fish oil. Krill are small shrimp-like crustaceans on which many fish feed. Krill oil is an increasingly popular source of omega-3: for instance the British eBay website lists well over 200 products and the American version some 450. However there are concerns that unrestricted krill trawling in the south Atlantic and other places will in time deplete the fish stocks. The researchers discovered that both krill oil and fish oil raised the level of EPA + DHA in the subjects' blood by a similar amount, but the krill oil dosage contained only 62.8% as much EPA + DHA as the fish oil dosage did.[121] Assuming that the fish oil used in the research was similar in its effects to pure cod liver oil this means that to supplement omega-3 from krill oil one has to consume about twice as much EPA + DHA as one would if one obtained it from fish.

(iii) Flaxseed oil

Flaxseed oil is an excellent source of omega-3 in the form of ALA, but only a small proportion of ALA is converted by our bodies into the EPA + DHA that they need, at least by men on a typical Western diet. The proportion is higher for women and for people who do not ingest a lot of omega-6 fatty acids. The measured conversion rate

---

119 Elvevoll EO et al. *Enhanced incorporation of n-3 fatty acids from fish compared with fish oils.* Lipids, December 2006; 41(12):1109-14.

120 Visioli F et al. *Dietary intake of fish vs. formulations leads to higher plasma concentrations of n-3 fatty acids.* Lipids, 38(4):415-8, April 2003.

121 Ulven S M et al. *Metabolic Effects of Krill Oil are Essentially Similar to Those of Fish Oil but at Lower Dose of EPA and DHA, in Healthy Volunteers.* Lipids, 46 (1): 37–46. January 2011.

varies from 0.2%[122] to 15%,[123] with 5% being the most commonly accepted figure.[124] All researchers report that the conversion rate for DHA, the kind of omega-3 needed by our nerve and brain cells, is much lower than for EPA.

Some researchers in North Dakota compared the effectiveness of flax oil and fish oil.[125] A company of firefighters, a group of men considered to be at risk of heart trouble due to stress and relatively poor diet, were given daily capsules of fish oil or flax oil over a period of 12 weeks. Both were effective in raising the levels of EPA, DHA and DPA in the blood, but the fish oil was much more effective than the flax oil, as shown in Table 3.

Table 3: Percentage increase in base level of EPA, DHA and DPA in the blood after 12 weeks of omega-3 supplementation among four experimental groups of men

Oil	No. of capsules per day	Omega-3 dose per day in milligrams	Percentage increase in blood EPA + DHA + DPA after 12 weeks
Fish	1	268mg EPA + DHA + DPA	123%
Fish	2	536mg EPA + DHA + DPA	187%
Flaxseed (linseed)	4	2,392mg ALA	54%
Flaxseed (linseed)	6	3,588mg ALA	71%

Using average values of the figures above it appears to obtain the same benefit from flax oil as from fish oil one needs 18.4 times as much ALA from flax seed oil as EPA + DHA + DPA from fish oil. This means that in order to produce a similar benefit from flax oil as from fish itself one needs 3 x 18.4 = 55 times as much ALA from flax oil as EPA + DHA + DPA from fish!

---

122 Pawlosky R J et al. *Physiological compartmental analysis of alpha-linolenic acid metabolism in adult humans.* Journal of Lipid Research, 2001; 42:1257–1265.

123 Emken E A et al. *Dietary linoleic acid influences desaturation and acylation of deuterium-labeled linoleic and linolenic acids in young adult males.* Biochemica et Biophysica Acta, 1994; 1213:277–288.

124 Gerster H. *Can adults adequately convert alpha-linolenic acid (18:3n-3) to eicosapentaenoic acid (20:5n-3) and docosahexaenoic acid (22:6n-3)?* International Journal for Vitamin and Nutrition Research, 1998(2); 68 (3):159–173.

125 Barceló-Coblijn G et al. *Flaxseed oil and fish-oil capsule consumption alters human red blood cell n-3 fatty acid composition: a multiple-dosing trial comparing 2 sources of n-3 fatty acid.* American Journal of Clinical Nutrition, September 2008; 88(3):801-9.

(iv) Milled flaxseed

Flax seeds have a hard shell, so in order to digest them they must either be toasted for 5 to 10 minutes in a skillet or in the oven at 190°C, or else they must be ground or milled. In the latter case they must be kept in an airtight container to protect them from oxidation.

(v) Required quantities of omega-3 supplements

Earlier, I said that for people on a typical British diet who have not experienced heart trouble SACN recommends a minimum consumption of 3,150mg of omega-3 a week from oily and non-oily fish, which is equivalent to a 140gm serving of salmon and a 140gm serving of cod. So to obtain a similar benefit from supplements you would need to consume two times as much omega-3 from krill oil, three times as much from fish oil, or 55 times as much from flaxseed oil. Table 4 shows the resulting minimum recommended amounts of each supplement for adults, together with the corresponding costs of typical products in the U.K. at the time of writing. As previously mentioned, it has been suggested that children should obtain a minimum of 1,400mg of omega-3 a week, so for children the quantities and costs shown in the table should be reduced by a factor of 1,400/3,150 = 0.44. The cost of some items may be considerably less in North America.

Table 4: Methods of obtaining a week's minimum recommended intake of 3,150mg EPA + DHA from fish or the equivalent benefit from oil, and some representative costs in the U.K.

Source	Description	Conversion factor	Amount required per week	Cost [1]
Oily fish + non-oily fish, fillets	Frozen salmon fillet + frozen cod fillet (Tesco)	1	One 140gm portion of each	£2.50
Oily fish + non-oily fish, canned	Sardines canned in brine + tuna canned in brine (Tesco)	1	One 120gm tin of sardines + one 185gm tin of tuna	£1.17
Cod liver oil	1,000ml costs £13.48. 10ml contains 1,400mg EPA + DHA. (Holland & Barrett (H & B))	3	67.5ml	£0.91

Cod liver oil capsules	240 Seven Seas high strength cod liver oil capsules cost £15.37. (H & B) 1 capsule contains 180mg EPA + DHA.	3	52 capsules	£3.33
Krill oil capsules	60 omega-3 krill oil capsules cost £20.23. (H & B) 1 capsule contains 120mg EPA + DHA.	2	52 capsules	
Flaxseed oil	946ml flaxseed oil costs £19.57. (H & B) 10ml contain 4,660mg ALA.	55	372ml	£7.69
Flaxseed oil capsules	240 flaxseed oil capsules cost £40.04. (H & B) 2 capsules contain 1,872mg ALA.	55	185 capsules	
Milled flaxseed powder	600gm costs £6.73 (H & B). 10gm contains 2,100mg ALA.	55	825gm	£9.25
Hemp oil	520ml of GranoVita hemp oil made from organically grown hemp seed costs £10.78 (H & B). 10ml contains 1,660mg ALA.	55 (Assumed the same as for flax oil.)	1,044ml	

[1] Based on some advertised prices in March 2013

The costs shown in Table 4 are per adult per week, so it's obvious that, apart from free vitamin drops, anything other than fish or bottled cod liver oil would be too expensive for the average family. For many people, even fish fillets are a luxury. And drinking 372ml a week of flaxseed (linseed) oil is unthinkable.

(vi) Omega-3 enriched foods

One other way of increasing one's intake of omega-3 in a small way is to eat foods that have omega-3 added to them. As previously mentioned, margarine manufacturers add omega-3 to make up for the excessive omega-6 in the margarine itself, and omega-3 is also added to some juice drinks, breakfast cereals, milk, cheese, eggs and even pet food! In most cases the words 'with added omega-3' are little more than an advertising gimmick, for the tiny amount added makes no significant difference whatsoever.

Flora Omega-3 Plus spread, for example, contains fish oil; hence it is advertised as containing two kinds of omega-3, EPA and DHA. But only 1.8% of it is fish oil. Nearly all the rest comprises vegetable oils in which the omega fatty acids are mainly omega-6. Therefore although it does contain omega-3 this hardly helps to redress the imbalance between the two kinds of omega fats.

Omega-3 is 'added' to some eggs by feeding the hens with canola (rapeseed) oil. This oil has a healthy O-6-3 ratio of 2:1, but because rapeseed is a plant, the omega-3 part is mainly ALA, and the amount of ALA in an egg that is converted to EPA and DHA in our bodies is so small that again it is of minimal benefit.

Some cows have fish oil added to their diet, so that dairy producers can advertise 'omega-3 enhanced' milk, butter or cheese and sell them at a premium. Doing this does increase the omega-3 content, but not by very much, and whether this is a good use of the world's dwindling stocks of fish is open to question. In any case natural milk from cows fed on grass has an excellent O-6-3 ratio of 1.5:1 so its omega-3 content needs no enhancing.

Birds Eye 'Omega-3 fish fingers' also contain a little added fish oil, and they are made from pollock, which contains twice as much omega-3 as cod does. However, pollock still contains only a quarter as much omega-3 as mackerel and herring, and even in these good quality fish fingers only 58% is actually fish. The remaining 42% is the surrounding crumb, and this contains omega-6 fats that offset the benefit of the omega-3 in the fish.

(vii) Omega-3 supplements: conclusions

Clearly the cheapest effective way to supplement your omega-3 supplement is not to pay extra for omega-3 enhanced foods, but to drink bottled cod liver oil or fish oil.

But is even that such a good idea? Fish itself contains protein (essential for growth and for the repair and regular replacement of nerves, tissues and bones, as well as combating infection), vitamin A (important for night vision and other things) and vitamin D (important for masses of reasons). Fish also contains selenium and other important minerals. Apart from a little vitamin D in cod liver oil, omega-3 capsules of all kinds contain almost none of these essential nutrients.

For only a little more than the cost of fish oil or cod liver oil you can buy the equivalent amount of canned fish and have it as part of a meal. A breakfast of half a tin of sardines on buttered toast would actually be cheaper than an equivalent dose of cod liver oil with a bowl of cornflakes and milk, and it would provide a better O-6-3 balance.

So don't take omega-3 supplements, eat fish instead! Cod liver oil capsules and krill and flaxseed oil are too expensive in the quantities required to be effective, and they are all nutritionally inferior to fish, whether fresh, frozen or canned. But much more than this, there is one reason why no responsible person should try to supplement his omega-3 intake from fish oil.

Fish *oil* isn't made from fresh air: it comes from fish. And as we have seen, in order to obtain the same amount of EPA and DHA in the blood from fish oil as from fish one has to consume *three times as much EPA and DHA*. That's why there is a factor of three against cod liver oil in Table 4. Now let's say that eating just the minimum recommended two portions of fish a week means killing two whole fish a month. If instead we obtain our minimum recommended omega-3 supplement from fish oil instead of fish, *six* fish will have to be killed every month! Currently, as I said, people in the U.K. eat on average only a little over one portion of fish a week, and even with that small amount the fish stocks in the North Sea are depleted. If we all supplemented our omega-3 by means of fish oil to obtain the same benefit as eating two portions of fish a week, then we would have to kill *six times* as many fish as at present, and obviously there would be none left within a year. Can it possibly be called responsible and unselfish to practise something that would create an environmental disaster if everybody did it?

So what on earth is the solution? How can we tip the omega scales in the other direction, if it can't be done by eating fish or by dietary supplements? The solution is very simple, but it is one our governments continually shy away from. It is this: we have to reduce our intake of omega-6.[126]

Solution 3: Eat less high omega-6 food

The only sensible way to reach a healthy balance of omega-3 and omega-6 fatty acids is to reduce our intake of omega-6: to get rid of some of those grey squirrels that are gobbling up all the red squirrels' food inside us. You would think this is obvious, but far from encouraging us to do it, the government tells us to use high omega-6 vegetable-based spreads and cooking oils instead of the traditional butter, lard and dripping in which omega-6 and omega-3 fats are in a healthy balance. On top of this they tell us to obtain most of our calories from starchy foods such as bread and breakfast cereals and potatoes and rice. Potatoes are fine and rice isn't too bad, but wheat flour, which is the

---

[126] Simopoulos A P et al. *Workshop on the Essentiality of and Recommended Dietary Intakes for Omega-6 and Omega-3 Fatty Acids.* Journal of the American College of Nutrition, Vol. 18, No. 5, 487–489, 1999.

basis of most bread and pastry and cakes, has a dreadful O-6-3 ratio of 17:1.

Food manufacturers introduce this same problem very early on in life. A popular toddler milk sold in the U.K. as 'nutritionally superior to cow's milk' has an O-6-3 ratio of 10:1, a rather strange claim if you recall that the ratio for natural cow's milk is a very healthy 1.5:1. Some toddler cereals that are widely used in the U.S.A. have ratios as high as 137:1![127] It is hardly surprising that diet-related health problems are affecting even children.

Bearing in mind that a healthy O-6-3 ratio lies between 1:1 and 4:1, Figures 17 and 18 clearly demonstrate why the ratios in our current Western diets are so unhealthily high.

Figure 17: Ratios of omega-6 to omega-3 for some common sources of fat[128]

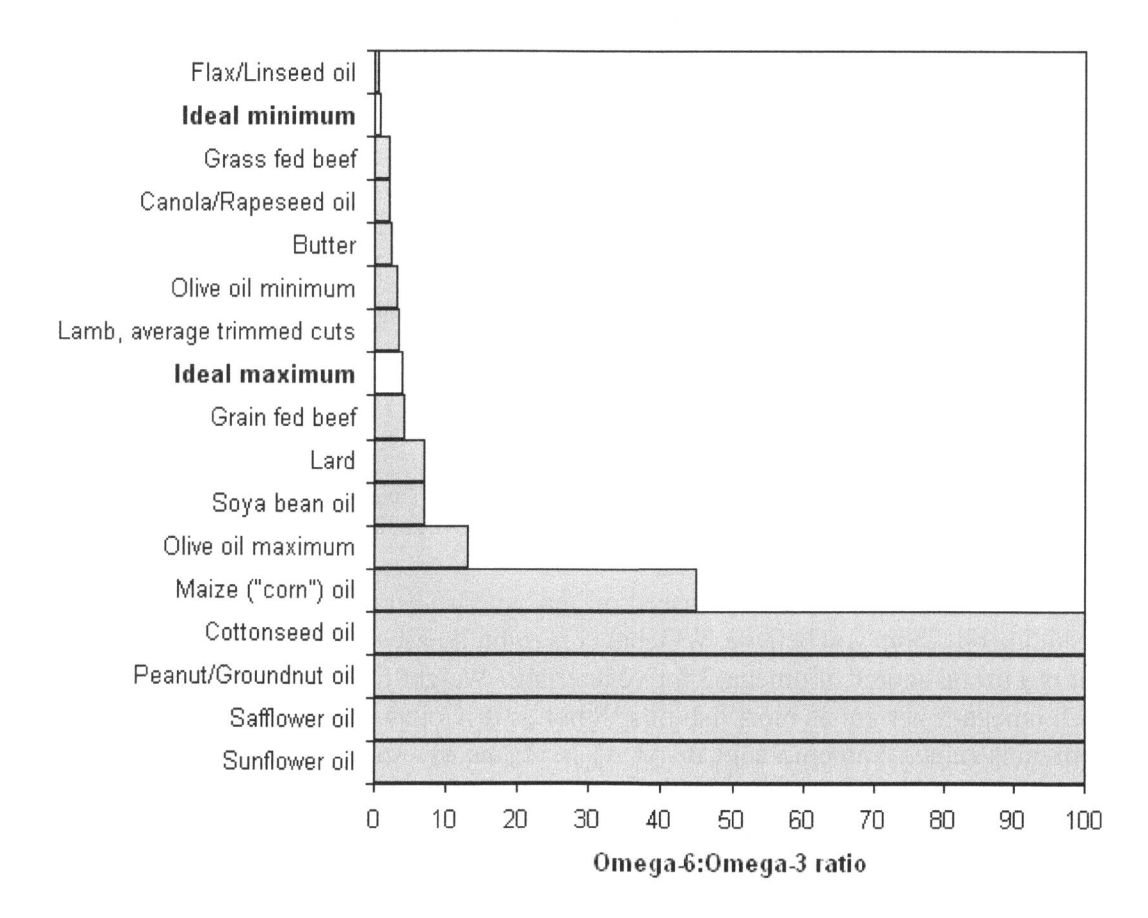

Source	Omega-6:Omega-3 ratio
Flax/Linseed oil	~0
Ideal minimum	~1
Grass fed beef	~2
Canola/Rapeseed oil	~2
Butter	~2
Olive oil minimum	~3
Lamb, average trimmed cuts	~3
Ideal maximum	4
Grain fed beef	~5
Lard	~7
Soya bean oil	~7
Olive oil maximum	~13
Maize ("corn") oil	~45
Cottonseed oil	>100
Peanut/Groundnut oil	>100
Safflower oil	>100
Sunflower oil	>100

---

127 *Babyfood cereal. Junior oatmeal cereal with apple sauce and banana.* Nutrition Tables, United States Department of Agriculture.

128 Various sources

Figure 18: Ratios of omega-6 to omega-3 for potatoes and some common cereals[129]

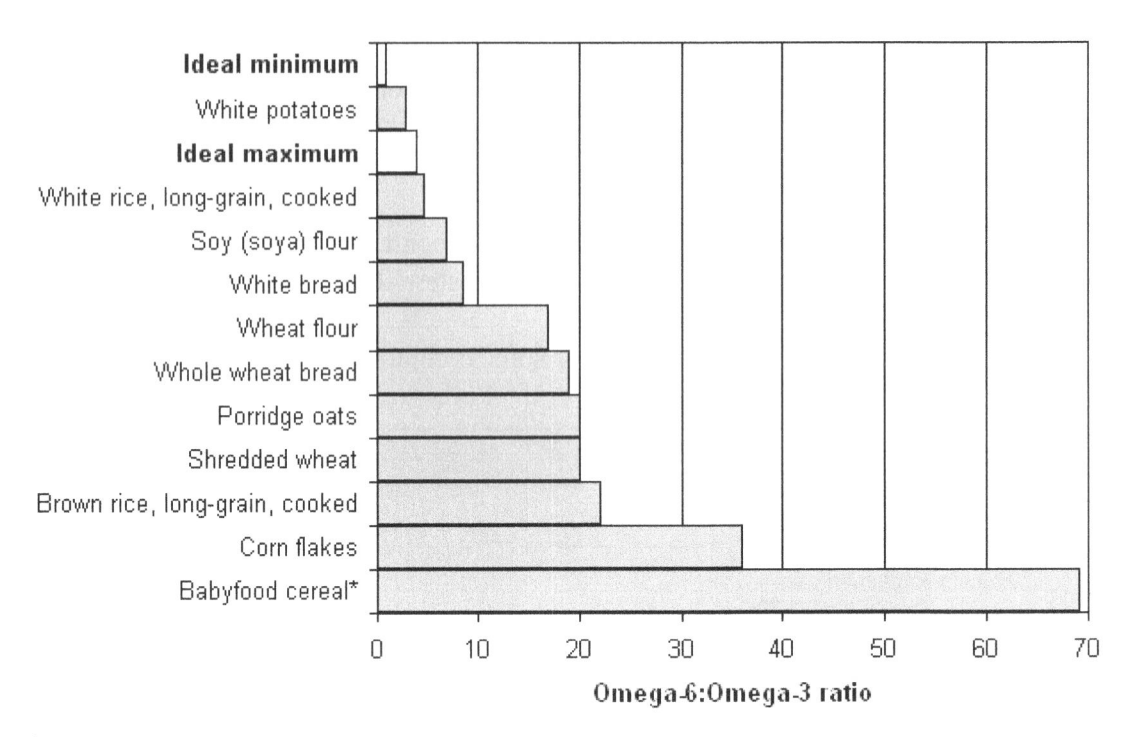

Food	Omega-6:Omega-3 ratio
Ideal minimum	~0
White potatoes	~2
Ideal maximum	~4
White rice, long-grain, cooked	~5
Soy (soya) flour	~7
White bread	~9
Wheat flour	~16
Whole wheat bread	~19
Porridge oats	~20
Shredded wheat	~20
Brown rice, long-grain, cooked	~22
Corn flakes	~36
Babyfood cereal*	~69

* Babyfood cereal. Junior oatmeal cereal with apple sauce and banana: O-6-3 ratio = 69:1 or 137:1. (USDA nutrition database. Two values are given.)

As you can see in Figures 17 and 18, some foods like beef and butter and potatoes do have omega-6 and omega-3 fats in a healthy ratio between 1:1 and 4:1. But let's look at a few others.

Flax oil, otherwise known as linseed oil, has an O-6-3 ratio of only 0.25:1 or 0.5:1, depending on whom you believe. Whichever is right, it has *more* omega-3 than omega-6, so it is a useful source of omega-3 for vegetarians. Weight for weight it has six times as much omega-3 per gm as most fish oils,[130] but as it is plant-based the kind of omega-3 it contains (alpha linolenic acid or ALA) is not nearly so nutritious as the kinds of omega-3 found in fish, meat and eggs. Assuming, as previously discussed, that only 5% of the ALA is converted to EPA and DHA, we would still have to drink three and a half times as much flax oil as fish oil to obtain a similar result. Added to that, ALA is probably not as effective as fish oil in preventing heart attacks or their recurrence, as previously mentioned, and the high proportion of polyunsaturated fatty acids in it makes it unsuitable for cooking purposes, because heating polyunsaturated fats makes them

---

129 Source: U.S. Department of Agriculture Food Database
130 Bartram T. *Bartram's Encyclopedia of Herbal Medicine: The Definitive Guide to the Herbal Treatments of Diseases*. Da Capo Press, September 2002, p. 271.

oxidize and produce harmful free radicals. It would however be fine used cold in a salad dressing.

Canola or rapeseed oil is generally labelled as 'vegetable oil' in the U.K. It is actually a modified form of rapeseed oil and, as shown on the first chart, it has a healthy O-6-3 ratio of 2:1. However 28% of the fat in rapeseed oil is polyunsaturated fat, as compared with 11% in lard and only 3% in grass-fed dripping (beef suet), so once again it isn't nearly so healthy for cooking purposes. And since the extraction process involves heating it to temperatures up to 260°C much of the polyunsaturated fat may be oxidized before you even purchase it, at least according to Mark Sissons, author of '*The Primal Blueprint*'.[131] It is obvious that the healthiest fats for frying and roasting are dripping and lard, because they consist primarily of saturated and monounsaturated fats, which do not easily oxidize and go rancid.

The contribution of beef to the omega balance depends very much on how the cattle are raised. In 2006-2009 the O-6-3 ratio for grass-fed Angus cross steers in the U.S.A. was measured as 1.65:1, while for grain-finished beef (beef fattened with grain prior to slaughter) it was 4.84:1.[132] The grass-fed beef had the same amount of protein in it, but more beta-carotene, B-vitamins and minerals; twice as much conjugated linoleic acid (which fights cancer); three times as much total omega-3; and nearly four times as much vitamin E!

For lard, the rather high 6:1 ratio shown in the first chart is very much an average value. The actual ratio again depends on what the poor old pig ate while it was alive. Lard from free-range pigs fed naturally on grass and roots, etc., has a healthy O-6-3 ratio of around 3:1. But lard from pigs kept in pens and fed on maize, soya and other industrially grown crops and offscourings can have a ratio as high as 33:1![133] However, only 11% of lard consists of polyunsaturated fat (the kind that contains omega fatty acids), whereas almost 70% of normal sunflower oil consists of polyunsaturated fat, mostly omega-6, so even the worst kind of lard contains far less omega-6 than sunflower and similar vegetable oils do. While most British supermarkets sell dripping made from British beef without any additives, supermarket lard in Britain generally comes from unspecified countries and its purity is not quite so certain. In Europe, the 2013 horsemeat saga demonstrated how hard it is to know for certain what ingredients supermarket food really contains. So why not ask your local butcher for advice on obtaining pure dripping, lard and other cooking fats from pasture-fed animals?

The last three oils shown on the fats bar chart are cottonseed, peanut and sunflower oil. These really have ratios of over 100:1 for they contain almost no omega-3 at all. There is a special type of sunflower oil called high oleic sunflower oil which is much

---

[131] www.marksdailyapple.com/healthy-oils/#axzz2MZckHjSf. Accessed March 2013.

[132] Duckett S K et al. *Effects of winter stocker growth rate and finishing system on tissue proximate, fatty acid, vitamin and cholesterol content.* Journal of Animal Science, 2009; 87 (9): 2961–70.

[133] Jaminet P and Jaminet S C. *Perfect Health Diet.* Scribner, 2012.

healthier, but it is not widely available and in Britain, at least, it is very expensive.[134]

Although nuts are a useful source of protein for vegetarians, with the exception of walnuts they have very high O-6-3 ratios and should therefore be eaten sparingly. Walnuts provide a fairly good balance of omega-6 and omega-3 fatty acids in a ratio of 5:1.

It is not only the widespread use of seed oils in spreads and cooked foods that has upset the balance in our diet. Dr. Mary Enig, author of '*Know Your Fats: The Complete Primer for Understanding the Nutrition of Fats, Oils and Cholesterol*', says that modern agricultural and industrial practices have reduced the amount of omega-3 fatty acids in commercially available vegetables, eggs, fish and meat. For example, organic eggs from hens allowed to feed on insects and green plants can contain omega-6 and omega-3 fatty acids in approximately equal quantities, but ordinary supermarket eggs can contain up to nineteen times more omega-6 than omega-3! (When I read this I was very glad that we've been buying organic free-range eggs for the last 3 years.) Nevertheless, apart from non free-range eggs I don't believe there is much of a problem with vegetables, fish and meat in the U.K. at least. Cattle here are mostly still fed on grass rather than maize and other cereals, and I find it hard to see why the O-6-3 ratio in vegetables and fish should have changed significantly, except perhaps in the case of farmed salmon and trout. So buy free-range eggs and keep eating fresh vegetables, fish (preferably wild) and good quality meat.

Reducing our consumption of omega-6 fatty acids

So now we come to the all-important question: how can we reduce our consumption of omega-6 fatty acids?

- Apart from high oleic sunflower oil (which you probably couldn't afford), avoid altogether corn/maize/sweetcorn, cottonseeds, sunflower seeds and peanuts/groundnuts, plus all oils and products made from them, including popcorn and peanut butter.
- Use flax/linseed oil or extra virgin olive oil in salads, or if you can't afford them use rapeseed/canola/vegetable oil.
- Cook with butter, dripping, lard or goose fat, preferably from pasture-fed animals or birds. Vegetarians should use butter, extra virgin cold pressed olive oil, or else organic virgin coconut oil, which has only about 4% omega-6[135]. Palm oil is also

---

[134] At the time of writing high oleic sunflower oil was being sold on the U.K. eBay website for £41.75 per litre.

[135] Mark Sissons, author of *The Primal Blueprint*. www.marksdailyapple.com/coconut-oil-health-benefits/#refined. Accessed March 2013.

stable at high temperatures, but should be obtained from a sustainable source – e.g. West African red palm oil.[136]
- Strictly limit your consumption of food made from seeds – including bread, pastry, pasta, breakfast cereals and rice.

Clearly if you buy any prepared foods such as cakes, biscuits, burgers, chips or ready meals there is a good chance that soya, cottonseed or other high omega-6 oils have been used to make them. That's why home-cooked food is so much healthier, and why it's so important to teach your children to cook and make home cooking a part of their lifestyle.

The website 180degreehealth.com says there are ten high omega-6 foods we really should avoid. Actually eleven foods are listed, not ten, so maybe the author was the same person who invented a baker's dozen. Anyway, here is the blacklist in detail:

- commercial peanut butter
- common oil-roasted snack nuts
- commercially fried potato fries (chips and crisps)
- other fried foods from restaurants
- commercially made salad dressings, including most vinaigrettes, Caesar dressing and coleslaw
- commercial mayonnaise and mayonnaise-based sauces
- doughnuts
- high-fat desserts
- margarine and foods often made with margarine, like cookies and brownies (cakes)
- vegetable oils, especially corn/maize/sweetcorn oil
- vegetable shortening (i.e. lard substitutes such as 'Trex', 'Cookeen' and 'Crisco') and foods made with it, such as biscuits, pie crusts and other pastries

So there we are. To defuse the obesity bomb ticking beneath every home in our nation we have to stop consuming so much omega-6. We have to stop stuffing our children with it. We have to make a radical change in our families' diets, and take a firm decision to banish the hoards of grey squirrels which enter our stomachs in seed oils from soya beans, sunflower seeds, maize and peanuts, and from all the products made with them – margarines and spreads, cooking oils, ready meals, fast foods, pastries and snacks of all kinds. We must revert instead to the traditional foods our grandparents and ancestors lived on, when there was no epidemic of obesity, coronary heart trouble and type 2 diabetes. We should use animal fats for cooking, drink full-cream milk, eat meat and fresh vegetables, and prepare our food at home without the preservatives and additives and other ingredients added by manufacturers to make money at the expense of a nation's health. We must ignore the alluring and deceptive advertisements of a multimillion

---

136 Mark Sissons. www.marksdailyapple.com/healthy-oils/#axzz2MZckHjSf. Accessed March 2013.

dollar food manufacturing industry, stop poisoning our kids with its profits, and nourish ourselves and our families with the food our bodies were designed for. That is how we and our children can remain healthy into a long old age. There is no other way.

It might sound as though that brings us to the end of dietary-related health problems, but I'm afraid it doesn't. In Victorian days, two wooden giants called Corineus and Gogmagog stood in Guildhall in the city of London. One held a mace and the other an axe: clearly they would have been formidable foes had they been alive. If we think of the mace-bearing giant as killing people with the wrong kinds of fat, the axe-bearing one is killing us equally effectively with something else. That something else is *sugar*.

CHAPTER 8: SUGAR – THE SWEET ASSASSIN

Sugar and spice and all things nice

Refined sugar, made either from sugar cane or sugar beet, provides us with nothing but calories. All the nutrients from the original plants, in the form of vitamins, minerals and enzymes are removed during the manufacturing process. That is why it is called 'refined'. The resulting sucrose is no more natural than a so-called artificial sweetener. It is a pure chemical, hardly a food at all.

In this chapter I am going to talk about the effects of sugar on:

- teeth
- obesity
- type 2 diabetes
- heart disease
- other health problems

But first I want to make some general comments on sugar in relation to children.

When children are small they don't have much choice about what they eat: we make their choices for them. Even when they grow bigger and start to choose their food they are likely to adopt similar eating patterns to the ones they have been brought up on. So it is essential, right from the start, not only to give our children healthy food but *not* to give them unhealthy food.

I once heard a British woman who had grown up in India tell how she and her small sister used to eat fruit before it was ripe because they liked the sour taste. Their mother told them, "*You should eat sweet things as well as sour things.*" Children don't necessarily prefer a sweet taste unless they are trained to do so. Their tastes in food develop when they are very young, and if they once get used to eating artificially sweetened foods they are very likely to prefer sweetened foods for the rest of their life. So parents and other carers should consider very carefully the wisdom of feeding their children on sweets, biscuits, sweetened cereals and other sugary foods.

I'm not saying that all sugar is harmful, for even milk and fruit have sugar in them. But most baked beans, cereals, cakes, biscuits, fruit pies, many drinks, sweetened desserts, chocolates and other confectionery all have sugar added to them artificially, and any food with sugar deliberately added to it is unnatural. Sugar as we know it wasn't around much at all until Elizabethan times, and our bodies are simply not designed to deal with a lot of it. So the more we can avoid it, the healthier we and our children shall be.

Sugar and teeth

'An apple a day keeps the doctor away' has a pip of truth in it, but 'No sugar each day keeps the dentist away' is almost totally true. If I'd known when I was a boy that it was only sweets and chocolates and sugary drinks that caused tooth decay I really might have thought twice about what I spent my pocket money on. When a graveyard in the mediaeval village of Wharram Percy was excavated, all the skeletons had very good teeth. Similarly excavations on the site of the Battle of Towton in AD 1461 revealed that the fighters '*suffered no major dietary deficiency diseases; moreover, because cane sugar, other refined carbohydrates and dried fruits could be afforded only by the nobility, their teeth, even if worn down, were in good condition and dental decay was rare.*'[137] In contrast, here am I in the twenty-first century with three teeth missing and half the remaining ones filled. There's progress for you.

Some sugars are more harmful than others. Sucrose is the worst, followed in descending order by high-fructose corn syrup (popular in the U.S.A.), glucose, fructose (from fruit), lactose (from milk), maltose (from barley), sorbitol and xylitol. The common kind of granulated sugar, called sucrose, is a 50-50 compound of glucose and fructose, so it is particularly harmful.

Honey consists mainly of glucose and fructose, so although it has some additional nutrients it is just as bad for the teeth as plain sugar is. By sticking to the teeth longer it might be even worse. Never sweeten a baby's dummy or pacifier with honey. You may think it's all right before any teeth appear, but you'll find it next to impossible to stop doing it once your little one starts teething and cries even more. And why give it a taste for sugar in the first place?

It's not the sugar itself that damages teeth: it's actually the acid produced by millions of tiny bacteria that feed on the sugar. The bacteria that cause tooth decay[138] need sugar to feed on and multiply, and they are especially partial to the sucrose extracted from sugar cane and sugar beet. Their waste products cause decay, because their waste products are acidic and dissolve the tooth enamel.[139] It is said that once tooth enamel is destroyed, it cannot be regenerated.

Sugar is even more harmful in a drink that is already acidic. The acidity of a liquid is

---

137 *Blood red roses: the archaeology of a mass grave from the Battle of Towton ad 1461.* Edited by Veronica Fiorato, Anthea Boylston and Christopher Knüsel. 2000. Oxbow Books, Oxford.
138 The principal bacteria which cause tooth decay are lactobacilli and mutans streptococci. They live within dental plaque.
139 Lactic acid is the primary waste product of dental bacteria.

measured by its pH value, with a lower value being more acidic. A pH value below 5.5 means a liquid is acidic, which is bad news for teeth. Tap water has a pH of around 6.0. According to Dr. Diane Johnson[140] Diet Coke has a pH of 4.0 and Coke Zero has a pH of only 3.0. Since pH values are logarithmic this means that Coke Zero is ten times as acidic as Diet Coke, and Diet Coke is 100 times as acidic as water!

Dr. Johnson analysed 48 common drinks, from tap water to draught Guinness, and she listed them in order of their harmfulness to teeth, based on their acidity and sugar content.[141] Of course there will be many other drinks as harmful to teeth as the ones she tested but here are the ten worst she discovered, starting with the most serious one. The order is based simply on the acid and sugar content of the drinks she tested, so while Tropicana grape juice, for example, turned out to be the worst for teeth, any other make of pure grape juice would probably have produced a similar result. And unlike colas, fruit juices do contain vitamin C.

- Tropicana 100% Grape Juice (and other brands of grape juice, no doubt)
- Tropicana Cranberry Juice Cocktail (and similar brands, no doubt)
- LiveWire Mountain Dew (orange)
- Mountain Dew (a nutrition drink)
- Coca-Cola Cherry Coke
- Pepsi Cola
- Coca-Cola Classic Coke
- Dr. Pepper
- Lemon juice
- Powerade Grape (a sports drink)

Perhaps the biggest surprise is that 'healthy' fruit juices top the list. I must say that when our milkman delivered a free 330ml bottle of pure orange juice the other day I was surprised to find that it contained 33gm of sugar – that's a heaped tablespoonful of sugar in a rather small bottle! And oranges are acidic, of course. However it did contain more than the recommended daily allowance of vitamin C, so I suppose I could have drunk a quarter of a bottle as part of a healthy breakfast.

The least harmful drinks on Dr. Johnson's list were milk drinks and water, although two versions of Starbucks' coffee also made it among the top ten safest drinks she tried. The *sweetest* by far was a liqueur called Limoncello di Capri made from lemons, and easily the most *acidic* was pure lemon juice, so the message seems to be, 'Avoid lemons!' And if you must know, draught Guinness came in at number nineteen, one worse than

---

[140] Dr. Johnson is a full-time practising orthodontist in the U.S.A. She obtained a doctorate from Northwestern University Dental School, and she writes reviews for the American Journal of Orthodontics and Dentofacial Orthopedics.

[141] The formula used by Dr. Johnson to determine harmfulness was $[10^{(5.5-pH)}] \times [(\text{sugar in mg/cl}) + 1]$.

Diet Coke and one better than a sweetened cup of tea, so it isn't too bad, for teeth at least.

Actually, the tooth issue is more relevant to children than adults because tooth enamel is softer when it is first formed and is much more easily damaged. If it is damaged during the growing period, and if it is true that it can never be replaced, then it's really important not to let youngsters drink any sweetened acidic drinks until they are well into their teens.

Many babies and small toddlers suffer from tooth decay, and in less well-off parts of the U.K. nearly two-thirds of children have one or more rotten teeth by the time they are five. So here's my advice for healthy toddler teeth, much of it based on information taken from an excellent Australian website:[142]

- Babies should never be left with a bottle in their mouth for long periods, because even the lactose in milk generates decay in time.
- Children more than a year old should drink from a cup.
- Don't let toddlers sip juice or milk for extended periods. Doing so prolongs the exposure of the teeth to sugar. (Water is fine, especially tap water. But some bottled water is actually acidic.)
- Don't give them honey or any sticky foods that are high in sugar.
- Limit or preferably exclude foods and drinks that have added sugar, including all sweets and chocolates.
- Restrict the consumption of all foods and drinks containing sugar to structured mealtimes, especially fruit juice because it contains both sugar and acid.
- Discourage snacking. Snacking throughout the day on foods containing starches such as crisps, corn snacks and cheese snacks also increases the risk of tooth decay and makes children put on too much weight.
- If possible brush your toddlers' teeth, or at least rinse their mouths with water, immediately after eating or drinking anything with sugar in it. Bacterial damage begins within minutes of eating sugary food.[143] Water might not dislodge bits of food as brushing does, but it will rinse out surface sugar and acid, and drinking plenty of water provides major health benefits. Concluding every meal with a glass of water is an excellent habit to instil in kids, by example as well as instruction!

If anyone wonders why there is so much tooth decay and childhood obesity, a peek at the snacks section of a typical supermarket will give a clue. One supermarket, for example, currently sells 138 'Kids' snacks', many of them with added sugar. I even saw a section headed 'Baby and Toddler Snacks'! If I were in government I would require all snacks to come in plain packaging with a health warning on them. Constant snacking never gives our digestive systems a rest. Children won't feel a need for snacks during the

---

142 www.meandmychild.com.au/toddler/health-care/teeth/
143 www.animated-teeth.com/tooth_decay/t2_tooth_decay_caries.htm

morning if they eat a proper breakfast such as a small bowl of porridge made with full-cream milk, and a slice of bread or toast with either a boiled egg, a good quality sausage or some reduced sugar baked beans. Nevertheless, if you really feel it is essential to pacify your baby or toddler with food, at least do an Internet search for 'baby and toddler snacks'. It will give you all kinds of ideas for healthy, sugar-free snacks that won't lead your children down the treacherous path to Caries Chasm or Pot Belly Pothole.

When children grow older it may be difficult to keep them off sweets, but it will be a lot easier if they are already used to living without them. I knew two dentists who adopted different approaches. One wouldn't allow his children to eat any sweets or chocolates at all until they were eighteen, when the enamel on most of their teeth was fully mature. They all had beautiful teeth as a result. The other one gave each of his two children a large sweet tin in which they had to put any sweets they had bought or were given. They were allowed to open their tin only once a week, on Sundays after lunch. Then they could eat whatever they wanted, so long as they brushed their teeth when they'd finished!

We all have to devise our own strategy for dealing with sweets. All I would say is that for the sake of our children and their teeth, it is important to have a strategy and to keep to it, except perhaps for special occasions such as birthdays and annual religious festivals like the Feast of Saint Cadbury, which takes place round about Easter time. Believe me, if you persevere in your crusade against decay your kids will thank you one day. If they don't kill you first!

It is just as important to discourage children and teenagers from drinking the most damaging soft drinks, especially the common kinds of sports drinks and energy drinks. If they genuinely need a glucose fix for immediate physical exertion it is best to take it in the form of a banana, as tennis players do, plain glucose tablets (avoiding the fructose in ordinary sugar), or a non-acidic sports drink, i.e. one in which the sugar is not dissolved in an acidic fruit juice![144]

Health food shops generally sell suitable drinks and the staff should be able to give advice about them. Diet Coke seems to be one of the less harmful ones, although even that isn't exactly tooth-friendly. I think that if I were a young teenager again I'd try to invent a sugar and acid-free drink that tasted so foul that nobody else would touch it. I'd pretend it was only for tough guys and that I loved it! When I was 13 or 14 I did try this once with cold tea, pepper and some other more worrying ingredients, but even I couldn't stand the taste of it. Richmal Crompton's William and his friends used to make liquorice water for themselves. Liquorice has some definite health benefits if it's not consumed in excess, but it's not very tooth-friendly either. Wine should definitely be off limits for teenagers with developing teeth, because grapes are highly acidic and wine has sugar in it as well.

---

144 One example of a non-acidic sports drink is Hammer Heed, available from various online and sports suppliers, but it is very expensive!

Whatever strategy you adopt on drinks, both parents (if there are two) should agree to enforce it and lead by example. Explain as clearly as possible to your kids why it is so important for them to avoid sugary and acidic drinks. If you think it would help, show them a photo of their favourite singer's perfect teeth, and then show them a photo of mine!

Dental decay is a serious problem, but it is not nearly as serious as other problems caused by sugary foods and drinks. For even if your children's teeth all decay they can have a complete set of false teeth and go on living normally. But if they can't walk because of joint problems arising from obesity, or if they go blind as a result of type 2 diabetes, or if they die because of coronary heart failure, then resuming normal life is going to be somewhat harder! I want to convince you that sugar is indeed a giant Gogmagog among the enemies of public health, and to persuade you to declare WAR ON SUGAR on behalf of your family!

Sugar and obesity

Let's start with *obesity*. Being merely overweight may not be a serious problem, although it will make physical activity more of an effort and make a person look less attractive in the eyes of many people. As a result it does sometimes lead to eating disorders in the teens, and for that reason alone it is a very bad idea to feed your family in a way that makes them put on too much weight. But I'm not really talking about being overweight. Being *obese* is much more serious, because it will, by definition, cause health problems. An obese person is someone who is so seriously overweight that sooner or later his health will suffer.

I've already listed the problems that obesity causes or at least exacerbates – heart disease, strokes, diabetes, cancer, arthritis, orthopaedic problems, asthma and sleep apnoea. An article in *The Lancet* in August 2011 said, '*As UN member states prepare to gather in New York in September, 2011, for the first High-Level Meeting of the UN General Assembly on non-communicable diseases (NCDs), the inexorable global rise of obesity will be the toughest challenge that they face. All countries are searching for answers about how to reverse the rising tide of adult and childhood obesity.*'[145] The article puts the problem down to the fact that we are simply eating more calories than we need. And one of the three main sources of calories is, of course, sugar.

It's difficult to obtain an accurate idea of how sugar consumption has increased in the last 60 years or so, because a lot of it is hidden in pastry, biscuits, cakes and snacks, but nationally it has at least doubled. The consumption of breakfast cereals manufactured with sugar in them, tinned fruit, sweets, chocolates, alcoholic drinks and fruit have all

---

[145] Boyd A et al. *The global obesity pandemic: shaped by global drivers and local environments.* The Lancet, Volume 378, Issue 9793, Pages 804 - 814, 27, August 2011.

increased. One particular new source of sugar is fruit juice. When I was a small child at the end of the war the only fruit juice we had was a tiny glass of orange juice once a day. It was made from small bottles of concentrated juice provided free of charge for children by the Ministry of Food, Agriculture and Fisheries. Nowadays many people have a large glass of fresh fruit juice for breakfast. Do you know how many oranges go into a 330ml glass of orange juice? The Tropicana website says at least four. Try to imagine sitting down and eating four whole oranges in quick succession. Wouldn't you regard that as both unnatural and greedy? Yet because the manufacture of fruit juice has become so cheap, many people are consuming all that fruit juice and more every day. A glass of milk at breakfast would be far healthier, with less sugar and more vitamins in it.

I'm not trying to say that fruit juice per se is unhealthy. Its vitamin C content is obviously good for you, and an occasional orange or apple or pear must be fine, otherwise God wouldn't have made them for us, or we wouldn't have evolved to enjoy and digest them, according to your point of view. However fructose, the sugar found in fruit, isn't nearly so friendly as one might think, and in any quantity it is positively dangerous. It is fructose that makes the sugar added to so much of our food harmful, as well as helping us to put on weight in just the wrong place.

In 2009 23 US scientists collaborated in an experiment involving 32 overweight men and women.[146] The research was devised and carried out very thoughtfully and thoroughly. Over a period of 10 weeks the subjects were asked to drink a measured quantity of sugar in a drink three times a day. Half of them had glucose and the other half fructose, with equal calorific values. Just to remind you, ordinary refined sugar is half fructose and half glucose. In both groups the research subjects put on about 3lb (1.5kg) of weight, because for the first 8 weeks the sugar drinks were in addition to their normal diets. However the fructose group put on *four times* as much weight around their stomachs as the glucose group did. This 'visceral adipose tissue', the so-called beer belly, is an alarm bell for the development of coronary heart disease and diabetes, so that was one major difference in the way that glucose and fructose affected the test subjects. Secondly, the fructose group suffered a worsening of blood glucose control and insulin sensitivity, in other words they experienced the beginning of diabetes. And thirdly, there was an increase in the small, dense LDL particles and oxidized LDL in their blood. Without going into detail, those are both factors that are strongly associated with the risk of a heart attack and may actually contribute to it. *None* of these changes occurred in the glucose group.

It is true that the amount of sugar they were given was at the high end of what most of us would drink in a day,[147] but most of us also consume substantial amounts of fructose

---

[146] Kimber L et al. *Consuming fructose-sweetened, not glucose-sweetened, beverages increases visceral adiposity and lipids and decreases insulin sensitivity in overweight/obese humans.* Journal of Clinical Investigation, 2009; 119(5):1322–1334.

[147] The research report says that the sugar dose provided 25% of their energy requirements. For most people that would be 500 to 750 kilocalories a day, equivalent to 125gm to 190gm of sucrose.

in sugar added to our food. Moreover the experiment lasted only 10 weeks, so if one drank even a quarter as much fructose year after year the results might be similar at least. Research carried out in 2011 demonstrated that even low to moderate amounts of fructose-sweetened drinks caused problems for the young men who were subjects in the research. Inflammation is a stepping stone to heart disease,[148] and it was found that, while all sugar-sweetened drinks increased inflammatory factors, fructose-enriched drinks increased them the most.[149]

In the light of such research, my advice would be to limit one's fruit consumption to one or two pieces a day – certainly not a full glass of fresh fruit juice, which is the equivalent of four oranges or a small bunch of grapes.

In fact my conclusion from the 2009 experiment is that the Five-A-Day advice we keep hearing needs to be amended. I would suggest that instead of 'Five Fruit and Veg', a better rule would be 'A Fruit and Five Veg', or even 'A Fruit and Seven Veg' for vegetarians. 'A Fruit and Five Veg' would more than satisfy the minimum recommendations of the World Health Organization,[150] although some countries recommend more than the WHO does.[151] In other words, I'm saying that many people should eat *less* fruit and drink *less* fruit juice, but most people should eat *more* vegetables.

Many studies have demonstrated the genuine health benefits of vegetables. Brassicas (broccoli, cabbage, sprouts, etc.) and small leaf salads (mustard, cress, rocket etc.) reduce the risk of bladder, colon and lung cancer,[152] and type 2 diabetes.[153] Eating eight portions of fruit and vegetables a day can reduce the risk of dying from heart disease by 22%.[154] And here's something really interesting: replies from recent censuses in England, Scotland and Wales indicate that the more fruit and vegetables people eat the better their mental health and the greater their happiness![155] So next time your little one pulls a face and spits out his Brussels sprout you can tell him, "Eat it up, dear. It will make you feel happy!" Speaking for myself, I'd much rather feel happy than have curly hair, which is

---

148 Hotamisligil G S. *Inflammation and metabolic disorders.* Nature, 2006; 444:860-867.

149 Aeberli I et al. *Low to moderate sugar-sweetened beverage consumption impairs glucose and lipid metabolism and promotes inflammation in healthy young men: A randomised controlled trial.* American Journal of Clinical Nutrition, 2011; 94:479-485.

150 In 1991 the World Health Organization recommended a minimum intake of 400g fruit and vegetables a day. One portion of fruit and vegetables is 80g, so five portions add up to 400g.

151 In Australia the recommendation is two fruit and five vegetables per day, and in France it is ten portions of fruit and vegetables a day.

152 *Cruciferous Vegetables, Isothiocyanates and Indoles.* World Health Organization, International Agency for Research on Cancer report, 2004.

153 Carter P et al. *Fruit and vegetable intake and incidence of type 2 diabetes mellitus: systematic review and meta-analysis.* British Medical Journal, 2010; 341, c4229.

154 Crowe et al. *The EPIC trial.* European Heart Journal, 2011; 32,1235.

155 Blanchflower D G, Oswald AJ & Stewart-Brown S. *Is Psychological Well-being Linked to the Consumption of Fruit and Vegetables?* Social Indicators Research, October 2012.

what I was told would happen if I ate my cabbage. In any case, I soon discovered that eating cabbage didn't work! Or maybe I secretly spat it out again. I can't remember now...

Actually that raises a rather important issue. If we tell our children curly hair stories to persuade them to eat food they don't like, the time will come when they realize that such stories are untrue. And when they make that discovery it is inevitable that they will assume, consciously or unconsciously, that we also made up true things we told them, like 'vegetables are good for you' or 'fish is good for the brain'. So they won't take seriously what we tell them about vegetables and sweets and doughnuts and alcohol, and as a result they may suffer severely. It's equally important not to tell 'rabbit food' stories that put children *off* eating something that's healthy. When my wife was a child her father wouldn't eat lettuce, calling it 'rabbit food'. The result was that she didn't consider it to be proper food either, and it wasn't until recently, some 60 years later, that she has started to eat lettuce – adequately laced with French dressing! It is very important that we always tell our children the truth.

Anyway, "Mind on the job in hand", as my chemistry teacher was always telling me. I was talking about sugar and obesity. Sugar, as I said, consists purely of calories, and all your body can do with them is either burn them up immediately as fuel for your muscles or brain, or convert them into fat. And since most of us don't spend our daylight hours hunting wild boar, or washing clothes with a scrubbing board and mangle like my mother used to do (washing clothes, I mean, not hunting wild boar), most of the sugar we eat is turned into fat. Most of us don't need sucrose added to our food: we get all the calories we need from natural sugars, carbohydrates, fats and even proteins. So sugar is the very worst cause of obesity: it makes us fat while doing no good at all.

There's another more subtle reason why sugar, especially fructose,[156] makes one put on weight. 100 calories from sugar don't make you feel as full as 100 calories from a starchy carbohydrate does, and even less full than 100 calories from fat or protein. So if your diet contains a lot of sugar and only a little fat, you will feel hungry, and if you feel hungry you will eat more, and if you eat more, you will put on more weight.

Sugar and type 2 diabetes

But obesity is only the beginning. I said sugar causes three major problems. Another major health problem in which sugar is involved is type 2 diabetes. In February 2009 the BBC reported that from 1997 to 2003 there was a 74% rise in new cases of diabetes in the U.K. By 2005, more than 4% of the population was classed as having diabetes –

---

[156] Stanhope K L & Havel P J. *Endocrine and metabolic effects of consuming beverages sweetened with fructose, glucose, sucrose, or high-fructose corn syrup.* American Journal of Clinical Nutrition, 2008; 88:1733S-1737S.

nearly double the rate of 10 years earlier. The increase, it said, was due to rising obesity rates. It also said that more children were being diagnosed with the condition, some as young as seven. According to Diabetes U.K., the NHS was spending £1m an hour – 10% of its yearly budget – treating diabetes and its complications.[157]

When our bodies detect sugar in the blood, our pancreas generates insulin, which tells our cells what to do with it. If we regularly consume more sugar than is good for us one of two things can happen: either our pancreas 'wears out' and stops producing insulin in the amounts we need it, or else our cells get so fed up with being told to take sugar in that they ignore the insulin when it knocks on their door, and the poor old pancreas has to generate even more to attract their attention so there is too much of it in our blood. The end result is that people with type 2 diabetes have to start taking tablets or inject themselves before every meal to maintain a safe insulin level in their blood, otherwise they risk horrendous damage to their eyesight, feet and kidneys, and may even fall into a life-threatening coma.

Diabetes – or susceptibility to diabetes – can be inherited genetically. Nevertheless there seem to be two independent causes of type 2 diabetes that may or may not be linked together: one is obesity and the other is fructose. Being obese greatly increases the risk, and it is thought the reason may be that, when one's body stores a lot of fat, the fat somehow generates hormones that tell the pancreas to stop producing so much insulin, because the cells don't want the insulin to order them to store yet more fat. However that can't be the whole story, because not everybody who develops type 2 diabetes is overweight. So another cause appears to be fructose, and this was pretty well proved in the following way.

I have already referred to the 'Nurses' Study', in which 91,249 nurses in the U.S.A., all young and middle-aged women, kept records of their diet, weight, and other medical information during the years 1991 to 1999. Initially they were all free of diabetes, but over the 8 years of the study 741 of them developed type 2 diabetes. It was found that those who daily drank one or more soft drinks such as colas sweetened with sugar had an 83% greater chance of developing diabetes within that 8-year period than those who didn't. For those who drank one or more sugar-sweetened fruit flavoured drinks the risk was 100% greater, i.e. they were twice as likely to contract diabetes![158] Almost certainly the sugar was causing diabetes. Ordinary sugar, as I said, is about 50% fructose. And, as I also said earlier, in the 2009 study with the 32 overweight men and women those who drank fructose-sweetened drinks suffered a worsening of blood glucose control

---

157 *Obesity diabetes time bomb.* BBC News, 24 February, 2009.

158 Schulze M B et al. *Sugar-sweetened beverages, weight gain, and incidence of type 2 diabetes in young and middle-aged women.* Journal of the American Medical Association, 25 August 2004; 292(8):927-34.

and a deterioration in insulin sensitivity, in other words the beginning of diabetes,[159] whereas those who drank glucose-sweetened drinks suffered no such harm. Combining the results of these two studies, it seems clear that fructose can cause type 2 diabetes.

This means that there is a major problem in the U.S.A., because a lot of Americans have started to replace sucrose with something called high fructose corn syrup, made from maize, in which more than half the sugar content is fructose. It is used by the manufacturers of many fizzy pops and processed foods to sweeten their products, as well as by individuals in their homes.

I'm speculating here, but since our bodies generate glucose from starchy foods, fats, and even proteins if necessary, and since the 2009 study suggested that raised levels of glucose do not increase the risk factors for diabetes, it may be that however much people eat and drink, and therefore however overweight they get, they don't increase their risk of contracting type 2 diabetes unless they are consuming too much fructose from ordinary refined sugar, high fructose corn syrup or fruit. Most people who consume too much sugar will of course end up overweight, which would explain the association of diabetes with obesity, but they wouldn't necessarily put on weight if at the same time they ate only a little starchy food or were very energetic. This would explain why some people who are not overweight also develop type 2 diabetes. While most scientists believe that obesity *per se* can lead to diabetes, I am not aware of any research which would disprove the idea that fructose is the only dietary culprit.

Whether sugar damages us just because of the fructose or because consuming too much of any sugar also makes us put on weight, consuming sugar puts us at greater risk of contracting type 2 diabetes with all its nasty consequences.

Sugar and heart disease

Moving on, sugar is, thirdly, a cause of heart disease. At about the time that the American scientist Ancel Keys was trying to prove that heart disease was caused by eating saturated fat, the British physiologist and scientist John Yudkin was demonstrating a far clearer association between hearts attacks and sugar consumption.[160],[161] 30 years later Yudkin was able to look back over another generation of research and state, '*There is no substantial and convincing evidence that dietary fat or cholesterol is a cause of coronary heart disease. However, this conclusion is not the same as saying that we must*

---

159 Kimber L et al. *Consuming fructose-sweetened, not glucose-sweetened, beverages increases visceral adiposity and lipids and decreases insulin sensitivity in overweight/obese humans.* Journal of Clinical Investigation, 2009; 119(5):1322–1334.

160 Yudkin J. *Dietary Fat and Dietary Sugar in Relation to Ischaemic Heart Disease and Diabetes.* Lancet 2: 4, 1964.

161 Yudkin J. *Dietary factors in atherosclerosis: sucrose.* Lipids, 1978; 13: 370–372.

abandon altogether the view that diet has nothing to do with causing the disease. There is indeed a dietary item other than fat for which there is now overwhelming evidence of its involvement in producing the disease. This item is sucrose ('sugar').'[162] Yudkin's famous book, '*Pure, white and deadly*', was republished in November 2012.

The fact that sugar causes heart disease was pretty well proved in 2012 when the results of a study on the effects of drinking sweetened drinks was published.[163] This study was based on a huge research project which began in 1986. Rather like the Nurses' Study, it involved 42,883 middle-aged men in the United States health profession who completed a dietary questionnaire every 4 years for 22 years or until they died. During that period 3,683 of them had heart attacks. After allowing for the effects of smoking, family history, alcohol consumption, use of multivitamins, exercise, calorie consumption, body mass index etc., it was found – wait for it! – it was found that just *one* drink a day sweetened with sugar increased the risk of a heart attack by 19%! A 'drink' was defined as a standard 355ml can or glass of cola or other fizzy pop or fruit-flavoured drink, whether caffeinated or caffeine-free. However the same drinks sweetened artificially (not with sugar) didn't increase the risk of a heart attack at all! So it is practically certain that it was sugar that was the culprit. The Nurses' Study, involving an even larger number of female nurses both young and middle-aged, had earlier produced a similar result. In this case one sugar-sweetened drink a day increased the risk of a heart attack by 15%.[164]

Sugar and other health problems

So we have sugar causing obesity, type 2 diabetes, and now heart disease. But even that isn't the end of the story. There is strong evidence that sugar is a major cause of gallstones[165] and many other health problems. Dr. Nancy Appleton lists no fewer than 49 ways in which sugar can damage our health or well-being, all with supporting references in the form of scientific papers or other published literature. In particular she cites the following effects that sugar can have on children:

- dental decay
- hyperactivity
- decreased activity

---

162 Yudkin J. *Diet and coronary heart disease: why blame fat?* Journal of the Royal Society of Medicine, September 1992; 85(9):515–516.

163 De Koning et al. *Sweetened Beverage Consumption, Incident Coronary Heart Disease and Biomarkers of Risk in Men.* Circulation, March 12, 2012. (Published online by the American Heart Association.)

164 Fung T T et al. *Sweetened beverage consumption and risk of coronary heart disease in women.* American Journal of Clinical Nutrition, 2009; 89:1037-1042.

165 Heaton K. *The Sweet Road to Gallstones.* British Medical Journal, April 14, 1984; 288:1103-4.

- anxiety
- difficulty in concentration
- drowsiness
- eczema
- general bad temper

No wonder she tells us to '*Lick the Sugar Habit!*'[166]

I wonder if some problems of teenage behaviour are caused by drinking lots of sugar-sweetened fizzy drinks or just eating sugary foods in general. If so, it's even more important not to give our sweet little kiddies a taste for sugar before they turn sour on us.

While the government has told us for years to obtain our calories from carbohydrates rather than fats, it does at last seem to be waking up to the troubles caused by that pure carbohydrate: sugar. In 2014 the U.K. government's Scientific Advisory Committee on Nutrition was instructed to reconsider the recommended levels of sugar intake, with a putative conclusion that no more than 10% of our calorie intake should be obtained from sugars, including naturally occurring sugars in fruit and other foods. The best recommendation it could come up with would be to avoid added sugar altogether, but this particular committee's recommendations often seem tempered by considerations of what is realistic and politically expedient rather than being based purely on scientific evidence.

Life after sugar

So let's do it! I know that while few of us would admit to sugar addiction, many would find the thought of a life without sugar, or at least without any added sugar, about as attractive as a dead mouse in a raspberry pavlova. But look on the positive side. Your life will actually be a lot sweeter if you and your children don't contract type 2 diabetes or coronary heart disease or gallstones or one of the other 49 health problems Nancy Appelton listed.

Food might not taste so sweet, it's true, but think how much tastier it can be in general! You can crunch roast chicken skin and munch pork chops and lunch on roast beef, knowing that in reasonable quantities these are good, not bad, for you. You can enjoy proper roast potatoes and roast parsnips again, cooked in dripping or lard instead of tasteless vegetable oil; or baked potatoes with melted butter and cheese and sugar-free baked beans. You can throw away all those bland, watery low-fat yogurts with added sugar (some Weight Watchers yogurts are sweetened with fructose syrup, or they were when I wrote this), and buy yourself instead some sucrose-free whole-milk yogurt such as Greek style yogurt flavoured with desiccated coconut or grated apple or banana,

---

[166] Appelton N. *Lick the Sugar Habit: How to Break Your Sugar Addiction Naturally.* Avery, 1997.

organic Yeo Valley live yogurt, or even creamy organic Rowan Glen fruit-flavoured yogurt if you live in Scotland. You can blow a raspberry at unappetizing fat-free cottage cheese and enjoy instead some mouth-watering full-cream Cheddar, Stilton or Double Gloucester. Or what about tasty fresh vegetables, steamed or sautéed in butter? They'll taste even nicer once your taste buds have been weaned off the idea that everything should taste sweet. You can treat yourself to an occasional slice of hot buttered toast or a buttered crumpet, and a dairy ice cream. Or eat fried bacon and eggs and sausages for breakfast. You can even fry fish and chips in beef dripping like they used to be cooked when we were kids. (So *that's* why they used to taste so nice!) And if you must spread jam rather than Marmite on your bread you can always buy the reduced sugar kind.

So don't look down your nose at a sugar-restricted diet. Instead, lift your nose up and snuffle up all those succulent smells steaming out of the stockpot. The aroma of proper food, the kind of food that you and your children were made to enjoy, the kind that does not make you ill or overweight or leave you perpetually hungry.

CHAPTER 9: CARBOHYDRATES – A WOMAN'S WORST FRIEND

Carbohydrates in food

So far we've talked about fats and sugars. Another main source of energy in our diet is what are commonly called carbohydrates. Actually sugar is also a carbohydrate, but when we say carbohydrates we usually refer to starchy carbohydrates, the kind of food that the government and other bodies tell us should make up the biggest portion of what we eat. Starchy carbohydrates come mainly from cereal crops, most commonly in the form of bread, pastry, pies, pasta, breakfast cereals and rice; and from root vegetables such as potatoes, carrots and parsnips. Potatoes, of course, are often eaten in the form of chips or crisps and similar snacks.

Carbohydrates and weight gain

Unlike sugar, starchy carbohydrates do have a lot of nutrients in them. They are all important and natural foodstuffs, so I don't want to dwell too much on the harm they can do or I'll be telling you that practically everything we eat is evil. However we have seen that eating too much of them makes us overweight, which explains why the current obesity epidemic started around the time that we were first told to eat more starchy foods, and when more of these foods became available at lower cost. The two reasons that starches make us put weight on are (a) that they are metabolized into sugar more quickly than fats and proteins are, so the resulting surge in blood sugar is more than we need to fuel our bodies and it gets stored as fat instead, and (b) they are less satiating. That means that, calorie for calorie, they don't make you feel as full as fats or proteins do, although they are better than sugar is in this respect. As a result someone whose diet is largely based on carbohydrates will generally end up eating more than he needs because when he has eaten the right number of calories for his weight and energy requirements he will feel hungry sooner and want to eat more.

Carbohydrates and heart disease

However there is more to the carbohydrate problem than that. Diets high in carbohydrates have now been clearly implicated as a major cause of coronary heart disease in women. This has been proved experimentally in a number of incontrovertible ways.

There are five or six different quantities scientists can measure in the blood to decide whether a patient could be heading for a heart attack. You could call them traffic lights, red meaning danger and green meaning safe. In a study made at Stanford University School of Medicine in 1995 five healthy women in their sixties were put on a *low* carbohydrate *high* fat diet for 3 weeks, while five more women were put on a *high* carbohydrate *low* fat diet for 3 weeks. Then for a further 3 weeks they all swapped diets and lived on the opposite one. All the different traffic lights turned green while they were on the *low* carbohydrate diet, and all the traffic lights changed to red while they were on the *high* carbohydrate one. The researchers looked at how the quantities they measured changed when women adopted the low fat, high carbohydrate diet, and concluded, *'Because all these changes would increase the risk of ischaemic heart disease*[167] *in post-menopausal women, it seems reasonable to question the wisdom of recommending that post-menopausal women consume low-fat, high-carbohydrate diets.'*[168] That was a diplomatic way of stating that a low fat, high carbohydrate diet is bad for older women.

Five years later scientists from the Stanford University School of Medicine, California, again compared the effects on blood fats of a low-fat, high-carbohydrate diet and a high-fat, low-carbohydrate diet, but this time their research subjects included both men and women. They found that subjects on the high-carbohydrate diet had significantly higher blood triglycerides and other indicators associated with heart disease. They concluded: *'Given the atherogenic potential of these changes in lipoprotein metabolism, it seems appropriate to question the wisdom of recommending that all Americans should replace dietary saturated fat with carbohydrate.'*[169] In plain English, they were saying that cutting down on good old saturated fat and eating starchy foods instead is likely to lead to heart trouble, so it's a BAD IDEA.

Both groups of researchers concluded that years of advice to cut down on fat and eat more carbohydrates were probably responsible at least in part for the epidemic of heart disease that has been around for the last 50 years or so.

While this research looked only at various measurements that are generally accepted as indicative of a potential heart attack, there have been at least two more investigations

---

167 Ischaemic heart disease is coronary heart disease.

168 Jeppesen J et al. *Effects of low-fat, high-carbohydrate diets on risk factors for ischaemic heart disease in post-menopausal women.* American Journal of Clinical Nutrition, 1997; 65:1027-33.

The two diets provided, as a percentage of total energy, were either 15% protein, 45% fat, and 40% carbohydrate, or 15% protein, 25% fat, and 60% carbohydrate.

169 Abbasi F et al. *High carbohydrate diets, triglyceride-rich lipoproteins, and coronary heart disease risk.* American Journal of Cardiology, 2000; 85(1):45.

in which a clear link was found between carbohydrate consumption and actual deaths from coronary heart disease. You see, by the turn of the century quite a few people were suggesting, as I am, that it would be healthier to eat fewer carbohydrates than the amounts currently being recommended. So some researchers in Boston set out to discover if this was true.[170]

They dug out the diet records of the nurses I told you about earlier and calculated from the kinds of carbohydrates that they had been eating and the quantities of these carbohydrates a value they called the glycaemic load. In simple terms, the glycaemic load is the amount of glucose a particular food generates in your bloodstream 2 hours after you have eaten it. Some kinds of carbohydrate like rice put much more glucose into your blood than others do. The initially healthy nurses started to record what they ate in 1984, and over a 10-year period 761 became victims of heart disease, with 208 of these actually dying. The researchers divided the nurses into five equal groups based on their average glycaemic load, the first group having the lowest glycaemic load, and the second group the next lowest, and so on. And they discovered that the nurses in the group that had the highest glycaemic load were nearly *twice as likely* to contract heart disease as those in the group with the lowest glycaemic load.

The foods that contributed most to their glycaemic load were not sugary drinks or fatty sausages, but mashed and baked potatoes and breakfast cereals. Other foods that contributed to a high glycaemic load were rice, pizza, bread, baguettes and chips. In other words, starchy carbohydrates. These nurses were all females between 38 and 63 years old at the beginning of the project, so this time we are not talking about a mere ten older women but thousands of women in their forties and upwards, and we are not talking about traffic lights but actual coronary heart disease being clearly associated with a high glycaemic load. So it looks very likely that eating a lot of starchy carbohydrate is not a good idea at all, for women at least.

Amazingly, a very different result was found for men. In April 2010 some Italian researchers decided that they should repeat this research on Italian people, whose diet is different from that of North Americans, and this time they included men as well as women.[171] They studied the dietary records of 47,749 volunteers comprising 15,171 men and 32,578 women, all aged between 35 and 74 years, who had been recruited for another project in the 1990s. 8 years after the year that their diets were recorded 463 of the volunteers had contracted coronary heart disease. In order to relate these cases to diet, they divided the subjects into four groups based on their glycaemic load. This time the women in the group with the highest glycaemic load had a risk of contracting heart disease 2.24 times as great as those in the lowest group. So among the women whose

---

170 Liu S et al. *A prospective study of dietary glycemic load, carbohydrate intake, and risk of coronary heart disease in US women.* American Journal of Clinical Nutrition, June 2000; 71(6):1455-61.

171 Sieri S et al. *Dietary Glycemic Load and Index and Risk of Coronary Heart Disease in a Large Italian Cohort. The EPICOR Study.* Archives of Internal Medicine, April 2010; 170(7):640-647.

diet produced a high glycaemic load, more than twice as many contracted heart disease as those whose diet produced a low glycaemic load. This more than confirmed what the American researchers had found from the Nurses' Study.

But the amazing discovery in the Italian study was that with the men their glycaemic load made no difference at all to their chances of contracting heart disease. Not even the total amount of carbohydrates that the men ate made any difference. Just as many men with a high glycaemic load contracted heart disease as those with a low one. And this wasn't a mistake, for similar tests carried out in the Netherlands[172] and in Sweden[173] produced the same result. Which only goes to show that men and women have very different metabolisms.

This means that for women, eating a bowl of manufactured cereal every day for breakfast is not the healthiest way to start the day. A healthier breakfast would consist of porridge or perhaps a fruit and nut muesli; a boiled egg with a thin slice of bread; something like cheese, baked beans or sardines on a thin slice of toast; or best of all good old fried egg and bacon with just half a thin slice of fried bread. Those are the kinds of breakfast that people ate before all the coronary heart disease started. As for potatoes, women should avoid too many baked and mashed potatoes and chips, and, whenever possible, eat boiled potatoes instead.

For men, the research raises a very interesting question. If eating a lot of starchy food doesn't increase a man's chance of suffering a heart attack, why do middle-aged men generally suffer more heart attacks than women? One explanation must be that more men than women smoke, and that middle-aged men tend to put themselves under more stress than women do. However there may also be diet-related causes that could affect men in the U.K. and the U.S.A more than the Continental and Scandinavian men who were studied in the research. We have seen that for both men and women consuming too much omega-6 polyunsaturated fat and fructose both increase the risk of a heart attack. The pies, burgers, crisps and chips made in factories and fast-food outlets and favoured by British men, particularly footballs fans, are mostly cooked with polyunsaturated fats high in omega-6. If starchy foods affect women more than men, perhaps polyunsaturated fats affect men more badly than women. Sugar certainly does. The two large studies of health workers described earlier showed that taking one sugar-sweetened drink a day increased the risk of a heart attack by 19% for a man, but only by 15% for a women. And many British builders and other manual labourers still use two spoonfuls of sugar to sweeten their frequent cups of coffee, which seems to have replaced tea as the beverage of choice, at least in the south of England where we live.

---

172 Van Dam R M et al. *Dietary glycemic index in relation to metabolic risk factors and incidence of coronary heart disease: the Zutphen Elderly Study*. European Journal of Clinical Nutrition, 2000; 54 (9):726-731.

173 Levitan E B et al. *Dietary glycemic index, dietary glycemic load, and cardiovascular disease in middle-aged and older Swedish men*. American Journal of Clinical Nutrition, 2007; 85 (6):1521-1526.

In any case the excessive glucose produced by eating too many starchy foods can cause type 2 diabetes in both men and women, and, it appears, age-related macular degeneration in the eyes.[174] Also too much starch makes both men and women put on weight, which can cause other health problems. So, even if starchy food that has not been cooked in polyunsaturated fat is safe for men, there are other very good reasons why men too should limit their consumption of starchy food. That won't please many men of course. How can you enjoy watching a football match on a chilly winter's day without stoking up your internal boiler with meat pies, burgers and fries? The only answer I can think of is to take a flask of hot soup and some cold chicken drumsticks or sausages cooked at home. After a match, when the fans of losing teams tend to eat more than the fans of winning teams, the best fast-food option is fish and chips. For even if the chips and fish batter are fried in a vegetable oil high in omega-6, the omega-3 in the fish will help to counteract its effects.

A food's glycaemic load and its associated GI value are both being taken seriously nowadays by many nutritionists. In this context GI is not an American soldier, nor a two-piece white garment worn in judo, nor a level 61 Warsong Gulch battlemaster located in the Vault of Lights in the Draenei capital of the Exodar (oh sorry! that's Jihi): GI stands for Glycaemic Index. This is a measure of how much glucose 1 gram of carbohydrate produces in the bloodstream of a healthy person within 2 hours of ingestion. The glycaemic load generated by your bowl of cornflakes or sun-dried organic lemongrass is simply its glycaemic index multiplied by the number of grams of carbohydrate in it.

For once I almost agree with the World Health Organization. In 1999, the World Health Organization (WHO) and the UN Food and Agriculture Organization (FAO) recommended that people in industrialized countries should base their diets on foods with a low GI in order to prevent coronary heart disease, diabetes and obesity. Some foods in Australia already show their GI rating on the nutrition information panel.

That statement by the WHO is amazing, because in most cases foods with a high GI, which they are now telling us we should avoid, are the very starchy carbohydrates that they were telling us 10 years earlier we should eat more of! The reason I say that I almost agree with them is that it was not the GI that was related to the incidence of heart disease in the Nurses' Study, but the glycaemic load. Watermelon, for example, has a very high glycaemic index, but because there is so little carbohydrate in a slice of watermelon it produces an almost negligible glycaemic load. Notwithstanding the association of heart trouble with glycaemic load found in the Nurses' Study, the Italian study found that food with a low glycaemic *index* didn't cause much of a problem at all, regardless of its glycaemic load. So it looks as though we should try to avoid foods with a high GI *and* try to keep down the total glycaemic load in our diet.

In Annexe 4 I've made a table that shows both the GI and the GL for typical servings

---

174 Chiu C J et al. *Informing food choices and health outcomes by use of the dietary glycaemic index.* Nutrition Reviews, April 2011; 69 (4): 231–42.

of some common starchy foods. The items shown in dark grey are the ones you should limit or avoid if possible.

Glycaemic loads and diabetes

Glycaemic loads are also related to the occurrence of type 2 diabetes. I've already explained why sugar causes extra insulin to be produced and how that can lead to type 2 diabetes. Eating a lot of food that produces a high glycaemic load has the same effect as eating sugar: it puts too much glucose into our bloodstream, which can eventually lead to type 2 diabetes.

Mitigate your munching

One obvious conclusion is to avoid munching snacks that consist largely of starch and sugar. Even more importantly, don't encourage your kids to do it, thereby training them to make such snacks part of their life.

If you must snack on carbohydrates, include some fat and protein as well, and teach your children to do the same. Fat and protein will lower your body's glycaemic response.[175] If you think about it, this is the way that people instinctively chose and ate food until fast food and factory-baked goods became so popular. People ate bread *and* butter, rice *and* meat, chips *and* fish. So a sausage sandwich in a thin slice of buttered bread, a slice of pork pie, a slice of quiche (which is made with eggs), or a biscuit accompanied by a glass of full-cream milk would all be healthier snacks than crisps, chips, doughnuts, bagels or popcorn eaten alone.

---

175 *Glycemic index*. Wikipedia.org.

CHAPTER 10: CHOLESTEROL – NOT THE BIG BAD WOLF

Forget cholesterol, it's not a problem

Any doctor who believes that cholesterol *causes* heart disease is at least 10 years out of date. I have a paper on my desk called *'A hypothesis out of date: the diet-heart idea'*.[176] It was published in the Journal of Epidemiology in 2002 by a Swedish doctor called Uffe Ravnskov, who published a similar paper in the *British Medical Journal* that same year.[177] Ravnskov spent over 10 years studying the evidence that linked saturated fatty acids and cholesterol to heart disease. He was particularly interested in why so many scientists were claiming that there was a link, and he found that in nearly every case they either ignored evidence that there is no causal link or else were claiming a link when their own research didn't really justify it. In his paper he cites 71 research papers on the subject, and concludes from them that high levels of cholesterol are not the cause of heart disease.

Cholesterol is good for oldies

At least one of the papers cited by Ravnskov[178] describes some research which discovered that old people die twice as often from a heart attack if they have a *low* cholesterol level rather than a high level of it. Another study[179] of more than a thousand elderly patients with severe heart failure found that within 5 years about 30% of those with high cholesterol levels (above 223mg/l of blood) had died, but 62% of those with low

---

176 Ravnskov U. *A hypothesis out-of-date: the diet-heart idea.* Journal of Clinical Epidemiology 55 (2002); 057-1063.

177 Ravnskov U. *Diet-heart disease hypothesis is wishful thinking.* British Medical Journal 2002; 324:238.

178 Krumholz H M et al. *Lack of association between cholesterol and coronary heart disease mortality and morbidity and all-cause mortality in persons older than 70 years. Journal of the American Medical Association, 1990;* 272, 1335-1340.

179 Horwich T et al. *Low serum total cholesterol is associated with marked increase in mortality in advanced heart failure. Journal of Cardiac Failure, August* 2002; 8(4):216-24.

cholesterol levels (below 129mg/l) had died. The investigators ensured that everyone involved was adequately fed to make sure that a low cholesterol level was not simply the result of undernourishment. The study made it clear that an old person with heart trouble and a low cholesterol level is twice as likely to die of heart failure in the next 5 years as one with a high cholesterol level. And Ravnskov found *eleven* different studies that came up with similar findings.[180] So at my age I am certainly not going to worry about keeping my cholesterol level down. I would rather have a high cholesterol level so that I can live as long as possible.

Cholesterol is good for ladies

For ladies there is even better news. A high cholesterol level means you are less likely to suffer a heart attack whatever your age may be. One of the most famous studies of cholesterol and heart disease is the Framingham Heart Study, which began in 1948 with 5,209 men and women between the ages of 30 and 62 living in the town of Framingham, Massachusetts. During the first 20 years of the study an association between high cholesterol levels and heart disease was indeed found in many of the subjects, but the researchers reported that in women over 50 '*cholesterol had no predictive value*'.[181]

Much more recently in Norway there was a huge study of over 52,000 Norwegians of both sexes aged 20 to 74. Over a period of 10 years their blood cholesterol levels were monitored, and if they died within that period the cause of their death was recorded. The results were published in the *Journal of Evaluation of Clinical Practice* in 2012.[182] The following amazing result was reported: '*Among women, cholesterol had an inverse association with all-cause mortality as well as CVD mortality.*' This means that as a woman, the *higher* your cholesterol level is, whatever your age, the *less likely* it is that you will die within the next 10 years. And those figures were corrected for smoking and high blood pressure, so they take into account the effects of cholesterol only. CVD stands for Coronary Vascular Disease and it includes such things as stroke and heart failure as well as coronary heart disease. They found that for women the chance that you will die of CVD if your cholesterol level is above 7.0mmol/l is only three-quarters of your chance of dying of CVD if the level is below 5.0mmol/l. So a *high* cholesterol level is good news for women of all ages!

---

180 Ravnskov U. *High cholesterol may protect against infections and atherosclerosis. Quarterly Journal of Medicine* 2003; 96, 927-934.

181 Kannel W B & Gordon T (editors). Framingham Monograph, Section 24. *An Epidemiological Investigation of Cardiovascular Disease.* U.S. Department of Health, Education and Welfare, National Institutes of Health, 1968.

182 Petursson H et al. *Is the use of cholesterol in mortality risk algorithms in clinical guidelines valid? Ten years prospective data from the Norwegian HUNT 2 study.* Journal of Evaluation in Clinical Practice, February 2012; 18(1):159-68.

It is true that, in the Norwegian study, the death rate from coronary heart disease alone was slightly higher for the highest concentrations of cholesterol (above 7.0mmol/l) than for the mid range. However the authors of the paper concluded, *'If our findings are generalizable, clinical and public health recommendations regarding the 'dangers' of cholesterol should be revised. This is especially true for women, for whom moderately elevated cholesterol (by current standards) may prove to be not only harmless but even beneficial'*. Clearly they were using some scientific caution in the wording of their conclusion, but their meaning is obvious. If you are a woman forget about your cholesterol – it's not a problem.

Part of the reason that the medical world still believes high cholesterol levels to be associated with heart trouble is that much of the earlier research was carried out on middle-aged men who are very prone to heart attacks, and in their case there does seem to be an association between the two. However, just as Ancel Keys did, they forget that an association between two things doesn't necessarily mean that one causes another. Most deaths occur in bed, but that doesn't mean that it is safer to sleep on the floor! When a water company van is parked at the roadside there is nearly always a damaged water main in the vicinity. But does that mean that water company vans drive around the countryside bursting our water mains? Of course it doesn't. The vans bring workmen along to repair the damage, not to cause it. And that's the reason that cholesterol turns up when there is a problem in our arteries.

One of cholesterol's jobs is to help reduce inflammation and repair damaged cell walls, problems that are caused by stress, smoking, or diet. So when our arteries become damaged the liver generates cholesterol to repair them. And that's almost certainly why people's cholesterol levels rise as they get older. They need more of it. In other words, cholesterol doesn't produce heart disease: it's heart disease that produces cholesterol!

Cholesterol is good for everyone

Cholesterol is a very important type of fat which is needed for a range of totally essential bodily functions. There is some cholesterol in food, but 80% to 85% of the cholesterol in our bodies is produced by our liver in whatever quantities it is needed. If we avoided foods with cholesterol in them then our liver would simply produce more of it to make up the shortfall, and vice versa.[183] One discovery in the Framingham Heart Study was that when subjects who had very high cholesterol levels (over 300mg/dl) were compared with those who had very low levels (under 170mg/dl) there was no difference in the overall amount of fat that they consumed in their diets. In other words, the amount of fat we eat has nothing at all to do with our cholesterol levels. Dr. Uffe Ravnskov once ate

---

183 Lecerf J M & de Lorgeril M. *Dietary cholesterol: from physiology to cardiovascular risk*. British Journal of Nutrition, 2011; 106 (1): 6–14.

59 eggs is 9 days to see if a cholesterol-rich diet would increase his blood cholesterol. It didn't: his cholesterol level actually fell by 11%.[184]

So our bodies make as much cholesterol as they need for various essential tasks. Here are some of those tasks that cholesterol carries out:

- Our bodies consist of trillions of cells. Cholesterol is an essential component of the cell membrane, the protective skin around a cell that allows nutrients, hormones and other substances into the cell and lets waste products come out. It is needed to build and rebuild these cells.
- Many essential bodily activities are controlled by messengers called hormones. Cholesterol is required to produce the hormones that regulate sexual functions, the body's response to stress, infection and inflammation, the digestion of protein and carbohydrates, and even some aspects of behaviour. Hormone deficiency makes our bodies susceptible to major disease and various kinds of malfunction.
- Cholesterol acts as an antioxidant, protecting us from heart disease and cancer.[185]
- Cholesterol is used in the production of bile, which the body needs in order to digest other fats.
- Cholesterol in conjunction with sunlight produces vitamin D (which is a hormone rather than a vitamin). Vitamin D is needed for the absorption of the calcium and phosphorus that our bones are made of. Insufficient vitamin D causes rickets and brittle bones.
- Cholesterol coats our nerve fibres and is one component of synapses, the connections between cells that enable them to pass messages from one to another. So it is an essential part of our nervous system and our brain.
- About a quarter of the brain's total weight consists of cholesterol. Mother's milk is especially rich in cholesterol and contains a special enzyme that helps the baby utilize this nutrient.[186] Babies and children need cholesterol-rich foods throughout their growing years for the proper development of their brains and nervous systems.[187]

---

[184] Ravnskov U. *The Cholesterol Myths*, p. 109. New Trends Publishing Inc, Washington DC, 2000.

[185] Cranton E M & Frackelton J P. *Free radical pathology in age-associated diseases: Treatment with EDTA chelation, nutrition and antioxidants*. Journal of Holistic Medicine, Spring/Summer 1984; 6(1):6-37.

[186] Jensen R et al. *Lipids of human milk and infant formulas: a review*. American Journal of Clinical Nutrition, 1 June 1978; 31 (6):990–1016.

[187] Alfin-Slater R B & Aftergood L. *Lipids*. Modern Nutrition in Health and Disease, 6th ed, p.131. R S Goodhart and M E Shils, eds, Lea and Febiger, Philadelphia, 1980.

The cholesterol delivery service

Cholesterol is cholesterol: there's no such thing as good or bad cholesterol. When people use these terms they are really talking about are the two different chemicals that carry cholesterol around the bloodstream. Cholesterol can't dissolve in blood because it is a fat, so it has to be carried around in special chemicals that can dissolve in blood. These chemicals are called lipoproteins, or fat-carrying proteins. The low density ones are thought to be bad for us, again because there always seem to be a lot of them around in people who have heart trouble, and the high density ones are thought to be good for the opposite reason.

When we eat carbohydrates in the form of starch or sugar, they are converted to glucose, which is either used immediately for energy purposes or is sent to the liver. The liver uses it for various things, including the manufacture of the all-important cholesterol, and any excess glucose it turns into fat that our body can store for use later. It does this by building fat molecules called triglycerides. It then has to transport these insoluble triglycerides and the cholesterol through the blood to the parts of our body that need them. In order to do this the liver does something else as well: it assembles some 'delivery lorries' called lipoproteins.

Low-density lipoproteins, or LDLs as they are usually called, are what I call the Low-loader Delivery Lorries. They transport cholesterol and triglycerides from the liver to the building sites and warehouses of our cells. High-density lipoproteins, or HDLs, are the High-sided Delivery Lorries, which are believed to carry back any used or spare cholesterol from the building sites to their factory in Liverpool for recycling or waste disposal.[188] It's LDL which is confusingly called 'bad cholesterol', and HDL which is confusingly called 'good cholesterol'. As I said, the reason people use those terms is that high levels of LDL in the bloodstream are associated with a high incidence of heart disease, whereas high levels of HDL are associated with a low incidence of it.

Incidentally, dietary fats, as distinct from carbohydrates, are also converted into triglycerides and cholesterol, but dietary fats are processed in the intestines and the resulting triglycerides and cholesterol are distributed, not by LDLs, but by great big container lorries called chylomicrons. 'Chylomicron' is Greek for 'small milky one'. Chylomicrons are very tiny milky-looking globules, which may be small compared with a raindrop, for example, but they are around twenty times bigger than LDL particles. So you can see that LDLs, which are associated with heart disease, have nothing to do with any fat that we eat. LDLs are created only as a result of eating carbohydrates!

Repairs and breakdowns

So if the body creates LDL, and if high levels of LDL are associated with heart disease, does that mean that our bodies are making something that is bad for us? No, it doesn't.

---

[188] Lewis G F & Rader D J. *New insights into the regulation of HDL metabolism and reverse cholesterol transport*. Circulation Research, June 2005; 96 (12): 1221–32.

One reason that people with heart trouble usually have large concentrations of LDLs in their blood is that when our cells are damaged they have to be repaired, and cholesterol is one of the main materials used to repair them. So if our arteries have suffered a lot of damage then the liver has to generate large amounts of cholesterol to repair them, which means making lots of LDLs to carry the cholesterol to the damaged cells.

However, it may be true that the LDL particles themselves contribute to arterial damage, at least when there are too many of them in our blood. The belief is that when an LDL lorry breaks down on an arterial roadway, a breakdown vehicle called a macrophage comes along and gobbles it up before driving off with it to the rubbish tip. Macrophages are the original Pac-Men, because 'macrophage' comes from two Greek words meaning 'big eater'! They are one kind of white blood cell. The trouble is that eating a whole lorry makes the macrophage so fat it gets stuck in the walls of a blood vessel, or it can do. And that can lead to the formation of plaque. When enough plaque has formed the blood vessel becomes so narrow that a blood clot can block it completely, resulting in a heart attack or a stroke. You won't find the process described in quite those terms in other literature, but in broad outline that is the story commonly presented.

An LDL hypothesis

I don't think anyone knows for certain why the LDL lorries break down, but perhaps this is the explanation.

The triglycerides that the liver makes are produced, as I said, from sugars and carbohydrates. These are transported along with cholesterol by the LDL lorries. But when we eat more sugar and carbohydrates than we need, the liver has to make so many triglycerides that some of the lorries leave the factory in Liverpool with only triglycerides in them, or at least only a little cholesterol. And since carbohydrates come mostly from plant sources, it may be that the triglycerides our liver makes contain mostly polyunsaturated fats, which are mainly the kind that come from plants. So the LDL lorries carry lots of polyunsaturated fat but relatively little cholesterol. However it is thought that cholesterol can protect polyunsaturated fat from oxidation. So if LDLs loaded with polyunsaturated fat and not much cholesterol hang around for a long time in the bloodstream because there are more of them than our bodies really need, then eventually the polyunsaturated fats oxidize. Once that happens white blood cells in the form of macrophages identify the LDL particles as carrying damaged goods and swallow them up.[189]

---

189 Steinberg D. *Low density lipoprotein oxidation and its pathobiological significance.* Journal of Biological Chemistry, 1997; 272:20963-20966.

An HDL hypothesis

Heart disease is associated with low levels of HDL as well as with high levels of LDL. This may be because HDL molecules are used to make LDL molecules. The liver doesn't actually make LDL directly to carry the triglycerides: it makes VLDL, or very low-density lipoprotein. When the VLDLs have delivered their triglycerides then HDL molecules turn them into LDLs, which are then carrying only cholesterol.

If a lot of VLDLs are made because there are a lot of triglycerides then a lot of HDL molecules will be needed to convert them to LDLs. Hence the supply of HDLs gets used up and the level of them in our blood falls. So the 'bad' LDL uses up the 'good' HDL, and heart trouble is then associated with low levels of HDL.

Whether that is the true explanation or not, your guess is as good as mine!

It's carbohydrates, stupid!

So LDL carrying oxidized polyunsaturated fats fur up our arteries because we eat too many carbohydrates. The LDL problem is nothing to do with eating saturated fat in foods like bacon and butter.

In reality there is an even closer association between triglycerides and heart disease than there is between LDL and heart disease. It's true that dietary fats also produce triglycerides, but the chylomicrons distribute these to our muscles and fat storing cells within about 5 hours of a meal, after which there is no trace of them in the blood,[190] whereas the triglycerides our liver produces from carbohydrates keep trickling out for many more hours after we have eaten. And, since fasting blood tests are usually carried out 12 hours after a meal, the triglyceride levels measured relate mainly to the carbohydrates we have eaten, not to fat.[191] Once again, since high triglyceride levels are associated with a higher risk of heart disease, it seems to be carbohydrates that are implicated.

Experiments with high fat/low carbohydrate diets

So here's a little test. If a man went on a diet in which most of his calories came from fats and only a very few from carbohydrates, what would happen to his levels of LDL, HDL, triglycerides and cholesterol? According to most doctors his LDL, triglycerides

---

190 Steinberg D. *Low density lipoprotein oxidation and its pathobiological significance.* Journal of Biological Chemistry, 1997; 272:20963-20966. (Also cited earlier.)

191 Chen Y D et al. *Why do low-fat high-carbohydrate diets accentuate postprandial lipemia in patients with NIDDM?* Diabetes Care, 1995; 18:10-16.

and cholesterol would all increase, being associated in most doctors' minds with heart disease and dietary fat, and his HDL levels would decrease. However, according to what I have been saying, the level of LDL and triglycerides in the blood would decrease on a high fat diet, and eventually cholesterol levels would decrease too because there would not be so much cell damage to repair if the fat was mostly saturated or monounsaturated fat. So what would actually happen?

In 2002 some scientists at the University of Connecticut got hold of twenty men of normal weight and with normal blood cholesterol levels.[192] (I am tempted to say that they had to search the whole of the U.S.A. to find twenty such men, but that would be cheeky!) They put twelve of these men on a very low carbohydrate, high fat diet for 6 weeks,[193] and allowed the other eight who didn't fancy the idea of such a diet to continue with their normal one as a 'control group'. The diet of the twelve high fat diet volunteers included moderate amounts of vegetables and salads as well as a daily vitamin and mineral supplement. What they found in the men on the high fat diet was that after 6 weeks their triglycerides had fallen by 33% and their 'good' HDL had risen by more than 11%. Surprisingly, there was no significant change in their LDL, although the kind of LDL measured (there are various kinds) did show an improvement. What most doctors and certainly most people would find even more surprising was that there was on average no change in their cholesterol levels at the end of the test period. A diet in which 61% of their energy was obtained from fat did not increase their cholesterol levels at all!

Not surprisingly the fasting insulin level of the men on the high fat, low carbohydrate diet fell by an average of 34%, which is a very healthy sign. They also lost on average just over 2kg in weight. Yes, that's right. *The men on a high fat diet lost weight.* In the control group the only significant change was that at the end of the investigation period they were all 6 weeks older!

The scientists who conducted this research rather cautiously concluded that in the short term a high fat, low carbohydrate diet is not harmful and may improve one's chances of avoiding 'atherogenic dyslipidemia', i.e. arterial damage caused by high fat levels in the blood. Why they didn't they have the courage to conclude that such a diet is healthy, I don't know!

All right, you might say, but 6 weeks isn't very long. Quite true, but listen to this. Following that study in Connecticut, doctors at Duke University, North Carolina, decided to conduct a study lasting 6 months to determine the longer-term effects of a

---

192 Sharman M J et al. *A ketogenic diet favorably affects serum biomarkers for cardiovascular disease in normal-weight men. Journal of Nutrition* 2002; 132:1879-1885.

193 *The energy distribution in the normal diet was* 17% protein, 47% carbohydrate and 32% fat. The distribution in the low carbohydrate diet was 30% protein, 8% carbohydrate and 61% fat. There were no restrictions on the type of fat.

low carbohydrate diet.[194] This was an amazingly brave piece of research, because they allowed 41 overweight or obese volunteers to eat as much fat as they liked, so long as they restricted their carbohydrate intake to 25 grams a day! Actually the project started with 51 volunteers, but ten had to drop out for work or other reasons, including two who couldn't keep off their doughnuts and bagels and pizzas. The remaining 41 volunteers, aged between 35 and 53, comprised both men and women, with the majority being white women. They all wanted to lose weight.

They attended regular meetings at which they were encouraged to take at least 20 minutes of aerobic exercise like walking, cycling or swimming three times a week. Blood samples were taken at these meetings. After they had lost 40% of whatever weight they were trying to lose they were allowed to increase their carbohydrate intake to 50 grams a day. That still isn't much – one thick slice of bread! The rest of their diet consisted of unlimited amounts of meat, fish and seafood (e.g. beef, pork, chicken, turkey, fish, shellfish), unlimited eggs, 4 ounces of cheese per day, 2 cups of salad vegetables per day, and 1 cup of low-carbohydrate vegetables per day. The subjects were told to eat as much meat and eggs as they liked until their hunger was relieved. How about that for a weight-loss diet?

So what happened? On average the dieters lost 9kg in weight. This time their LDL decreased on average by 7%, a small improvement, and their cholesterol level fell by 5%. Their average HDL increased by 19%, a substantial improvement, and finally their triglyceride level, a major warning sign for the development of heart disease, fell by an enormous 43%! The effect on their insulin levels was not reported.

Hence after 6 months' eating unlimited amounts of fat and protein, but strictly limited amounts of carbohydrate, these participants lost weight, lowered their LDL, cholesterol and triglyceride levels, and substantially improved their HDL. These were similar changes to those found in the shorter study, but were even greater in magnitude over the longer period! All these changes were in accordance with what I was predicting, and they were all the complete opposite of what generally accepted wisdom would predict. But these are facts. They prove that fat is good for you, and that the amounts of carbohydrates we are currently encouraged to eat are bad for us.

I'm not recommending a diet as extreme as either of those described above, partly because of the cost and partly because they do seem to be somewhat unnatural. However it's very hard to argue against the following conclusions:

- Eating more fat does not increase your cholesterol level if you keep your carbohydrate consumption down and include vegetables and salads in your diet.
- Eating more fat and less carbohydrate decreases the risk factors for a heart attack.
- It is possible to lose weight by restricting one's carbohydrate intake without restricting one's intake of fat.

---

194 Westman E C et al. *Effect of 6-month adherence to a very low carbohydrate diet program. American Journal of Medicine,* 2002; 113: 30-36.

From what I have said earlier, it seems most likely that it was decreasing their carbohydrate intake rather than eating more fat that decreased the risk factors for the project participants. So if you are already eating enough fat don't get the idea that simply adding more will improve your health, especially if you are already overweight!

The final proof

Now here's my final shot at anyone who claims that high cholesterol levels cause heart disease or are even associated with it. The world's largest ever study to monitor trends in heart disease was started by the World Health Organization in the early 1980s and ended in 2003.[195] Some 10 million people in 21 countries in Europe, Australia, North America, China and Russia participated in 'MONICA' (Multinational *MONI*toring of trends and determinants in *CA*rdiovascular disease). When the data were examined in 2003 no overall relationship whatever was found between national blood cholesterol levels and incidences of cardiovascular disease or death.[196] Figure 19 illustrates this very clearly!

---

195 Tunstall-Pedoe H et al. *World's largest study of heart disease, stroke, risk factors, and population trends 1979-2002.* World Health Organization, MONICA Project.

196 Tunstall-Pedoe H. *MONICA Monograph and Multimedia Sourcebook.* World Health Organization, Geneva, Switzerland, 2003.

Figure 19: Relationships between percentage of national population with high cholesterol levels and death rates from coronary heart disease[197]

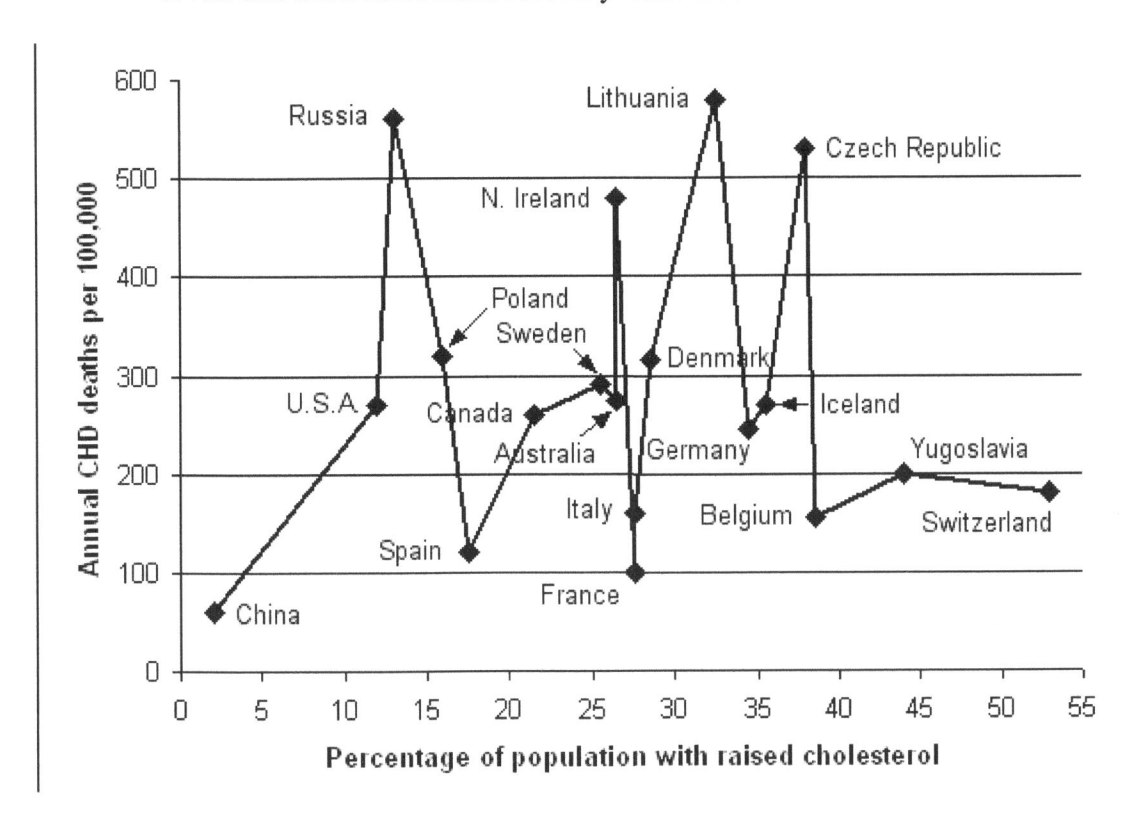

---

[197] High cholesterol levels were defined in the Monica study as greater than 6.5mmol/l (260mg/dl.) Data for the figure was extracted from the previous reference by Dr. Malcolm Kendrick, author of *The Great Cholesterol Con*.

CHAPTER 11: VITAMINS – CAN'T LIVE WITHOUT THEM

What is a vitamin?

A vitamin is an organic substance (one containing carbon) that is necessary in tiny amounts for life. The body cannot make it so it must be obtained from food. Some vitamins are fat-soluble, which means that the body can store them in its fat for use when needed. Others, like vitamins B_6, B_{12} and C, are water-soluble. The body cannot store these so they must be replenished regularly from food that contains them. Vegetables should not be cooked by boiling them in water, because the water soluble nutrients will dissolve in it and be lost when you drain the vegetables, unless of course you are making soup or a stew, or you save the water for use another time as vegetable stock. A deficiency of any vitamin can cause serious health problems, but so long as you eat a varied diet that includes fresh vegetables, preferably organically grown or at least home grown, you should get all the vitamins you need with one possible exception: vitamin D.

Vitamin D, the special one

Vitamin D is not strictly a vitamin because our bodies can make it, but only with the help of sunlight. Just as the chlorophyll in plant leaves uses the energy of sunlight to generate plant cells from carbon dioxide, so our liver and kidneys use the energy in ultraviolet light to generate vitamin D from cholesterol. Small quantities of vitamin D can be obtained from:

- the oil of fatty fish (especially cod liver oil)
- egg yolks
- milk, cheese and butter in Canada and the U.S.A., where milk is fortified with vitamin D
- meat and poultry liver
- blood sausage
- mushrooms
- any other foods that are artificially fortified with vitamin D

However most of the vitamin D we need has to be generated by our own bodies on exposure to ultraviolet light, or else be provided by a supplement.

Vitamin D enables the body to absorb the calcium that is needed to build and maintain our bones and teeth. Consequently a lack of it in children and young people results in rickets, a condition in which the bones soften and deform producing bowed legs and spinal curvature. A deficiency in older people results in osteomalacia or osteoporosis, a condition in which the bones weaken and break easily. In recent years however doctors have learned that insufficient vitamin D produces a sheaf of other health problems too.

Satheesh Nair, a specialist in liver disease, tells us that vitamin D plays an important role in reducing the risk of type 2 diabetes mellitus, cardiovascular diseases, cancers, and several autoimmune and infectious diseases.[198] All these are more likely to occur if we don't have enough of the vitamin. Dr. Nair says that a deficiency of it also causes muscle weakness, and that low levels of it are associated with frequent falls. Uffe Ravnskov, whose work I quoted previously, agrees with this, and adds autism and rheumatoid arthritis to the list of problems caused by a lack of this essential vitamin.[199] In an article in the *New York Times*, published in March 2012, Dr. Jane Brody explained that nearly every bodily tissue has receptors for vitamin D, among them the intestines, brain, heart, skin, sex organs, breasts and lymphocytes, as well as the placenta. She says that the vitamin, which acts as a hormone, is known to influence the production of more than 200 genes. No wonder a deficiency of it spells trouble!

Life on the dark side

All three doctors tell us that most people, in the Western world at least, don't receive nearly enough exposure to sunlight to produce an adequate amount of vitamin D. In latitudes greater than 35°, which means anywhere north or south of Africa, the human body can produce little or no vitamin D from November to February.[200] Likewise, people who cover their skin completely when outdoors, or always use sunscreen, or who rarely venture outside at all, are likely to experience vitamin D deficiency. There is reliable evidence that all Muslim women who cover themselves fully in the street and do not take supplementary vitamin D are vitamin D deficient.[201] All black people living far from the

---

198 Nair S. *Vitamin D Deficiency and Liver Disease.* Gastroenterology and Hepatology, August 2010; 6(8): 491–493.

199 Ravnskov U. *The Cholesterol Myths.* Newtrends Publishing, Inc., October 1, 2000.
(This important book is now out of print, but the author has published a simpler version of it under the title, *Fat and Cholesterol are good for You!*)

200 Nair S. *Vitamin D Deficiency and Liver Disease.* Gastroenterology and Hepatology, August 2010; 6(8): 491–493. (Also cited earlier.)

201 Mishal A A. *Effects of Different Dress Styles on Vitamin D Levels in Healthy Young Jordanian Women.* Osteoporosis International, 2001; 12(11): 931-935.

equator are at risk of vitamin D deficiency diseases because the melanin in their skin acts as a natural sunblock.

These views are supported in a startling manner by statistics on the incidence of renal cancer (cancer of the kidneys) published by the World Health Organization's Globocan 2008 project.[202] The statistics are presented in graphical form in Figure 20. The two graphs shown come from a paper by Dr. C F Garland and colleagues. This paper demonstrates clear associations between low levels of vitamin D and many forms of cancer, including renal, colorectal and breast cancer, as well as multiple sclerosis, rickets and the more serious type 1 diabetes; and it provides evidence that supplementary doses of vitamin D can significantly reduce the incidence of many of these diseases.[203]

Figure 20: Rates of renal cancer by latitude, 2002

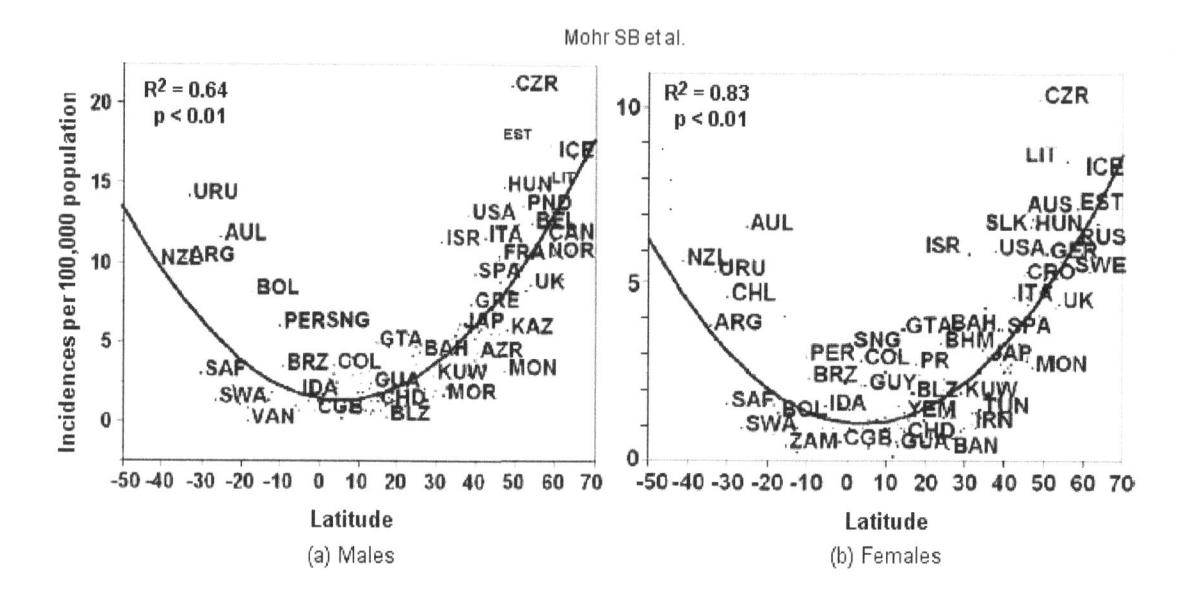

To put it simply, the two figures demonstrate that people living near the sunny equator, in the countries shown in the middle of each graph, have very low incidences of renal cancer, almost zero in some cases; whereas in countries like New Zealand and Iceland and the U.K., which are further from the equator and where there is much less sunlight, people have relatively high levels of the cancer. This shows how important it is for us to have adequate exposure to sunlight, or at least to ensure that our bodies get all the

---

202 *Cancer Incidence and Mortality Worldwide: IARC CancerBase No. 10.* [GLOBOCAN 2008 v2.0. Internet].

203 Garland C F et al. *Dose-Response of Vitamin D and a Mechanism for Prevention of Cancer.* Department of Family and Preventive Medicine, UCSD School of Medicine; and Moores UCSD Cancer Center. December 2, 2008.

vitamin D that we need. It also shows that many people in the more extreme northern and southern latitudes don't have enough of the vitamin.

Of course, going back to our old discussion on associations versus cause and effect, an alternative explanation might be that renal cancer is connected with low external temperatures rather than lack of sunlight. But if this were the case the figure for the U.S.A., where people keep warm with central heating and get their car out to visit someone in the next block, would appear below the curved line, indicating a lower than average occurrence of cancer at that latitude. And I'd expect the figure for a poorer country like Montenegro, where people keep warm with woollen underwear and have to go out to the yard to pump up some water, would come above the line, showing a higher than average occurrence of renal cancer. In fact the opposite is true. People in the U.S.A. who keep warm have twice as much renal cancer as people in Montenegro who live at the same latitude. So it is lack of sunlight rather than warmth that is almost certainly the cause of the higher rates of renal cancer further from the equator.

There is no doubt that vitamin D deficiency is a problem in countries like the U.K. and the U.S.A. In a study carried out in Boston in 2008,[204] 7.5% had rickets and 32.5% showed demineralization of bone tissue! Overall, 40% of infants and toddlers were found to be vitamin D deficient, using 30nanograms/millilitre as the cut-off point. And in 2011 the BBC reported that over 20% of children tested for bone problems at Southampton General Hospital showed signs of rickets. Vitamin D deficiency is evidently a dreadful reality for some youngsters. Part of the problem is that a mother's milk is a poor source of vitamin D when the mother herself is deficient in it. When a mother's own vitamin D level is normal her breast milk is an excellent and adequate source.

Another cause of vitamin D deficiency is the growing problem of obesity. This particular vitamin is stored in body fat, and for some reason obese people are more likely to be deficient in it, perhaps because they need more.

But the main reason, of course, is that nowadays people in our country don't go out in the sun enough, or if they do, they cover their skin with clothing or sunblock. Kids used to play in the street or wander off to parks on their own. I can remember sitting on the pavement for what seemed like hours as a small child digging moss out from between the paving stones and trying to make ants go where I wanted them to and setting up totally unsuccessful snail races. Nowadays children are kept indoors for safety reasons or they prefer to stay inside and play computer games. Adults used to walk or cycle to work and spend free time in their garden or allotment, but now those things don't happen much either. Most of us travel to work by car, bus or train, we work indoors all day long and we spend next to no time out of doors in the sunshine. Medium wavelength ultraviolet light or UVB, the kind our bodies need to generate vitamin D, cannot penetrate glass.

---

[204] Gordon C M. *Prevalence of vitamin D deficiency among healthy infants and toddlers.* Archives of Pediatric & Adolescent Medicine, June 2008;162(6):505-12.

So even if we spent every day in a sunny conservatory or office we would acquire little or no vitamin D.

How to get enough vitamin D

According to Uffe Ravnskov we should aim for at least 15 to 20 minutes of exposure to sunlight without sunscreen during the middle of the day on a regular basis. Michael Holick says that sensible sun exposure (which he defines as 5 to 10 minutes of exposure of the arms and legs or the hands, arms and face, two or three times per week), and increased dietary and supplemental vitamin D intakes are reasonable approaches to guarantee vitamin D sufficiency.[205]

Supplemental vitamin D means taking vitamin pills, or preferably capsules with liquid vitamin D in them. The difficulty is in deciding whether one really needs to do this and if so how much one should take. Garland's paper describes experiments carried out over a number of years to determine the benefit of supplementing one's vitamin D intake artificially, typically by supplying experimental subjects with 2,000 international units of vitamin D_3 a day in liquid capsule form. His conclusions were as follows:

- People living in sunny regions with minimal clothing that doesn't limit vitamin D synthesis have 54 to 90 nanograms/millilitre of $25(OH)D_3$ in their blood.[206] ($25(OH)D_3$ is vitamin D in the form in which it is made by the liver.)
- A good target is 60ng/ml of blood.
- For every 100 IU (international units) of vitamin D_3 ingested as a food supplement, one's serum (blood) vitamin D level will increase by 1ng/ml. Therefore if a patient's current level is 20ng/ml he needs to take 4,000 IU per day to raise it to 60ng/ml.[207]
- Families living further than 30° north or south of the equator should supplement their vitamin D intake with a minimum of 1,000 IU of vitamin D_3 per day for infants, 2,000 IU per day for children from 1 to 12 years old, and 2,000 to 2,400 IU per day for adults.

---

[205] Holick M F. *Sunlight and vitamin D for bone health and prevention of autoimmune diseases, cancers, and cardiovascular disease.* American Journal of Clinical Nutrition, 2004; 80(suppl):1678S–88S. (I consider this particular paper to be the ultimate source of knowledge on this subject. It can be read free of charge on the Internet at ajcn.nutrition.org/content/80/6/1678S.full.pdf+html)

[206] Hollis B W. *Circulating 25-hydroxyvitamin D levels indicative of vitamin D sufficiency: implications for establishing a new effective dietary intake recommendation for vitamin D.* Journal of Nutrition, 2005; 135:317-22.

[207] Heaney R P et al. *Human serum 25-hydroxycholecalciferol response to extended oral dosing with cholecalciferol.* American Journal of Clinical Nutrition, 2003; 77:204-10.

D_3 is one of three forms of vitamin D, and the best one to take as a supplement. It's called cholecalciferol. Some researchers discovered that when elderly women in care homes took it as a supplement they didn't die so often. Sorry, I couldn't resist writing that! What they actually found was that vitamin D_3 supplements made them live longer, but the other two forms of vitamin D didn't make any difference.[208] So for that and several other reasons D_3 is the kind one should take.

Garland's 60ng/ml does sound like a good level to aim at, but the American Institute of Medicine recommends minimum serum levels of only 20ng/ml, while many bone specialists and vitamin D researchers consider 30ng/ml to be a desirable level. Stephan Guyanet, an independent food researcher whose work I respect, says that 30ng/ml of $25(OH)D_3$ is required to normalize parathyroid hormone levels, and 35ng/ml is required to optimize calcium absorption, so he says it's probably best to maintain at least 35ng/ml $25(OH)D_3$.[209]

Because of the uncertainty over the required levels of vitamin D supplementation, a long-term placebo-controlled clinical trial called VITAL began in 2011 to assess the effects of a daily supplement of 2,000 IU of vitamin D and 1gm of omega-3 fatty acids on the risks of developing cancer, heart disease, stroke and other illnesses.[210] The trial involves 20,000 middle-aged and older men and women with no prior history of the three main diseases. At the time of writing it is still in progress, so I'm afraid I can't tell you the results.

Meanwhile the U.S. Endocrine Society recommends that anyone who is likely to be deficient in vitamin D should have a blood test to check his vitamin D level. People at risk include:

- those suffering from bone disease, chronic kidney disease, liver failure, overactive parathyroid and granuloma-forming disorders, or malabsorption syndromes resulting from cystic fibrosis, irritable bowel disease, weight-reduction surgery or abdominal radiation
- those taking drugs like anticonvulsants, glucocorticoids, antiretrovirals, antifungals and cholestyramine
- older adults with a history of falls or non-traumatic fracture
- people with dark skin

---

208 Bjelakovic G et al. *Vitamin D supplementation for prevention of mortality in adults*. Cochrane database of systematic reviews (Online) (7): CD007470, July 2011.

209 Guyanet S. *Vitamin D: It's Not Just Another Vitamin.* wholehealthsource.blogspot.co.uk/2008/10/vitamin-d-its-not-just-another-vitamin.html

210 VITAL (the Vitamin D and Omega-3 Trial), is funded by the U.S. National Institutes of Health and is being run by Harvard Medical School in conjunction with Brigham and Women's Hospital. See www.vitalstudy.org.

- obese children and obese adults
- pregnant and nursing women

In Canada and the U.S.A. all milk has to be fortified with vitamin D by law, but that doesn't happen in the U.K. Here the government provides free drops containing vitamins A, C and D for children up to their fourth birthday, but you have to apply for them, and unless you live in Northern Ireland you have to collect them yourself every 8 weeks from a special distribution centre, which may not be local.[211] Parents in High Wycombe, where we live, have to travel 15 miles to Slough and collect them between 2 pm and 4 pm on a Wednesday afternoon, not exactly a helpful NHS service! And poorer families, who are probably more in need of them but don't have a second car, would have to go by bus, an expensive 3 hour bus journey there and back if they don't live in the town centre. You can imagine how many of them are claiming their free vitamin drops! In any case vitamin D is just as important for older children and adults, so we have to take action for ourselves one way or another.

As I child I had to attend a 'sun-ray' clinic, where we undressed to our underwear, put dark glasses on, and sat in a circle round a lamp which emitted ultraviolet light. My mother told me that when my sun-ray treatment finished I would be strong enough to blow the house down. So the day that it finished, being of a scientific turn of mind even before I started school, I decided to test the truth of what she said by blowing as hard as I could – but at our neighbour's house, not our own, in case it worked!

Certainly, in the days just after the war, there was an awareness that children needed to supplement their intake of vitamin D, both with ultraviolet light and with the cod liver oil which was supplied to us free of charge by the government. These measures brought to an end the disease of rickets that had been widespread in the U.K. and the U.S.A. But exactly the same disease is now returning among families who are doing nothing to keep rickets and all the other vitamin D deficiency health problems at bay.

Personally I take 2,000 units of vitamin D_3 a day in the darker half of the year, and throughout the year I go out for a 40 minute walk in the lunch hour 5 days a week, without sunscreen. I believe that this supplies my vitamin D_3 needs. Children could get by with half the same dose, but the more they can be encouraged to play in the garden or recreation ground or get out into the fields the better.

If you decide to buy vitamin D_3, the cheapest source I have found is the American Internet store www.iherb.com. Even paying for delivery to the U.K. (by the cheapest means) the overall cost of the capsules they sell is only half the cost of most kinds available in this country. IHerb also sells at reasonable prices a multitude of other health products such as omega-3 fish oil capsules and magnesium tablets. If you quote the discount code PUB014 you will receive $5 off your first purchase.

---

211 Ask your health visitor about 'Healthy Start' vitamin vouchers, or go to www.healthystart.nhs.uk/healthy-start-vouchers/healthy-start-vitamins/.

One word of warning: any goods ordered from the U.S.A. with a value exceeding £15 are subject to import V.A.T. on arrival in the U.K., and both DHL and the Royal Mail will charge an additional administration fee for dealing with this. So it is best to keep the value of your goods below £15.

CHAPTER 12: MINERALS IN MELTDOWN

What are minerals?

Minerals are inorganic (carbon-free) substances such as calcium, magnesium, phosphorus and iron. Like vitamins, minerals are essential in tiny amounts for life. They all perform different functions inside us so we need them all. Our bodies can't make them so they have to be obtained from food. Once again, a varied diet with raw or properly cooked vegetables should supply all the minerals you need, but unfortunately that may no longer be true, particularly in the case of magnesium.

A dangerous decline

Ever since 1940, '*The Composition of Foods*' by McCance & Widdowson has reported the nutritional contents of well over 2,000 kinds of food available in the U.K. In 2001 a Sussex food researcher, David Thomas, visited the British Library. He compared the mineral contents of foods reported in the 1940 edition with those in the then current edition. He was startled to discover dramatic declines in the mineral content of fruit and vegetables during the previous 60 years. On average calcium was down 46%, sodium 49%, copper 75%. More specifically, carrots had lost 75% of their magnesium, broccoli plants 75% of their calcium, and sodium had disappeared entirely from runner beans.[212] The *Guardian* reporter Matthew Engel who wrote this up commented, '*This is not going to go down well with at least one eight-year-old I know. The answer is not that we can give up broccoli. On the contrary, we now have to eat four or five times as much!*'

During a similar period meat and dairy products lost minerals too. Between 1940 and 1991 the magnesium content of meat declined by 15% and cheeses by 26%.[213]

In the U.S.A. the nutrient contents of crops declined by up to 40% between 1950 and 1999.[214] The authors of that report attributed this to the breeding of new varieties that

---

[212] Matthew Engel. The Guardian, Tuesday 20 February 2001.

[213] Thomas D. *The Mineral Depletion of Foods Available to Us as a Nation (1940-2002)*. Nutrition and Health, 2007; 19:21–55.

[214] Davis D et al. *Changes in USDA Food Composition Data for 43 Garden Crops, 1950 to 1999.* Journal of the American College of Nutrition. 2004;23(6):669-682. Available at: www.jacn.org/cgi/content/full/23/6/669. Accessed November 11, 2009.

grow faster and bigger but do not have the ability to make or absorb nutrients at the same faster rate. For example, if asparagus grows twice as big but its iron content remains the same then it has only half the iron per gram as it used to. David Thomas believes it is the widespread use of nitrogen, phosphorus and potassium that increases the amount of vegetable matter without increasing the mineral content. Yet another factor may be that growing fruit and vegetables repeatedly in the same soil depletes the mineral content of the soil and therefore of the food it produces.

In Chapter 13 we shall look at the serious results produced by deficiencies in two particular minerals, zinc and magnesium.

Where have all the minerals gone?

As we shall see later, there is evidence that many British and American people are deficient in certain minerals, but this is not only due to the declining mineral content of food. There are five clear reasons for a dietary deficiency of these nutrients, which point us to solutions to the problem.

(i) Food production

As previously explained, modern horticultural and agricultural practices have drastically depleted the mineral content of the fruit, vegetables and cereal crops that we eat, and feeding livestock and poultry on material grown intensively reduces the mineral content of the resulting meat, milk and eggs as well. J.I. Rodale carried out an experiment with two groups of chickens.[215] He fed one group from birth with food grown organically, and the other with commercial mash. When they began laying eggs, he sent some to a laboratory in Philadelphia for analysis. The eggs laid by the organically fed chickens had twice the amount of magnesium in them that the others did.

The reported reductions in nutrient content are not due simply to a change in the methods of measurement, as some food manufacturers have claimed. In the U.S.A. a comparison of the USDA food tables between 1963 and 1998 showed that the vitamin and mineral content of crops that continued to be grown in traditional ways did not change, whereas the vitamin and mineral content of crops produced by more intensive, industrialized farming practices decreased significantly.[216]

---

215 See the earlier reference to *Magnesium - the nutrient that could change your life.*
216 Wallach J. *Our Food is Deprived of Minerals: the Proof.* Longevity Institute Newsletter 16, 2006; Available at: www.longevinst.org/nlt/newsletter16.htm. Accessed November 11, 2009.

(ii) Food refining

A second cause of a shortage of magnesium in our diet is the food refining process. Oils produced from seeds have increasingly replaced animal fats in the food we eat, but although raw seeds contain high levels of magnesium this mineral is removed during the refining process.[217] Similarly the refined white flour used in commercial baking that is favoured by many people for bread contains very little magnesium. At least twenty nutrients are removed in the process of refining flour. Only five are replaced, and magnesium is not one of them.[218] You could probably obtain more magnesium by eating a firework than a whole loaf of white bread. Even natural sugars contain nutrients, including magnesium, but refined sugar contains no nutrients at all: it is a purely organic chemical.

(iii) Food choices

Vitamins and minerals are mainly found in fruit and vegetables, although a few of them such as vitamin B can also be obtained from meat, poultry or dairy products. The four main groups of food that contain magnesium, for example, are:

- beans, peas and nuts
- whole grains such as brown rice and wholewheat bread
- green leafy vegetables, carrots and celery
- fish and seafood

On the whole these are not the kinds of food that people in the U.K. spend their money on, with the exception perhaps of sugary baked beans, mushy peas and fish fingers! In 2011 people on average incomes ate less than four 80gm portions of fruit and vegetables a day.[219] In spite of the government's 'Five a day' mantra, the average consumption per head of fresh green vegetables halved between 1978 and 2008,[220] and between 2008 and 2011 the consumption of fruit and vegetables continued to fall![221]

---

217 Seelig M & Rosanoff A. *The Magnesium Factor*. Avery, New York, 2003.
218 Lieberman S & Bruning N. *The Real Vitamin & Mineral Book*. Avery, New York, 2007.
219 *Family Food 2011*. U.K. Government Department for the Environment, Food and Rural Affairs. www.defra.gov.uk/statistics/files/defra-stats-foodfarm-food-familyfood-2011-121217.pdf
220 Rabbani N & Thornalley P J. *Vegetables and Health – the Nrf2 Connection*. University Hospital, Coventry and Warwick Systems Biology Centre, University of Warwick, U.K. July 2012.
221 Family Food 2011. See the earlier reference.

(iv) Food cooking

One 80gm serving of organically grown broccoli contains 100% of an adult's daily requirement of vitamins C and K, along with smaller amounts of seven other vitamins, eight minerals and several other goodies such as glucosinolates, which are believed to be protective against cancer. However vitamin C, most B vitamins and the glucosinolates in broccoli and other green vegetables are soluble in water, which means that if they are boiled a lot of these important substances dissolve into the cooking water and are washed away through the colander and down the sink.

In 2007 two food researchers at Warwick University cooked broccoli, cauliflower, Brussels sprouts and cabbage in four different ways – up to 20 minutes of boiling, up to 20 minutes of steaming, up to 5 minutes of stir-frying and up to 3 minutes of microwaving.[222] (In order to microwave the vegetables they put them into sealed plastic bags with 10% added water.) While the vegetables were cooking they measured the amount of glucosinolates left in them at various time intervals to see what was happening. After 10 minutes of boiling broccoli its glucosinolate content was down to about 65% of its original value, and after 20 minutes less than 50% of it remained. Nearly all the rest had dissolved into the water. But with stir-frying only 5% to 10% was lost from the broccoli, and with the other two methods of cooking hardly any glucosinolate was lost at all. The results were similar for all four vegetables.

So simmering vegetables is not a good way to cook them, unless you can also drink the liquid in which they are cooked, as in a stew, casserole or vegetable soup. The best way to eat vegetables is not to cook them at all, but to eat them raw, for then all the vitamins and minerals are retained, in particular vitamin C, which is fairly quickly destroyed when heated. Some children like the taste of raw broccoli stalks, and several raw vegetables such as carrots and cabbage taste nice when they are shredded. But if you must cook them then either steam them, stir-fry them, or microwave them with just enough water to be fully absorbed after about 10 minutes on a high setting.

(v) Inadequate vitamin D

Vitamin D enables the body to absorb calcium, and it improves the body's ability to absorb magnesium,[223] so both calcium and magnesium deficiency may simply be due to a lack of vitamin D. I've talked about this already, so I don't need to say more here.

---

222 Song L & Thornalley P J. *Effect of storage, processing and cooking on glucosinolate content of brassica vegetables.* Food and Chemical Toxicology, Volume 45, 216–224, 2007.

223 Hardwick L L et al. *Magnesium Absorption: Mechanisms and the Influence of Vitamin D, Calcium and Phosphate*. American Institute of Nutrition, 1991; 0022-3166/91.

Restoring the magic

An adequate intake of all the minerals the human body uses is essential if you and your family are to remain healthy. But due to modern methods of food production, food choices and lifestyle it is more than likely that you are currently deficient in one or more of these minerals, at least if you live in the U.K. or the U.S.A. To remedy the situation and keep yourself healthy, take the following steps:

- Choose plenty of food that contains vitamins and minerals. Spinach and chard leaves, halibut, herbs, cocoa and most nuts are some particularly good sources of magnesium.
- So far as possible grow your own food or buy food that has been produced organically, especially eggs and poultry. Avoid genetically modified food.
- Buy wholemeal bread, or better still bake your own using organically produced flour.
- Make sure that all your family members have adequate vitamin D, either by regular exposure to the sun or by taking vitamin D capsules or cod liver oil.
- Consider taking a combined multivitamin and mineral supplement, or just a magnesium supplement, on a regular basis. Magnesium is the mineral most likely to be lacking in our diet, and supplementing it is especially important for people who drink a lot of alcohol, for older people and for certain other groups.[224]

The dietary supplements I personally take are:

- one 2,000 IU vitamin D_3 capsule a day during the darker half of the year
- two 100mg tablets of absorbent magnesium daily
- one 300mg omega-3 fish oil capsule (180mg EPA + 120mg DPA) daily

The cost of all these in the U.K. when bought from the U.S.A. is about 20p per day including postage; less if ordered within the U.S.A or Canada for use there.

Is salt bad for you?

Throughout history salt has been of major, major importance. Many wars have been fought over it, great roads have been built in order to transport it, cities such as Munich have been founded in order to trade it, and it has even been used as currency because of its high value. According to the Wikipedia article on 'The History of Salt', caravans consisting of as many as 40 thousand camels traversed 400 miles of the Sahara bearing

---

[224] *Fact sheets: Magnesium.* U.S. National Institutes of Health: Office of dietary supplements.

salt to inland markets.

Salt's principal uses have been for the preservation of food during the months when it was not available fresh, for disinfection and for flavouring. However it is also required for at least twenty bodily functions, including perspiration, digestion, the transmission of electrical signals for thought and internal communication, the clearing of air passages in the nose, throat and lungs, and the prevention of osteoporosis. The chlorine in salt is used to generate the dilute hydrochloric acid that the stomach uses to digest food. The body cannot function without salt. So why are we constantly told that eating salt is bad for us? Is this true? As usual in matters of nutrition, scientists are not united in their reply.

The theory is that an increase in the salt content of blood will increase blood pressure through a process called osmosis, and that since high blood pressure is associated with heart disease, heart attacks and strokes, the risk of all these will be reduced by eating less salt. But is this theory true in practice?

The gold standard for assessing research evidence about health matters is something called a Cochrane Review.[225] Cochrane Reviews are systematic reviews of primary research in human health care and health policy, and according to the Cochrane Library they are internationally recognized as the highest standard in evidence-based health care. The authors of one Cochrane Review concluded in 2009 that *'there was not enough information to assess the effect of changes in salt intake on health or deaths'*.[226] Another review of 167 separate studies concluded that while a reduced salt intake lowered normal blood pressure by 1% and high blood pressure by 3.5%, it might have some other harmful consequences in the long-term.[227] A third review concluded that reducing the salt intake of people with normal or high blood pressure provided 'no strong evidence of benefit' in terms of reducing the chance of dying from cardiovascular disease, and that it actually '*increased* the risk of all-cause death in those with congestive heart failure'.[228]

On the other hand a further Cochrane Review published in the *British Medical Journal* in 2013 criticized the method of one of the earlier reviews and concluded that lowering population salt intake would '*likely lower blood pressure and thereby reduce cardiovascular disease*'.[229] However it did not include a review of any evidence for this

---

225 www.cochrane.org/cochrane-reviews.

226 Hooper L et al. *The long term effects of advice to cut down on salt in food on deaths, cardiovascular disease and blood pressure in adults.* Cochrane Database of Systematic Reviews, 2004, Issue 1, Art. No. CD003656.

227 Graudal N A et al. *Effects of low sodium diet versus high sodium diet on blood pressure, renin, aldosterone, catecholamines, cholesterol, and triglyceride.* Cochrane Database of Systematic Reviews, 2011, Issue 11, Art. No. CD004022.

228 Taylor R S et al. *Reduced dietary salt for the prevention of cardiovascular disease.* Cochrane Database of Systematic Reviews, July 2011, Issue 7, Art. No. CD009217.

229 He F J et al. *Modest salt reduction lowers blood pressure in all ethnic groups at all levels of blood pressure without adverse consequences.* Cochrane Database of Systematic Reviews, 2013, Issue 4. Art. No. CD004937.

claimed reduction in cardiovascular disease, so I question how objective its conclusion really was. Nevertheless its authors recommended that one's salt consumption should be no more than 3gm a day, half the amount currently recommended in the U.K. and the U.S.A., and hardly the '*modest reduction*' described in its title.

One problem with all this is that in many of the reviewed studies the research subjects themselves had previously lived on a typical modern diet of fast food and prepared meals that are artificially high in salt, with the result that reducing their salt consumption experimentally might well have proved beneficial; whereas for someone who is on a healthy diet of largely home-made food a reduction in salt consumption may not be beneficial and may even be harmful if it means that one's intake of sodium falls too low. Another problem with such research is while all the reviewed studies measured the effect on blood pressure of reducing one's salt intake, few were able to examine properly the long-term health effects of doing this by means of salt reduction.

For people with type 2 diabetes, a low-salt intake is associated with a *higher* risk of premature death, particularly from cardiovascular disease.[230] While it is important to treat high blood pressure in people with diabetes, reducing their salt intake in order to do this may be wrong or even dangerous. Just 7 days on a reduced salt diet increased the insulin resistance of 152 healthy experimental subjects.[231] Insulin resistance is a leading cause of both diabetes and obesity.

In conclusion there is currently no clear consensus in the scientific community that lowering one's salt intake conveys any significant health benefit. Yet in spite of that we continue to be told to restrict how much salt we eat. The NHS Choices website recommends the following maximum amounts of salt per person per day:

- under 1 year old – less than 1gm, and don't add any to a baby's milk or food
- 1 to 3 years – 2gm
- 4 to 6 years – 3gm
- 7 to 10 years – 5gm
- 11 years and over – 6gm

There is one point to watch out for if you want to know the salt content of a particular food or drink. Common salt is a compound of sodium and chlorine, and while most food labels specify the amount of salt in a serving, some simply specify the amount of sodium. You must multiply the amount of sodium by two and a half to find out how many grams of actual salt there are.

Actually the NHS target levels are perfectly easy to reach if shop and factory-made

---

[230] Ekinci E I et al. *Dietary Salt Intake and Mortality in Patients With Type 2 Diabetes.* Diabetes Care, March 2011; Vol. 34, no. 3:703-709.

[231] Gard R et al. *Low-salt diet increases insulin resistance in healthy subjects.* Metabolism - Clinical and Experimental, July 2011;Vol. 60, Issue 7:965–968.

foods are avoided. The 3 days of recipes in Annexe 2 for meals prepared at home use no 'low salt' ingredients, and three of them even ask for 'a little salt' to be added, yet the total ingredients contain only 1.7gm of salt per adult per day. (In calculating the 1.7gm salt content it was assumed that 'a little salt' means half a teaspoonful for four people, or 0.6gm each. The bread was taken to be home-made bread containing 0.42gm of salt per slice.)

Contrast this with a typical 335gm Italian margherita pizza for two from the supermarket and you immediately hit 1.5gm of salt per person. Or eat a single serving 220gm 'Everyday Value Cheeseburger and Chips' and at the time of writing you will have consumed 2gm of salt, more than an entire day's salt provided by the home-made food recipes shown in Annexe 2. Some plainer foods are particularly salty too. Two typical rashers of bacon contain 1.5gm of salt; a 15ml tablespoon of soy sauce may contain 1.7gm; and a typical 100gm kipper fillet contains 2.5gm.

Having said that, the fact remains that there is little reliable evidence that eating such salty foods is unhealthy, or that adopting a low-salt diet will significantly improve one's health. Food prepared at home will generally be low in salt anyway. So keep salting your vegetables, rice and boiled eggs to taste, confident that in reasonable quantities at least salt is good for you.

CHAPTER 13: DIETARY DEFICIENCIES

Am I missing something?

Since each vitamin and mineral carries out particular but essential functions in our bodies, it seems likely that the reduction in our intake of these vital substances since 1940 must explain to some extent the increase in a whole range of ailments that has occurred during that period. Quite apart from obesity, diabetes, heart disease and some of the cancers we have already considered, all kinds of common health problems can be caused, not by infection or some congenital condition, but by deficiencies in our diet.

Consider stainless steel, the kind that table knives are made of. Stainless steel is strong, flexible and rust resistant. It is made from iron with small quantities of chromium, nickel and manganese added to it. Iron without these additional elements is not bright and shiny like stainless steel is: it is dull brown in colour. It rusts on exposure to moisture and air, it is weaker than steel in tension, and cast iron at least is brittle and breaks when it is dropped. "Very interesting, but what has all this got to do with diet?" you ask. Well in many ways our bodies are like iron. To be disease resistant, strong and supple they must be supplied with regular small quantities of various vitamins and elements. A shortage of vitamin C and we can no longer fight colds and other infections; a shortage of calcium and our bones grow weak; a shortage of magnesium and they become brittle and break when we fall.

So a shortage of any essential mineral, vitamin, or macronutrient will cause all kinds of health problems and even behaviour issues. Rickets in Southampton General Hospital due to vitamin D deficiency and the disruptive behaviour of young prisoners in Aylesbury who were deficient in omega-3 both demonstrate that nutrient-deficient health problems really do occur in our land.

Annexe 3 lists most of the various health problems that a lack of each essential nutrient can produce. It also lists problems that an *excess* of each nutrient can produce. On a normal diet we are unlikely to consume too much in the way of essential minerals and vitamins, but major problems are being caused by consuming too much starch, sugar, omega-6, polyunsaturated fat and alcohol, as we have already discussed at great length.

What's up, Doc?

The shortage of a nutrient in our diet can have various causes. The two most obvious causes are not consuming enough of the foods that contain it, or consuming only intensively grown or manufactured foods which contain very little of it. Less obvious causes are an inability to assimilate the nutrient properly, the presence of substances that decrease its effectiveness ('antagonists'), excreting it before it can be fully assimilated, or an increased need for it.

A shortage of zinc, for example, could be due to any of the causes just mentioned:

- Insufficient consumption. Anorexics are likely to consume too little zinc as well as other nutrients.[232] Vegetarians may not consume enough zinc-rich food, because the foods that contain most zinc are seafood and meat.[233] The process of refining flour involves the removal of zinc, so diets relying on processed food are likely to be zinc deficient.
- Inadequate assimilation. Zinc assimilation is inhibited by many medical conditions, including diabetes, chronic diarrhoea, ulcerative colitis and disease of the liver or kidneys. Gastrointestinal surgery can impair zinc absorption. It is inhibited by the alcohol in beers, wines and spirits and by phytates in whole grains and legumes (although soaking them in water for some time before use can solve this problem). The assimilation of zinc requires the presence of vitamins A, E, D and B_6, and of magnesium, calcium and phosphorus, so a shortage of any of these substances can hinder zinc's assimilation too.
- Antagonists. An excess of calcium, iron and particularly of copper[234] reduces the nutritional effectiveness of zinc.
- Excessive excretion. Alcohol, stress and certain medications such as diuretics increase the excretion of zinc by urination before the body can utilize it properly.
- Increased requirement. Pregnant and lactating women need more zinc than normal, although the zinc level in breast milk itself appears to be unaffected by a mother's diet.[235],[236] Sugar needs zinc for its metabolism, so sugary foods and drinks increase one's zinc requirements.

---

[232] One effect of a zinc deficiency is loss of appetite, which exacerbates anorexia.

[233] Hunt J R. *Bioavailability of iron, zinc, and other trace minerals from vegetarian diets.* American Journal of Clinical Nutrition, 2003; 78 (3 Suppl):633S-9S.

[234] Gittleman A L. *Why Am I Always So Tired? Discover How Correcting Your Body's Copper Imbalance Can Keep Your Body From Giving Out Before Your Mind Does.* HarperSanFranciso, 1999.

[235] Parker P H et al. *Zinc deficiency in a premature infant fed exclusively human milk.* The American Journal of Diseases of Children, 1982; 136:77–78.

[236] Weymouth R D et al. *Symptomatic zinc deficiency in a premature infant.* Australian Paediatric Journal, 1982; 18:208–210.

There isn't space in this book to consider in detail the consequences of consuming too little or too much of every single nutrient listed in Annexe 3. But as examples of nutrient deficiencies I'd like to hold a magnifying glass, as it were, over zinc and magnesium, since it does appear that some people don't have enough of these two minerals. Then we'll learn how to find out if a health problem is due to some dietary deficiency, and, if it is, how to put it right.

No zinc, no zing!

Sources of zinc

According to the U.S. National Institutes of Health and other sources, the best sources of zinc per serving, in approximate order, are:

- oysters and other seafood (oysters contain at least ten times as much per serving as any other food)
- beef, lamb, pork and poultry
- vitamin-fortified breakfast cereals

Smaller quantities are found in:

- beans, peas and nuts
- pumpkin seeds
- egg yolks
- oatmeal
- yogurt, milk and cheese

Why we need it

Among other functions, zinc is required for normal growth and cognitive development, especially during infancy, sexual development and procreation, resistance to infection, healing of wounds, the ability to digest carbohydrates, and for the senses of smell and touch. Although many people consume enough of this important metal, many more do not.

The zinc shortage

Since our bodies cannot store zinc we have to replenish it regularly from our diet. So how common is zinc deficiency? Nearly half the world's population is estimated to suffer health problems because of zinc deficiency,[237] but in developed countries it is likely to be a problem mainly for older people and for some babies and young children. According to the U.S. National Institutes of Health, 35% to 45% of U.S. citizens over the age of 60 are zinc deficient.[238] Infants need relatively large quantities of zinc, and breastfed babies whose mother's milk is zinc deficient can experience severe problems,[239] but in general zinc deficiency is more common in babies fed on cow's milk or infant formula milk than breast milk, since zinc in human milk is more absorbable.[240]

In 1997 a sample of infants aged from 2 to 24 months from middle and upper-income families in urban Tennessee were found, on average, to ingest less than the recommended daily requirements of zinc and vitamin D.[241] Two years later the same researchers found that most children aged 2 to 5 years among similar families had less than the recommended daily allowances of zinc, folate, and vitamins D and E.[242] Among poorer families it is likely that there were even greater deficiencies in zinc, due to a lack of zinc-rich foods in the diet and a shortage of the vitamins A and D, which are needed for its absorption.

In all people groups the excessive consumption of alcohol or sugar increases the likelihood of zinc deficiency, for the reasons already given.

The effects of zinc deficiency

Annexe 3 will tell you that a shortage of zinc can produce all kinds of problems, in particular lethargy, mental depression, and a loss of interest in food and sex. So no zinc, no zing!

Infants need large quantities of zinc during the first months of their lives, to support growth, immune function, and cognitive development. A zinc deficiency in an infant results in red and inflamed patches of dry and scaly skin, particularly around body openings such as the mouth, anus, and eyes. This can be caused by a congenital deficiency

---

237 Brown K H et al. *The importance of zinc in human nutrition and estimation of the global prevalence of zinc deficiency.* Food & Nutrition Bulletin, June 2001; Vol. 22, No. 2, 113-125(13).

238 *Zinc - Fact Sheet for Health Professionals.* National Institutes of Health, Office of Dietary Supplements, 2014.

239 Kelleher S L et al. *Mammary gland zinc metabolism: regulation and dysregulation.* Genes and Nutrition, Jun 2009; 4(2):83–94.

240 *Acrodermatitis enteropathica.* http://www.dermnetnz.org/systemic/acrodermatitis-enteropathica.html. Accessed June 2014.

241 Skinner J D et al. *Longitudinal Study of Nutrient and Food Intakes of Infants Aged 2 to 24 Months.* Journal of the American Dietetic Association, May 1997; Vol. 97,Issue 5,496-504.

242 Skinner J D et al. *Longitudinal Study of Nutrient and Food Intakes of White Preschool Children Aged 24 to 60 Months.* Journal of the American Dietetic Association, December 1999; Vol. 99,Issue 12 ,1514-1521.

of zinc in a mother's milk.

In both infants and young children a deficiency can also produce:

- conjunctivitis
- sensitivity to light
- loss of appetite
- diarrhoea
- irritability (babies cry and whine incessantly)
- depressed mood
- stunted growth

In older children and adults a shortage of zinc can cause a range of symptoms[243],[244], including:

- lethargy
- poor appetite
- diarrhoea
- reduced resistance to infection
- retarded healing of wounds
- loss of the senses of smell and touch
- retarded growth
- retarded sexual development
- reduced testosterone production and fertility in men and women[245],[246]
- problems with ovulation and pregnancy[247]
- impaired night vision
- depression[248]

More severe deficiencies can result in loss of hair and damage to the brain, nerves and eyesight.

Older people are more likely to be zinc deficient than most. This may be due to a

---

[243] www.patient.co.uk/doctor/zinc-deficiency-excess-and-supplementation. Accessed May 2014.

[244] *Risk Assessment – Zinc*. U.K. Food Standards Agency. Expert Group on Vitamins and Minerals, 2003.

[245] El-Tawil A M. *Zinc deficiency in men with Crohn's disease may contribute to poor sperm function and male infertility*. Andrologia, December 2003; 35(6):337-41.

[246] Prasad A S et al. *Zinc status and serum testosterone levels of healthy adults.* Nutrition, May 1996; 12(5):344-8.

[247] Sandstead H H. *Is zinc deficiency a public health problem?* Nutrition, Jan-Feb 1995; 11(1 Suppl):87-92.

[248] Yary T & Aazami S. *Dietary Intake of Zinc was Inversely Associated with Depression*. Biological Trace Element Research, September 2011.

decreased ability to absorb zinc as the result of declining levels of acid in the stomach. Helicobacter pylori (H. pylori) hinders the production of stomach acid, and more than a quarter of people in the U.K. become infected with this bacterium at some time in their life,[249] while in the U.S.A. it is thought that half the population is affected.[250] H. pylori is often not diagnosed and in this case it remains in us for life, hence it is more common in older people. One effect of the resulting zinc deficiency, in older people particularly, is a decline in resistance to infection, particularly respiratory infections such as pneumonia.[251]

Some results of zinc supplementation

The reality of the zinc shortages can be demonstrated by the remarkable results of zinc supplementation for some sufferers:

- Zinc-deficient infants who suffered horrendously from red, inflamed and scaly skin were cured almost completely after only 5 days of zinc supplementation.[252]
- Six months of zinc supplementation for a group of marginally zinc-deficient elderly men doubled their testosterone levels![253]
- Zinc supplementation significantly reduced liver damage and the long-term outcome of patients with chronic hepatitis C and liver cirrhosis.[254]
- A review of three independent trials concluded that zinc acetate doses of more than 75mg a day reduced the average duration of a cold by 42%.[255]

A cure for colds?

Colds and flu are the recorded causes of 40% of industrial sick leave, both in the U.K.[256]

---

249 http://www.patient.co.uk/health/helicobacter-pylori-and-stomach-pain. Accessed June 2014.
250 Sardi B. http://knowledgeofhealth.com/modern-day-zinc-deficiency-epidemic/. Accessed June 2014.
251 Barnet J B et al. *Low zinc status: a new risk factor for pneumonia in the elderly?* Nutritional Review, January 2010; 68(1):30-7
252 DermNet NZ. Acrodermatitis enteropathica. http://www.dermnetnz.org/systemic/acrodermatitis-enteropathica.html. Accessed June 2014.
253 Prasad A S et al. *Zinc status and serum testosterone levels of healthy adults.* Nutrition, May 1996; 12(5):344-8.
254 Matsumura H et al. *Zinc supplementation therapy improves the outcome of chronic hepatitis C and liver cirrhosis.* Journal of Clinical Biochemistry and Nutrition, November 2009; 45,292–303.
255 Hemilä H. *Zinc lozenges may shorten the duration of colds: a systematic review.* Open Respiratory Medicine Journal, 2011;5:51-8.
256 *The Sick Report.* BreathHR, U.K. November 2013.

and the U.S.A.[257] Adults typically have from two to five infections a year, while children have from six to twelve.[258] Therefore the possibility of reducing the duration of a common cold by 42% as a result of zinc acetate supplementation is both significant and exciting. However most zinc capsules and lozenges do not contain zinc in the form of zinc acetate, and according to George Eby nearly all zinc-based cold remedies on sale are useless, due to added substances that react adversely with the zinc they do contain.[259] He concluded a published research paper with the words, '*Zinc (acetate) lozenges slowly dissolving in the mouth over a 20 to 30 minute period releasing more than 18mg of ionic zinc (iZn) and used every 2 hours shorten common colds by 6 to 7 days, which is a cure for the common cold. However, due to inadequate iZn, very few of more than 40 different brands of zinc lozenges on the U.S. market are expected to have any effect on the duration or severity of common colds.*'[260]

It appears that to obtain reliable relief from colds one must order zinc acetate lozenges from Mr. Eby's company, coldcure.com, costing about US$10 per cold plus postage. It might be a good idea to buy a small pot on a trial basis if your children are particularly susceptible to colds and important school exams or other events are due. Having said that, the British Medical Research Council's Common Cold Unit closed in 1989 after concluding that there was probably no practical cure for colds other than rhinovirus colds, which they found could be alleviated somewhat using zinc gluconate lozenges.[261]

The magic of magnesium

Sources of magnesium

The best sources are:

- green vegetables
- some pulses (beans and peas)
- some nuts and seeds
- whole grains (e.g. wholemeal bread)
- hard tap water

---

257 Kirkpatrick G L. *The common cold.* Primary Care, December 1996; 23 (4):657–75.

258 *Common cold.* Wikipedia. Accessed June 2014.

259 Eby G A. *Zinc Lozenges as a Common Cold Treatment.* George-eby-research.com, revised May 2014.

260 Eby G A. *Zinc lozenges as cure for the common cold – A review and hypothesis.* Medical Hypotheses, 2010; 74 (2010) 482–492.

261 Al-Nakib W et al. *Prophylaxis and treatment of rhinovirus colds with zinc gluconate lozenges.* Journal of Antimicrobial Chemotherapy, December 1987; 20 (6): 893–901.

Why we need it

A fact sheet produced by the United States government informs us that magnesium helps the muscles and nerves to function, steadies the heart rhythm, and keeps the bones strong by enabling the body to assimilate calcium and stops them becoming brittle. It also helps the body to create energy and make proteins.

The magnesium shortage

Most people in the U.K. and the U.S.A. have less magnesium in their diet than people in other countries,[262] and many consume less than the recommended amounts of it.[263]

The effects of magnesium deficiency

Leg cramps, foot pain or muscle twitches are usually the first signs of magnesium deficiency. Other early signs include loss of appetite, nausea, vomiting, fatigue, and weakness.[264] Insufficient magnesium can cause:[265]

- irritability
- nervousness
- hyperactivity
- depression
- dizziness
- muscle weakness, twitching and cramps
- arthritis
- type 2 diabetes
- coronary vascular disease
- osteoporosis

Insufficient magnesium can also cause:[266]

- abnormal heart rhythm

---

[262] Seelig M S. *The Requirement of Magnesium by the Normal Adult.* American Journal of Clinical Nutrition, June 1964.

[263] Fact sheets: *Magnesium*. U.S. National Institutes of Health: Office of Dietary Supplements.

[264] Rude R K. *Magnesium deficiency: A cause of heterogeneous disease in humans.* Journal of Bone and Mineral Research 1998; 13:749-58.

[265] As above.

[266] www.calmnatural.co.uk/magnesium-deficiency. (Admittedly this website has a commercial interest, but it does quote research reports in support of the statements it makes.)

- premenstrual problems and various other hormonal imbalances
- kidney stones
- fatigue
- insomnia
- headaches
- anxiety

Magnesium deficiency is more likely in older adults, for whom it can be particularly harmful.[267]

I should point out that many of the symptoms listed above are related to a variety of medical conditions, so if you ever do find yourself suffering from any of them consult a doctor in the first instance.

I want to highlight in particular two health issues associated with magnesium deficiency. The first is the problem of brittle bones; the second is the problem of depression, particularly when it is severe and does not respond to conventional antidepressants.

Magnesium and brittle bones

Back in 1950 an orthopaedic surgeon, Dr. Lewis Barnett, became aware that his patients from the Dallas region were suffering many more factures of the cervical neck of the femur than patients from the Hereford region were; they were occurring on average nearly 20 years earlier in a patient's life and were taking three times as long to heal. When he analysed the water in the two regions the only major differences he discovered were that the Dallas water contained considerably *more* calcium than the Hereford water but only half the quantity of magnesium. He wondered if a lack of magnesium was the problem in Dallas, so over a period of time he analysed the magnesium content of the bones of 500 female patients with an average age of 55 who were undergoing lumber and cervical vertebrae surgery. The results were startling: the average magnesium content in the bones of his Dallas patients was only 0.05% as compared with a content of 1.76% in his Hereford patients. To find out if this was the cause of their problems he then compared the magnesium content of healthy people with that of people who were suffering from severe osteoporosis. He found little difference in the calcium, phosphorus, and fluoride content of their bones, but the magnesium content of the osteoporosis victims was only half that of the healthy people.[268]

It is difficult to avoid the conclusions that brittleness in the bones of older people is caused by a lack of magnesium rather than a lack of calcium, and that if there is

---

267 *Dietary Reference Intakes: Calcium, Phosphorus, Magnesium, Vitamin D and Fluoride.* Institute of Medicine, Food and Nutrition Board. National Academy Press, Washington, DC, 1999.

268 Rodale J I with Taub H J. *Magnesium - the nutrient that could change your life.* Pyramid books, New York, 1968.

insufficient magnesium in the diet this can be caused by a lack of magnesium in the drinking water.

Magnesium and depression

When we look at depression we find once again that it is a relatively modern disease. Only 1% of Americans born before 1905 developed depression before they were 75 years old, whereas 6% of Americans born in 1955 developed depression by the time they were only 24 years old. By 2007 in one U.S. state at least 13.6% of the adults had suffered a major depression of one kind or another![269],[270] In England the percentage of teenagers suffering from irritability, general worry, sleep disturbance, fatigue or panic increased by 50% between 1986 and 2006, by which time 6% of boys and 20% of girls had experienced such problems to a significant extent at one time or another.[271]

There may be several reasons why depression is becoming more common, but decreasing magnesium intake is a major contender. A paper published by George and Karen Eby in 2006 reported several cases of adults with severe depression who had either not responded to conventional antidepressants or had found its side effects unbearable. In each case they were given a magnesium supplement at mealtimes and at bedtime, and they all recovered within a week! The supplements took the form of magnesium glycinate or magnesium taurinate, in doses ranging from 125mg to 300mg per meal.[272] Having studied 47 other papers on the subject the Ebys came to the startling conclusion, *'It is likely that magnesium deficiency causes most major depression and related mental health illness, IQ loss and addictions'*!

More recently Dr. Emily Deans has explained that magnesium may reduce the body's production of the stress hormone cortisol, which is widely believed to be the cause of depression and other mental health problems.[273] While she is still uncertain whether magnesium deficiency causes depression or depression causes magnesium deficiency, she concludes that most people would be wise to supplement their diet with 200mg to 350mg of magnesium a day, albeit with a doctor's approval if they have kidney disease or are elderly.

---

269 Meyer J S & Quenzer L F. *Psychopharmacology, Drugs, the Brain and Behavior.* Sinauer Associates, Sunderland, Massachuesetts, 2004.
270 *Trends in depression: shedding light on the darkness.* L A Health, January 2011.
271 Collishaw S et al. *Youth Trends: 20-year trends in depression and anxiety in England.* MRC Social, Genetic and Developmental Psychiatry Centre, King's College, London, 2006.
272 Eby G A & Eby K L. *Rapid recovery from major depression using magnesium treatment.* George Eby Research, Austin, U.S.A., January 2006.
273 Deans E. *Magnesium and the Brain: the Original Chill Pill.* Evolutionary Psychiatry, June 2011.

Obtaining the magnesium we need

Dealing with a deficiency of magnesium without taking a supplement is not entirely straightforward. On the one hand nuts, seeds and whole grains are good sources,[274] and one study found eating such foods increases bone density;[275] on the other hand we are told that the phytic acid found within the hulls of nuts, seeds and grains combines with magnesium and other minerals such as calcium, iron and zinc rendering them insoluble, a process which can lead to dietary *deficiencies* in these minerals.[276],[277],[278] Similarly hard water generally contains high levels of calcium and magnesium, which are both good for bones, but several laboratories have found that increasing the amount of calcium in a person's diet reduces the absorption of magnesium,[279],[280] a fact which suggests that high levels of calcium in water or food might actually produce osteoporosis!

Magnesium deficiency is therefore one dietary problem which may most reliably be solved by taking tablets, in the form of magnesium glycinate, magnesium citrate or magnesium taurinate, but not magnesium aspartate or magnesium glutamate, which can be toxic to people suffering from depression.[281]

The National Health Service recommends total daily magnesium intakes (if possible from food and drink) of 300mg for men and 270mg for women. For people over 14 years old, the Dietary Reference Intake for the U.S.A. and Canada recommends 420mg a day for men and 320mg a day for women, with decreasing amounts for younger ages. Dr. Barnett, the orthopaedic surgeon I mentioned, suggested 600mg day on the basis of his research. I don't think anyone knows for certain how much *supplemental* magnesium one needs, for the amount of supplement you need depends on what you are eating and

---

274 *USDA National Nutrient Database for Standard Reference, Release 24.* U.S. Department of Agriculture, Agricultural Research Service, 2011. Nutrient Data Laboratory Home Page, www.ars.usda.gov/ba/bhnrc/ndl.

275 López-González A A et al. *Phytate (myo-inositol hexaphosphate) and risk factors for osteoporosis.* Journal of Medicinal Food, December 2008; 11(4):747-52.

276 Hurrell R F. *Influence of vegetable protein sources on trace element and mineral bioavailability.* The Journal of Nutrition, September 2003; 133 (9): 2973S–7S.

277 Oberlees D. *Phytates.* Chapter 17, pp. 363–371, of *Toxicants Occurring Naturally in Foods.* Committee on Food Protection, Food and Nutrition Board, National Research Council, 1973. National Academy of Sciences.

278 Rodale J I with Taub H J. *Magnesium - the nutrient that could change your life.* Pyramid books, New York, 1968. (Also cited earlier.)

279 Clarkson E M et al. *The effect of a high intake of calcium on magnesium metabolism in normal subjects and patients with chronic renal failure.* Clinical Science, 1967; 32: 11-18.

280 Norman D A et al. *Jejunal and ileal adaptation to alterations in dietary calcium: changes in calcium and magnesium absorption and pathogenic role of parathyroid hormone and 1,25-dihydroxyvitamin D.* Journal of Clinical Investigation, 1981; 67: 1599-1603.

281 Eby G A & Eby K L. *Rapid recovery from major depression using magnesium treatment.* George Eby Research, Austin, U.S.A., January 2006. (Also cited earlier.)

whether it is organically produced or not. I feel that a daily supplement of 200mg of magnesium should compensate for any shortfall in my food and keep my bones strong. Having fallen 10ft down a mountainside at the age of 70 without any serious damage, I think that this policy has worked for me! The kind of tablets I use are 'Doctor's Best' high absorption magnesium glycinate tablets. These are in a form that is easily digested.

Finding the missing ingredient

What should you do then, if you or your child develops some health problem that might have a dietary cause? In the first instance, if there is any chance that the problem is caused by an infection or some more serious disease you should consult a doctor. (Consulting a doctor is particularly important in the case of ear infections, for these can damage hearing permanently if they are not treated immediately – it happened to me!)

However if a persistent problem is caused by a dietary deficiency then a general practitioner may not diagnose this, or at least not until all other avenues have been explored. For one thing most doctors are not trained nutritionists, so they are more inclined to look for a cure using medication rather than a change of diet. Secondly the received wisdom is that a normal diet provides adequate quantities of all the essential nutrients, so if the answer to the question, "Are you eating all right?" is "Yes" then that is usually as far as the topic will go. Thirdly, hunting for a dietary cause can be very time-consuming, so a busy doctor will naturally prefer a quick fix with some tablets if a quick fix works. Fourthly some essential substances such as zinc and magnesium are stored mainly in the tissues and bones rather than in the blood, so if a doctor orders a blood test the result may be totally misleading.[282],[283] And finally, even where the amount of some nutrient in our body can be measured reliably and is found to be at a normal level, we shall still experience health problems if our bodies are not fully utilizing it for some reason.

Medication can treat some of the problems arising from a poor diet – for example high blood glucose levels in people with type 2 diabetes caused by eating too much sugar – but it is far better to deal with the cause itself. For one thing medical drugs can produce undesirable side effects, and for another they cost the health service a lot of money, which could be better spent on other things. NHS Scotland spent nearly £230 million on drugs to treat diabetes and obesity during the 3 years 2010 to 2013, in a population of little more than 5 million. So if there is any possibility that diet may be at the root of a health problem, it makes all the sense in the world to investigate this possibility. But how can we discover whether a dietary deficiency is what is causing the trouble, and how can

---

282 Haigney M C P. *Noninvasive Measurement of Tissue Magnesium and Correlation With Cardiac Levels*. Circulation, 1995; 92:2190-2197.

283 In the U.S.A. it is possible to obtain tissue samples by means of a scrape inside the mouth, by hair analysis or by X-ray analysis of the tissue beneath the tongue, but even there these procedures are not standard. So far as I know they are not available at all in the U.K.

we discover what that deficiency is?

Food disappearing from the larder every night might be due to ants, rodents or even a small, sleepless and hungry child. How can we find out which of these is responsible? One way is to deal with each possibility in turn. If we put a lock on the door and the nibbling stops then we can be pretty sure that the thief must have been a child, assuming our spouse isn't the culprit! We can adopt a similar approach to discover whether a nutritional deficiency is responsible for a health problem. Here is the procedure:

- Look at Annexe 3 for a list of potential suspects. If your health problem is listed there as a potential result of a deficiency in a particular nutrient, and if you can increase your intake of that nutrient by taking a dietary supplement in the form of tablets, capsules, powder or liquid, then supplement your diet for 1 to 3 months with the nutrient required. If this corrects the problem then you can be reasonably sure that your body did need more of this particular nutrient.
- Next, look at Annexe 3 again to see which *foods* provide the required nutrient or nutrients. Can you change your diet in order to increase your consumption of these foods? If so, try doing that for another 3 months instead of taking the supplement. If this does the trick, well and good: you have solved the problem. If it doesn't work, revert to taking the supplement on a more permanent basis.
- Finally, inform your doctor what happened. If taking a supplement cured your health problem, it may be that your body needs more of this nutrient because of some medical condition that needs addressing, in which case the information you give to your doctor may enable him to identify what it is. If on the other hand a supplement did not solve the problem and the problem persists, then your doctor still needs to know this so that he can look for the true cause of the problem.

If your health problem is listed under more than one kind of nutrient deficiency, investigate each nutrient in turn, one at a time, until you discover which one has been causing the problem. Don't try to deal with them all at once, for even if the problem is solved you won't know which of the nutrients you were supplementing was the one that was lacking.

One word of warning: when supplementing a nutrient be careful not to exceed its maximum recommended daily intake, unless you are under medical supervision, since many nutrients can be harmful when taken in excess.

Too much of a good thing?

Annexe 3 also lists health problems which can be caused by consuming too much of each particular nutrient. If you think this might be the cause of a health problem all you can do is to reduce your intake of the foods containing that nutrient to see if it helps.

Some health problems are caused, in whole or in part, not by too little or too much of a particular nutrient, but rather by particular foods, and sometimes even by very small amounts of them. The tiniest quantity of peanut oil can cause a violent reaction in some people, particularly children, and in extreme cases it can lead to death. So in the next chapter let's have a look at food allergies and similar related problems.

CHAPTER 14: ALLERGIES, INTOLERANCES, COELIAC DISEASE AND IBS

A case of mistaken identity

The word 'allergy' was invented in 1906 by an Austrian paediatrician, Clemens von Pirquet, from two Greek words best translated as 'strange activity'. Food allergies are bad reactions to particular kinds of food. They occur when the body's immune system mistakenly identifies a food as some kind of hostile invader and produces antibodies to deal with it. The antibodies associated with the commonest food allergies are called Immunoglobulin E or IgE antibodies, but there are some less common allergies, including coeliac disease (CD), which involve other kinds of antibody. These are called non-IgE-mediated food allergies. Food allergies can cause all kinds of distressing reactions, ranging from eczema to panic attacks and even to death.

Strictly speaking we should distinguish between a food *allergy* and a food *intolerance*. The symptoms produced by a food allergy are caused by antibodies that our own bodies generate, whereas food intolerances have a variety of other causes, mainly in the foods themselves. With most food allergies only a small quantity of the food is required to trigger it; and the reaction can be very serious and even life-threatening. A reaction to the allergenic food usually occurs within a few seconds or minutes of swallowing the food, although symptoms of the less common non-IgE allergies may take hours or even days to appear. With a food intolerance, however, the bad reaction nearly always takes several hours to develop, its degree depends on the amount of food eaten, and while the effects may be distressing or painful they are never life-threatening. Food intolerances are far more common than food allergies.

A worsening problem

According to the medical charity Allergy UK, there has recently been a significant increase in the incidence of food allergies, particularly amongst children. The NHS states that about 2% of the population and 8% of children under the age of three are affected.[284] It also states that allergies in general have increased over the last 10 years,

---

284 http://www.nhs.uk/conditions/food-allergy/pages/intro1.aspx. Accessed June 2014.

and that around 25% of the British population suffers from an allergy of some kind. The situation is similar in the U.S.A. and other developed countries.[285]

While genuine food allergies affect relatively few people, it has been reported that up to 45% of the population suffers from some kind of food intolerance.[286]

No one knows why allergies and food intolerances are increasing. One theory is that excessive hygiene is responsible; another that the increased use of antibiotics has something to do with it. It is also believed that agricultural pesticides in drinking water and other forms of environmental pollution may be contributing to the problem.[287] This last suggestion sounds like a very good reason for filtering drinking water, since pesticides and herbicides can be removed by filtration with activated carbon, as explained in Chapter 16.

Strange activities

Consequently, if you or your child has a recurring health problem that isn't due to an infection, it might be caused by something in the diet. However many allergies are due to causes other than food and drink, such as pollen, dust mites and cats. Some people might want to list reality TV shows too! Since the symptoms of some of these other allergies are similar to those of some food allergies, the root of the problem may not be immediately obvious. But to help you to dig it out, here is a list of the more common symptoms of food allergies and intolerances.

Von Pirquet's 'strange activities', in the form of IgE allergic reactions, may take the form of:[288]

- an itchy or tingling sensation inside the mouth, throat or ears
- sneezing or itchy eyes
- a raised itchy red rash
- swelling of the face, around the eyes, lips, tongue and the roof of the mouth, or sometimes other parts of the body
- difficulty in swallowing
- vomiting
- wheezing or shortness of breath
- feeling dizzy and light-headed

---

285 UCLA Health. http://fooddrugallergy.ucla.edu/body.cfm?id=40. Accessed June 2014.
286 *Stolen Lives 3, The Food Allergy and Food Intolerance Report.* Allergy UK Report, 2007.
287 Jerschow E et al. *Dichlorophenol-containing pesticides and allergies: results from the US National Health and Nutrition Examination Survey 2005-2006.* Annals of Allergy, Asthma and Immunology, December 2012; Vol. 109, Issue 6,420–425.
288 Abstracted from *Food allergy – Symptoms.* NHS Choices website. Accessed June 2014.

- abdominal pain or diarrhoea
- feeling sick or vomiting

Non-IgE allergy reactions:

- redness and itchiness of the skin – not a raised rash
- itchy, red, dry and cracked skin
- colic in babies, causing extended periods of inconsolable crying for no apparent reason*
- heartburn and indigestion caused by stomach acid leaking up out of the stomach into the oesophagus
- frequent loose stools
- blood and mucus in the stools
- constipation
- redness anywhere under the bottom
- unusually pale skin
- retarded growth

*While colic is very distressing it usually stops by the age of 4 months, or by 6 months at the most. It is not thought to cause any permanent harm, at least to the baby! Nevertheless a doctor should be consulted in case the crying is due to some more serious ailment. While there is no known cure for colic, the NHS Choices website[289] does provide some advice on alleviating it to some extent.

See http://www.nhs.uk/conditions/Colic/Pages/Introduction.aspx.

A severe allergic reaction is called anaphylaxis. It begins with the typical symptoms of an allergic reaction but these rapidly worsen and can produce:

- increased breathing difficulties, such as wheezing and coughing
- an intense feeling of anxiety or fear
- an abnormally rapid heartbeat
- a sharp and sudden drop in blood pressure, causing light-headedness, dizziness or confusion
- unconsciousness

If anyone in your family displays symptoms of anaphylaxis you should phone 999 or another emergency phone number immediately.

As for food intolerances, it seems that they can be responsible for almost any non-fatal health problem! The charity Allergy UK lists the following symptoms that can

---

289 http://www.nhs.uk/conditions/Colic/Pages/Introduction.aspx.

indicate a food intolerance:[290]

- abdominal pains
- aches and pains
- acid reflux
- asthma
- arthritis
- autism
- bloating
- constipation
- chronic fatigue syndrome
- diarrhoea
- eczema
- fatigue
- fibromyalgia
- IBS (irritable bowel syndrome)
- headaches
- lethargy
- ME (myalgic encephalomyelitis)
- migraine
- nausea
- rashes
- rhinitis (inflammation of the nose)
- sinusitis
- skin problems (e.g. acne, psoriasis)
- stomach cramps
- tension
- urticaria (hives)
- weight loss
- wheezing

Rheumatism, and psychological disturbances such as depression, panic and ADHA (attention deficit hyperactivity disorder) have also been postulated.[291]

The chief villains

Among *allergenic* foods the chief villains are:[292],[293]

For children

- peanuts
- cow's milk
- soya
- nuts*
- eggs
- fish
- shellfish
- wheat

For adults

- citrus fruit
- nuts*
- fish
- peanuts
- shellfish
- wheat

* Hazelnuts, walnuts, almonds, and Brazil nuts.

The wives of the allergenic villains are the foods that are commonly associated with food *intolerances*. These comprise:[294]

---

290 http://www.allergyuk.org/food-intolerance/symptoms. October 2012 update.
291 http://www.yorktest.com.
292 *Common Food Allergies*. Medical News Today, August 2013. http://www.medicalnewstoday.com.
293 NHS Choices website: http://www.nhs.uk/conditions/food-allergy/pages/intro1.aspx. Accessed June 2014.
294 *Food Sensitivities*. The World's Healthiest Foods. http://www.whfoods.com/genpage. php?tname=faq&dbid=30. Accessed June 2014.

- cow's milk and dairy products
- gluten
- fructose
- eggs
- yeast
- alcohol
- fermented, pickled, aged, marinated and any other foods that contain the chemicals tyramine or phenylalanine
- wheat

Intolerance to wheat is commonly called 'wheat sensitivity'.

Food intolerances have various causes, for example an intolerance to dairy products is caused by a lack of the enzyme lactase, which is needed to digest them.

One of the best free sources of further information on the subject of food intolerance and food allergy is The World's Healthiest Foods website, www.whfoods.com.

Making an arrest

How can one identify the villain that is stealing one's health in order to arrest it? In most cases, the recommended method is simply trial and error. If you suspect that a particular food is producing a bad reaction then try cutting it out of your diet. If the symptoms cease, reintroduce the same food into your diet to see if they return. If they do return then you can be reasonably sure that you have caught your villain.

This raises two questions: how can you decide which food or foods may be the troublemakers, and how long should you try eliminating them from your diet if there is no immediate improvement in your health?

With certain common (IgE) allergenic foods, particularly those that are not eaten every day, the offending items may be obvious, since the reaction to them will occur almost as soon as the food is ingested. Two obvious examples of such foods are peanuts and shellfish. But more often it is far from obvious which foods one should try eliminating from one's diet. In this case the first step is to keep a food and symptom diary, recording everything you eat and drink, and the nature and severity of your symptoms, with the associated dates and times. In this way you should eventually be able to match the occurrence of your symptoms with particular foods or drinks and thereby draw up a list of suspects.

You can then find out what happens if you eliminate one of the suspect foods from your diet. There is evidence that eliminating a food to which one is intolerant normally produces a noticeable benefit within 3 weeks, but it can take up to 8 weeks before one's health improves.[295] So even if you don't notice a benefit continue to eliminate a suspect food for up to 8 weeks before deciding that the cause of your health problem lies elsewhere.

If you suspect that more than one food may be a troublemaker you could save time by removing several suspects from your diet at once. If the health problem then clears up, reintroduce each food one at a time, 6 to 8 weeks apart, to see if the symptoms return. If they do then eliminate that food permanently from your diet.

Cutting out too many foods at a time is not recommended because this may deprive your body of essential nutrients, and that would muddy the waters with additional health problems. If you are in any doubt about the best plan of action, arrange an appointment with a nutritionist.

If you suspect that you or your child cannot tolerate lactose (the sugar in cow's milk and its products) you should consult a doctor because there is a reliable test for this.

Gluten intolerance

There is a particular issue with wheat and other cereals that contain gluten, and with all the products made from such cereals including flour, bread, pastry and pasta. Commercial flour and its products contain many chemical additives, which may include preservatives, whiteners, pesticides, hormonal residues and bactericides. It seems to me that any health problems connected with flour are as likely to be caused by these various chemicals as by the wheat or gluten itself. In my opinion these chemicals are far more likely to be responsible for the reported increases over the last 50 years in the prevalence of wheat sensitivity, wheat allergy, coeliac disease and irritable bowel syndrome, than some strange biological change in humanity during that period which has made it harder for us to digest natural foods such as naturally grown wheat.

Therefore, if you think that bread, pastry or other foods containing wheat flour or gluten are causing a health problem, I would recommend the following three-stage approach:

- First try baking all your own bread and pastries from organic flour. Most supermarkets sell both organic flour and organic bread flour. Baking bread at home is very quick and easy using a bread maker. Adequate bread-making machines can be purchased for as little as £40, and since home-made bread is cheaper than all but the cheapest kinds of supermarket bread you will soon recover the cost of such a machine. During your trial period don't eat any other foods such as pastas, cakes and biscuits that are made from wheat or other glutinous cereals, unless they have

---

295 Hardman G & Hart G. *Dietary advice based on food-specific IgG results.* Nutrition & Food Science, 2007; Vol.37, Issue 1.

been produced entirely organically.
- If this doesn't solve the problem then you may truly be wheat intolerant or have a wheat allergy, so try eliminating wheat altogether.
- Finally if that doesn't work then you may indeed have a problem with gluten, so try a totally gluten-free diet.

Gluten

Gluten is a compound of two proteins found in wheat, rye, barley and some similar cereals. It is what makes dough sticky and enables it to rise. It is found in anything made from wheat, rye or barley, including bread, pastry, pasta, couscous and beer. Maize, rice, soya beans and oats, and products made from them, do not contain gluten, although oats may be contaminated from other cereals unless they are produced very carefully.

Gluten does seem to cause health problems for many people, principally CD (coeliac disease) and, more commonly, gluten sensitivity.

CD is the more serious. It involves the degeneration of the intestines, and it can lead to death. A sufferer's immune system identifies gluten as an enemy that has to be destroyed, but while doing this, the gut is severely damaged too. The damaged gut results in nutritional deficiencies, various digestive problems, diarrhoea, anaemia, osteoporosis and fatigue, and an increased risk of more serious autoimmune diseases such as type 1 diabetes and rheumatoid arthritis. During the first 2 years of a child's life the main symptoms of CD are a failure to thrive, diarrhoea, abdominal pain and distension.[296]

One study concluded that during the 50 years preceding 2009 deaths from undiagnosed CD increased fourfold in the U.S.A.,[297] and another study concluded that the prevalence of the disease increased fivefold during only 15 years between 1974 and 1989.[298] As with wheat, it seems far more likely to me that this apparent increase in gluten intolerance was produced by the concurrent changes that took place in agriculture and bread manufacture rather than any change in the way the human immune system functioned during that period.

Fortunately CD is still fairly uncommon. In Europe and North America it appears to affect about 0.75% of the population,[299] although the Food Standards Agency quotes a

---

296 Barker J M & Liu E. *Celiac Disease: Pathophysiology, Clinical Manifestations and Associated Autoimmune Conditions.* Advances in Pediatrics, 2008;55: 349–65.

297 Rubio-Tapia A. *Increased Prevalence and Mortality in Undiagnosed Celiac Disease.* Gastroenterology, July 2009;Volume 13u7, Issue 1, 88-93.

298 Catassi C. *Natural history of celiac disease autoimmunity in a USA cohort followed since 1974.* Annals of Medicine, October 2010;42(7):530-8.

299 Fasano A. *Prevalence of celiac disease in at-risk and not-at-risk groups in the United States: a large multicenter study.* Archives of Internal Medicine, February 2003;163(3):286-92.

figure of only 0.33% for the U.K.,[300] which is about one in every 300 people. However, only one in six of these people are aware of their condition, creating a serious problem.[301] So if your food elimination trials show that only a gluten-free diet will relieve your symptoms then you ought to consult a doctor, because you may have CD. Undiagnosed CD can eventually lead to death, and since there is a reliable test for it then you should ask for a test if you believe it is appropriate.

It is more likely, however, that you are suffering from gluten sensitivity, which is six times as common as CD, according to the National Foundation for Celiac Awareness.[302] Gluten sensitivity does not involve damage to the intestines. Its symptoms are similar to those of CD, albeit less serious. However they are usually accompanied by other symptoms not directly related to the intestines, such as headache, mental fuzziness, joint pain, and numbness in the legs, arms or fingers.[303] The symptoms typically appear hours or days after the gluten has been ingested.

For both CD and genuine gluten sensitivity the only cure is to eliminate gluten totally from your diet.

Don't adopt a gluten-free diet merely for general health reasons. The food industry has latched on to the fact that there is profit to be made in selling gluten-free food, and it is doing what it can to persuade us that gluten-free food is good for the health. Don't fall for such propaganda unless you have diagnosed coeliac disease or gluten sensitivity, because cereals in small quantities are good for most people, and what is the point of paying more than necessary for your food, and unnecessarily having to quiz the waiter about ingredients every time you go out for a meal?

Irritable Bowel Syndrome

More common than any of the above is IBS or irritable bowel syndrome. IBS is a collection of bowel-related symptoms, which may include any of abdominal pain, wind, bloating, incontinence, alternating diarrhoea and constipation, fatigue, backache, nausea and gynaecological symptoms. According to the IBS Network the condition is estimated to affect around a third of British people at some time in their lives, but only one in ten of these people seek the help of a doctor. Similarly IBS is estimated to affect 14% of the U.S. population, but only about one in seven of these have had their condition

---

300 *Common Food Allergies*. Medical News Today, August, 2013.

301 Rubio-Tapia A et al. *The prevalence of celiac disease in the United States*. American Journal of Gastroenterology, October 2012;107(10):1538-44.

302 http://www.celiaccentral.org

303 Sapone A et al. *Spectrum of gluten-related disorders: consensus on new nomenclature and classification.* BMC Medicine, February 2012

diagnosed.[304]

IBS may have one or more different causes, including diet, stress, bacterial imbalances, inflammation, or even abnormal sensitivity to pain.[305] A number of researchers have concluded that IBS and inflammation of the intestinal lining are caused or exacerbated by gluten.[306],[307] Consequently IBS has no simple cure, but in most cases the symptoms can be alleviated and patients can be helped to cope better with whatever symptoms remain. Diarrhoea can be controlled by loperamide, while the anti-emetic ondansetron has also proved helpful.[308] Constipation can be controlled by lactulose, or by senna for diabetics, while tegaserod also appears to be helpful in alleviating IBS with constipation.[309] In some cases paracetamol, antispasmodic agents or even small doses of tricyclic antidepressants can help. Medication for pain, diarrhoea and constipation may work better if taken before eating rather than waiting for the problem to surface afterwards, or else taken in small doses on a regular basis. Everyone who suffers from IBS should eliminate, so far as possible, sources of stress and their own stressful reactions to it.

However, since this is primarily a book on nutrition and health, I want to add a few things about some dietary causes of IBS.

Many doctors tell IBS patients to eat more fibre, but according to Professor Peter Whorwell insoluble fibre is the worst kind of food for someone suffering from an already irritated colon.[310] Professor Whorwell is one of the world's leading experts on the treatment of IBS, and his treatment centre in Manchester receives referrals from all over the U.K. In an interview recorded at an international symposium on the subject he said:

'A high fibre diet is a disaster for a lot of patients. Leave fibre out of your diet for three months, every single bit, not a trace of cereal fibre. You can have other forms of fibre such as soluble fibre in fruits and vegetables, but no bran and that sort of insoluble

---

304 Hungin A P et al. *Irritable bowel syndrome in the United States: prevalence, symptom patterns and impact.* Alimentary Pharmacology and Therapeutics, June 2005;21(11):1365-75.

305 Whorwell P J. *What is irritable bowel syndrome?* Therapeutic Advances in Gastroenterology, November 2012; 5(6):379-380.

306 Biesiekierski J R et al. *Gluten causes gastrointestinal symptoms in subjects without celiac disease: a double-blind randomized placebo-controlled trial.* American Journal of Gastroenterology, March 2011;106(3):508-14.

307 Carroccio A. *Non-Celiac Wheat Sensitivity Diagnosed by Double-Blind Placebo-Controlled Challenge: Exploring a New Clinical Entity* American Journal of Gastroenterology, December 2012; 107, 1898-1906.

308 Garsed K et al. *A randomised trial of ondansetron for the treatment of irritable bowel syndrome with diarrhoea.* Gut, December 2013. Medscape Gastroenterology

309 *Management of IBS With Constipation: An Expert Interview With Peter Whorwell, MD.* Medscape Gastroenterology. 2004;6(1)

310 *Eating fibre may NOT be so good for your stomach.* Article by Jane Feinmann, Daily Mail, January 2010.

fibre. Do that for three months, and see what happens.'[311]

This means eating white bread, white pasta and no wholegrain cereals of any kind, especially bran cereals – practically the opposite of normal advice about healthy food!

If a 3-month bran fast makes no improvement, Whorwell recommends omitting chocolate and coffee in turn, for he has found these to be the next two most common dietary causes of IBS in the U.K. If these don't prove to be the problem, I would recommend trying wheat next, and then gluten.

Eating a daily serving of probiotic yogurt may also alleviate IBS symptoms. Since bacterial imbalances are thought to cause or exacerbate IBS in some patients, the ingestion of live, beneficial bacteria may help to solve the problem. That was certainly the belief of Nobel Prize winner Elie Metchnikoff. The cheapest way to obtain such yogurts is to make your own from long-life milk and a little added milk powder in a simple yogurt-making machine. A small carton of live yogurt will start the process off and many subsequent batches can then be made using a teaspoonful or two from each preceding batch as a starter.

Whorwell's advice to eliminate bran for 3 months before looking for another cause tells us that tracking down a cause of IBS may take a long time. I suffered from IBS for over 30 years, experiencing alternating constipation and diarrhoea, and painful wind that woke me a couple of times each night. During this period we ate frozen, chilled and even tinned meals, and factory or shop-produced bread and cakes. My wife and I then adopted the kind of diet recommended in this book, and 16 months later one major symptom of my IBS finally and rather suddenly came to an end. I am not aware of any other major changes in my lifestyle during those 16 months, so I rather think that it was something in our previous diet that was partly responsible for my IBS.

If you are an IBS sufferer perhaps following the dietary advice given in Chapter 22 will help you, too.

---

311 Whorwell P J. *Irritable Bowel Syndrome: An Approach to Treating Patients*. 7th International Symposium on Functional Gastrointestinal Disorders, April 2007. (At the time of writing videoed talks by Professor Whorwell on this subject can be found at http://www.iffgd.org/site/learning-center/video-corner.)

CHAPTER 15: ARE ORGANIC FOODS BETTER?

There are five issues involved in any discussion about the superiority of organically produced food and drink:

- its nutrient content
- its freedom from possibly harmful chemicals
- its freedom from genetic modification
- environmental considerations
- its flavour

Nutrient content

A widely publicized 2010 literature review funded by the U.K. Food Standards Agency (FSA) concluded, '*On the basis of a systematic review of studies of satisfactory quality, there is no evidence of a difference in nutrient quality between organically and conventionally produced food-stuffs.*'[312] That is very clear, but it did contradict several earlier studies, including one based on published values of nutrients that observed, '*Organic crops contain significantly more vitamin C, iron, magnesium, and phosphorus.*'[313]

2 years later researchers at Stanford University came to a similar conclusion to the FSA. They wrote, '*The published literature lacks strong evidence that organic foods are significantly more nutritious than conventional foods.*'[314] However, these researchers did admit that '*Studies were ... limited in number, and publication bias may be present.*' They also concluded that, '*Consumption of organic foods may reduce exposure to pesticide residues and antibiotic-resistant bacteria.*' A spokesman for the Soil Association pointed out that none of the studies included in their review lasted more than 2 years, making it impossible to draw any conclusions about the long-term effects of eating organic or non-

---

312 Dangour A D et al. *Nutritional quality of organic foods: a systematic review*. American Journal of Clinical Nutrition, July 2010; 92(1):203-10.

313 Worthington J. *Nutritional Quality of Organic Versus Conventional Fruits, Vegetables, and Grains*. The Journal of Alternative and Complementary Medicine. April 2001; 7(2):161-173.

314 Smith-Spangler C et al. *Are Organic Foods Safer or Healthier Than Conventional Alternatives? A Systematic Review*. Annals of Internal Medicine, September 2012; Vol. 157, No. 5.

organic food. Of course the BBC reported the study under the heading, '*Organic food will not make you healthier.*'[315]

In Chapter 12 we saw from public records that the mineral contents of fruit and vegetables both in the U.K. and the U.S.A. fell by 40% or more during the 60 years following 1940. Even the mineral content of meat and cheese declined significantly. We saw that these falls were not due to changed methods of analysis, for a comparison of the USDA food tables between 1963 and 1998 showed that the vitamin and mineral content of crops that continued to be grown in traditional ways did not change, whereas the vitamin and mineral content of crops produced by more intensive, industrialized farming practices decreased significantly.[316] We also saw that some eggs from free-range hens fed naturally had double the magnesium content of battery raised hens.

So if it is true that organic food is no more nutritious than non-organic food, either:

(i) the public records of the nutritional contents of a wide range of conventionally grown fruit, vegetables, meat and dairy products published in both the U.K. and the U.S.A. over the last 60 or 80 years are wrong. and there has been no decline in the nutritional content of conventionally grown food, or

(ii) organically grown foods, grown now in the same way as they were grown in 1940 or 1963 respectively, have also for some unfathomable reason lost 40% of their nutritional content in the intervening period, otherwise they would now be more nutritious than conventionally grown food

Neither of these options appears credible.

A serious omission in the FSA review was that it didn't consider the total antioxidant contents of the foods studied. Antioxidants, as we have seen, have a prime role in protecting our bodies from inflammation and disease, in particular cardiovascular disease, neurodegenerative diseases and certain cancers. A more recent and more comprehensive study published in 2014 by Newcastle University concluded that the organic food content of the six[317] major antioxidants is, respectively, from 19% to 69% greater than that of industrially grown food.[318]

A further omission of both reviews was an analysis of the relative amounts of omega-3 and omega-6 fatty acids in the foods studied. As we have seen, a dietary imbalance in these essential fatty acids has been responsible for many significant health problems.

---

315 BBC News; 4 September, 2012.

316 Wallach J. *Our Food is Deprived of Minerals: the Proof.* Longevity Institute Newsletter 16, 2006. Available at: www.longevinst.org/nlt/newsletter16.htm. Accessed November 11, 2009.

317 Phenolic acids, flavanones, stilbenes, flavones, flavonols and anthocyanins.

318 Baranski M et al. *Higher antioxidant concentrations and less cadmium and pesticide residues in 2 organically grown crops: a systematic literature review and meta-analyses.* British Journal of Nutrition, 2014; 112, 794–81.

Chapter 12 reported a very healthy O-6-3 ratio of 1:1 for some organically produced hens eggs, compared to a very unhealthy ratio of 19:1 for the eggs of some hens fed entirely on cereal crops. The omega ratios of beef and pork are also significantly better for cattle and pigs that graze or forage naturally than for animals fed artificially. Milk from organically raised animals contains higher levels of omega-3 fatty acids and conjugated linoleic acid.[319] Yet the reviewers reached their conclusions about the nutritive values of organic and non-organic food without considering their omega contents.

Finally, although the authors of the FSA review stated under 'Conclusions' that there was no difference in the nutrient content of organic and non-organic foods, the table of results in the body of their report stated that organic food had 8% more phosphorus than conventionally grown food, and this was flagged with the word 'difference'.[320] Phosphorus helps to form healthy bones and teeth. It helps the body to turn carbohydrates and fats into energy and to make protein for the growth and repair of cells and tissues. It is also needed for the correct operation of muscles, heartbeat, kidneys and nerves. It is therefore a beneficial nutrient, and there is more of it in organically grown food. The omission of this difference from the FSA's published conclusion suggests to me that the report's authors didn't want to publicize any advantages of organically grown food. If that is so then their impartiality must be questioned. Certainly other scientists immediately questioned the way that they had selected the relatively small number of papers that they eventually included in their study.

In the first 10 years of this century ten review papers were published comparing the nutritional contents of organic and non-organic food. Eight of these found some evidence that organic food was more nutritious, while two of them (one being the FSA report), found no such evidence. These reports are listed in an incredibly detailed study on Californian grown strawberries, which found that organically grown strawberries had 9.7% more vitamin C than similar strawberries grown conventionally.[321] Similarly tomatoes grown organically in Brazil had up to 57% more vitamin C than similar tomatoes grown nearby with the help of inorganic fertilizers and the pesticide FASTAC 100.[322]

I have little doubt that organically grown food is generally more nutritious than food as it is commonly grown in the Western world.

---

319 Huber M et al. *Organic food and impact on human health: Assessing the status quo and prospects of research.* NJAS - Wageningen. Journal of Life Sciences, 2011.

320 It also found that organic food contained higher levels of other important minerals, but the evidence was not considered reliable enough to be counted.

321 Reganold J P et al. *Fruit and Soil Quality of Organic and Conventional Strawberry Agroecosystems.* Public Library of Science ONE, September 2010; 5(9):e12346

322 Oliveira A B et al. *The Impact of Organic Farming on Quality of Tomatoes Is Associated to Increased Oxidative Stress during Fruit Development.* Public Library of Science ONE, February 2013; 8(2):e56354.

Harmful chemicals

(i) Nitrates

The FSA review did acknowledge that industrially grown foods contain a higher concentration of nitrogen. This isn't surprising, since nitrogen is one of the three principal elements added to the soil in industrial agriculture. A higher concentration of nitrogen probably means that conventionally grown crops have higher levels of nitrates in them, which could be bad news. When we consume sodium nitrate or other nitrates, bacteria in our mouths convert them to nitrites, releasing nitric oxide which helps to keep our blood pressure down. But the acid in our stomachs then converts the nitrites to compounds known as nitrosamines. Most nitrosamines are considered to promote the growth of cancers, especially cancers of the stomach[323] and oesophagus.[324] Green vegetables naturally contain nitrates, but because they also contain lots of antioxidants these counteract any nasty effects of the resulting nitrosamines. And vitamin C, which they also contain, tends to prevent the formation of nitrosamines in the first place. It follows that non-organic produce, which contains more nitrogen, fewer antioxidants and less vitamin C than organically grown produce, is almost certainly less healthy.

(ii) Pesticides, etc.

The Newcastle University study found that conventional crops were *four times more likely* to contain pesticide residues than organically grown crops. Pesticide residues were not considered in the FSA review. Exposure to pesticides has been found to diminish the cognitive abilities of adults who regularly use them in their work, and to pose a greater risk for pregnant women and all adults of reproductive age.[325],[326],[327] It also affects the brain development of young children. Children living in an area with heavy pesticide usage were compared with children in a similar area where very few pesticides were used. The children exposed to pesticides had strikingly impaired hand to eye coordination, less physical stamina, reduced short-term memory and impaired drawing ability, compared with the less exposed children. Furthermore, observers of the exposed children noticed

---

[323] Larsson S C et al. *Processed meat consumption, dietary nitrosamines and stomach cancer risk in a cohort of Swedish women.* International Journal of Cancer, August 2006; 119(4):915-9.

[324] *Nitrosamine.* Wikipedia, August 2014.

[325] Jolles J et al. [The Maastricht aging study (MAAS). The longitudinal perspective of cognitive aging] (Article in Dutch.) Tijdschrift voor Gerontologie en Geriatrie, June 1998; 29(3):120-9.

[326] *Pesticides matter. A primer for reproductive health physicians.* University of California, Program on Reproductive Health and the Environment, December 2011. (Includes 118 supporting references.)

[327] *Trouble on the Farm. Growing Up with Pesticides in Agricultural Communities.* Natural Resources Defense Council, October 1998.

more aggressive and antisocial behaviour compared to their less exposed counterparts.[328]

Most non-organic fruit and vegetables, as well as the barley and hops used to make beer, are treated with various pesticides, bactericides, fungicides, nematicides and herbicides. Residues of some of these substances are regularly found in some foods and drinks by the Pesticides Residues Committee (www.pesticides.gov.uk/prc_home.asp), but nearly always at levels which the government considers unlikely to be harmful to human health. Although it is known that these substances are harmful in any quantity, it is very difficult to determine what a safe level is, if indeed a completely safe level exists. These products are not used in organic horticulture and agriculture, so with organically grown foods the question doesn't arise.

Fruits such as oranges and apples that are grown for fruit juice do not have to be free from blemishes, so they are generally grown more naturally and are therefore less likely to contain chemical residues. There seems little reason to pay a premium for organically produced fruit juice, but beer and milk are another story.

(iii) Cadmium

The Newcastle study also found that organic crops had on average 48% less cadmium, weight for weight, than conventional crops. Cadmium is a highly toxic metal that can cause kidney failure, bone softening and liver damage. It can accumulate in the body, so even at low levels chronic exposure is dangerous. This is further evidence that organic foods are healthier than non-organic foods.

(iv) Growth regulators and antibiotics

Some crops are treated with growth regulators. In the European Union the use of growth hormones for animals is banned, but this is not the case in North America, where recombinant bovine growth hormone is used to promote milk production; and oestrogen, testosterone and progesterone are used to promote growth. I would not like to drink milk in the U.S.A!

There is also a worry that the use of antibiotics in non-organically reared animals may be making those same antibiotics ineffective to fight infections in human beings.

Genetic modification

Genetically modified crops, or 'GM crops', are produced by artificially altering the DNA of agricultural plants to introduce some beneficial property that doesn't occur

---

328 Guillette E A et al. *An anthropological approach to the evaluation of preschool children exposed to pesticides in Mexico.* Environmental Health Perspectives, 1998; 106:347-53.

naturally. This might be resistance to pests, diseases, drought, deluge, herbicides or other chemicals. It might even be an improvement in the nutritional content. Most scientists and producers of GM crops support their development and use (particularly those who own the patent rights), but in Britain, France, Russia and several other countries there is substantial opposition to venturing into such uncharted territory. The histrionic opposition by American GM food producers to the identification of GM material on food labels in California does make me wonder what they have to hide. At the very least it indicates that there is a substantial amount of opposition to GM food in the U.S.A. too, otherwise labelling the food as such would not affect its sales there.

A 2-year French study on the effect of GM maize on rats was first published in the *Journal of Food and Chemical Toxicology* in 2012. This maize was produced to resist a particular herbicide called Roundup. Although the paper successfully passed 4 months of what are called 'peer reviews' by knowledgeable independent scientists, the Journal's editorial staff withdrew it almost as soon as it was published, under pressure from the manufacturers of the maize and its accompanying herbicide. Happily it was republished in 2014 in the journal *Environmental Sciences Europe, beginning with a convincing rebuttal of previous criticisms and including yet further evidence for its conclusions.*[329]

Over a period of 4 years the GM-fed rats developed all kinds of serious health problems which did not develop in a control group of rats fed with ordinary maize – severe kidney deficiencies, a two to threefold increase in mortality, large mammary tumours in the females, and in the males four times as many large tumours as in the control group and starting 2 years earlier. The research team concluded that long-term trials are required to evaluate thoroughly the safety of GM foods and pesticides in their full commercial formulations.

If the study had been carried out earlier, the U.S. Food and Drug Administration would not have approved the sale of this particular product, at least until further investigations had been made.

On the basis of the research report the Russian Prime Minister Dmitry Medvedev *immediately banned the importation of all GM foods. "If the Americans like to eat GMO products, let them eat it then. We don't need to do that; we have enough space and opportunities to produce organic food," he said.*[330] *A large group of Russian scientists had already called for a 10-year moratorium on the use of GM crops until their long-term effects on human health had been properly evaluated – using Americans as the guinea pigs!*

Presumably GM crops, even if they were grown organically, would not qualify for an 'organic' label. While it has not yet been proved that they are harmful to humans

---

329 Séralini G-E et al. *Republished study: long-term toxicity of a Roundup herbicide and a Roundup-tolerant genetically modified maize.* Environmental Sciences Europe, 2014; 26:14.

330 http://rt.com/news/russia-import-gmo-products-621. Accessed August 2014.

it has certainly not been proved that they are safe. Personally I intend to avoid them altogether, at least until I die!

Environmental considerations

Serious concern has been raised about the health effects of the artificial fertilizers used for conventional crop production. For example, researchers at Rhode Island Hospital reported that they had found a substantial link between increased levels of nitrates in food and the environment, and increased deaths from diseases including Alzheimer's, diabetes mellitus and Parkinson's disease.[331]

One problem is that nitrogen-containing fertilizers, even if they are not applied as ammonium nitrate, can be converted to nitrates by bacteria in the soil, and nitrates are water-soluble, which means that they can find their way into drinking water.

Cancer

A recent study in Oxford of the diet and health of 623,080 middle-aged U.K. women found no overall benefit in eating organic food in relation to the incidence of various cancers common to women. One or two types of cancer were found to be more common among women who said they usually or always ate organic foods, while other types were less common.[332] Studies like this based on population studies are called 'epidemiological' studies. The problem with them is that while they can examine associations between two variables they cannot tell whether one causes the other. In this particular case the women who always ate organic food were likely to have had very different lifestyles from those who never ate it, so there could have been a number of other reasons or 'confounding factors' why women who regularly ate organic food were more or less likely to develop a particular form of cancer.

Flavour

According *The Organic Center*, organic fruit and vegetables don't necessarily taste better than their non-organic neighbours, except in the case of apples, strawberries and tomatoes. However, 43% of organic food customers cite 'better taste' as their reason

---

[331] De la Monte S et al. *Epidemiological Trends Strongly Suggest Exposures as Etiologic Agents in the Pathogenesis of Sporadic Alzheimer's Disease, Diabetes Mellitus, and Non-Alcoholic Steatohepatitis*. Journal of Alzheimer's Disease, July 2009; Vol. 17:3: 519-529.

[332] Bradbuy K E et al. *Organic food consumption and the incidence of cancer in a large prospective study of women in the United Kingdom*. British Journal of Cancer, April 2014; 110, 2321-2326.

for choosing organic food.[333] From my personal experience, the peaches and apricots I once bought in a Chilean street market tasted ten times as nice as any I have bought in a British supermarket.

The increasing numbers of organically grown products sold in supermarkets as well as the growing success of companies like Abel and Cole, which deliver organic vegetables and fruit to the door, demonstrate that more and more people believe organic foods are healthier and tastier, and that it is worth paying extra for them.

To learn more about organic food, what its benefits are and how to obtain it at minimum cost visit www.soilassociation.org.

---

333 http://www.organic-center.org/reportfiles/Taste2Pager.pdf. Accessed August 2014.

CHAPTER 16: WATER – A SPRING OF LIFE OR A LOW-LEVEL POISON?

Water is even more important than food! A healthy person can go without food for a week without any noticeable effects, but a week without water in some form would probably kill him. Unfortunately much of the water we drink contains very low levels of unhealthy contaminants that may harm us in the long term. While waterborne infections such as cholera or typhoid are unlikely to occur in the drinking water of developed countries, contaminants from agriculture and other industries are more likely to be present, and even bacterial infections such as E. coli and legionnaires' disease are not unknown.

We need water

Water is essential for life and many people don't drink enough of it. Thirst, dry skin, smelly breath and dark coloured urine can all be symptoms of dehydration. According to Dr. Mercola, a Fellow of the American College of Nutrition, chronic dehydration can lead to weight gain and the following problems:

- fatigue
- digestive disturbances such as heartburn and constipation
- urinary tract infections
- autoimmune diseases such as chronic fatigue syndrome and multiple sclerosis
- premature ageing

To avoid dehydration, the NHS follows the European Food Safety Authority in recommending that men should drink 2 litres of fluid a day and women 1.6 litres. All drinks count, including tea and coffee, but we are quite rightly advised to choose healthy drinks such as water, milk and fruit juice rather than sugary or alcoholic drinks. These recommendations are strongly supported by the U.K.'s Natural Hydration Council and Europe's Hydration For Health Initiative, which both talk almost entirely about drinking water. (*'Consumption of water in preference to other beverages should be highlighted as a simple step towards healthier hydration.'*) Their support is hardly surprising, given that all the members of the Natural Hydration Council are producers of bottled water

(Danone, Highland Spring, Nestlé, etc.), and that the Natural Hydration Council was set up by the French company Danone, which produces Volvic, Evian and Badoit bottled waters.

What is surprising, however, is a paper published in the *British Medical Journal* in 2011 which examined very thoroughly the evidence put forward by the Natural Hydration Council in support of this well-known recommendation, as well as other papers that appeared to support it. The author concluded that the recommendation has no sound scientific basis whatsoever: it is little more than an urban myth.[334] There is no evidence that adding eight cups of water to everything else you eat and drink will do you any good and it could even do you harm.[335] A survey in Australia concluded that the diet of an average adult provides more than enough fluid for his daily requirements.[336]

Drinking a lot may not be important even in endurance sports. Fairly recent research has shown that dehydrated cyclists on a hot day in Western Australia performed just as well as fully hydrated cyclists;[337] while warnings have been issued to amateur long-distance runners that drinking too much water can lead to a dangerous condition known as hyponatremia, or water intoxication.[338] Of course modest amounts of drinks containing glucose and mineral salts will help to maintain energy and salt levels in a long-distance event, so I'm not suggesting that one should drink nothing. But the amount one truly needs depends on the air temperature and one's energy expenditure, perspiration rate and body weight.

I once cycled all along the north coast of Fuerteventura, an island off the west coast of Africa. The temperature in the shade was around 30°C, but there was no shade where I was. For some miles the rough track was covered in sand blown over the sea from the Sahara desert. Have you ever tried cycling through sand? Needless to say, when I finally reached a small town on the west coast I was thirsty. I bought two 1.5 litre bottles of fizzy pop and drank both of them, more or less straight off!

So how much should we drink? It is no more possible to answer that question in terms of litres per day than it would be to specify how much we should breathe. Several sources, including the NHS Livewell website, tell us that drinking water with or after a meal aids digestion and softens stools, helping to prevent constipation, and that website recommends drinking a glass of water with each meal. However other fluids would work as well as water, except drinks containing alcohol. That's because the brain communicates

---

334 McCartney M. *Waterlogged?* British Medical Journal, 2011; 343:d4280.

335 Valtin H. *Drink at least eight glasses of water a day. Really? Is there scientific evidence for "8x8"?* American Journal of Physiology - Regulatory, Integrative and Comparative Physiology, November 2002; 283:R993-1004.

336 Tsindo S. *What drove us to drink 2 litres of water a day?* Australian and New Zealand Journal of Public Health, June 2012; Vol.36 Issue 3:205-207.

337 Wall B A. *Current hydration guidelines are erroneous: dehydration does not impair exercise performance in the heat*. British Journal of Sports Medicine, September 2013.

338 *Runners at risk from too much water*. BBC News Channel, June 2003.

with the kidneys through the posterior pituitary gland and tells them either to excrete water as urine or if necessary to hold on to it for reserves. Alcohol interferes with this communication process, causing excess fluid excretion that can lead to dehydration.[339]

If you are in normal health and are not taking any medication that makes you feel thirsty, your body will have several ways to tell you if you need to drink more.

(i) Urine colour. Normally urine should have a light straw colour. Orange means you need to drink more: white means you are drinking more than you need to or you have been drinking alcohol.
(ii) Lips and mouth. If they feel dry you need a drink.
(iii) Thirst. Surprise, surprise! You need to drink something when you feel thirsty!

Assuming that at both breakfast and lunch you have at least one drink of something non-alcoholic, I would recommend drinking a full glass of water with your evening meal and additional water whenever you feel you need it. Actually green or black tea is even more beneficial than water – see under 'The fluorine controversy' later in this chapter.

For babies, of course, human breast milk is the best drink, for as well as nutrients it contains various substances to combat infection and aid digestion.[340] Failing that, cow's milk is normally the best alternative, preferably organic.

Is public water safe to drink?

Contaminants in drinking water are generally limited to only a few parts per million. For example, the maximum concentration of trihalomethanes (THMs) permitted by the U.S. Environmental Protection Agency is only one part in 10 million. However because we drink so much water and other liquids containing water, the cumulative effect of even tiny amounts of some substances can be harmful. So it is important to ensure that you and your children drink water as free as possible from harmful substances.

In the U.K. at least water from the mains supply is considered to be safe to drink provided that its original source is fairly pure. Such sources can be underground aquifers, springs, rivers, natural lakes and reservoirs, or a combination of these. Before distribution the water is filtered for solid impurities and then disinfected, usually by treatment with chlorine gas or some chemical compound of chlorine that kills most types of bacteria.

However, one problem with chlorine and its compounds is that if the original source contains certain impurities they can react with the chlorine to form harmful trihalomethanes

---

339 Guest S, Stanford University. Accessed at http://www.webmd.com/diet/features/6-reasons-to-drink-water, August 2014.
340 Goldman A S & Smith C S. *Host resistance factors in human milk*. The Journal of Pediatrics, June 1973; Vol. 82, Issue 6:1082–1090.

and haloacetic acids.[341] A report by a non-profit body called the Environmental Working Group concluded that, from 1996 to 2001, more than 16 million Americans consumed tap water containing dangerous amounts of such substances. Several studies in the U.S.A. have linked a high consumption of chlorinated water by pregnant women living in certain areas with increased rates of miscarriage and birth defects. One study from North Carolina showed that women in the highest exposure group were 2.8 times as likely to suffer a miscarriage as those in the lowest group,[342] while a study in California showed that women who drank cold tap water were nearly 5.0 times as likely to suffer a miscarriage as women who drank mostly bottled water very low in trihalomethanes.[343] These are only associations of course, and other factors such as income might have been responsible, but with such large differences in the rates of miscarriage I think that if I were pregnant in one of the localities studied I'd stick to bottled or suitably filtered water, wouldn't you? Less serious problems with chlorinated water are that some people find it distasteful, and a few people find that it irritates their eyes or nose.

For these reasons some European countries and U.S. states use ozone gas instead of chlorine to disinfect their water supply. Ozone is generally used to disinfect most bottled water. This is mainly for reasons of taste, but it could easily explain the results of the Californian study.

Nevertheless chlorine-disinfected water is considered safe to drink so long as the source of the water is relatively pure.

The Endocrine Disruptor Hypothesis

In 2014 some researchers in France studied the data on falling sperm counts recorded in a study of 26,000 generally healthy Frenchmen over a period of 16 years. By correlating the figures with changes in local agriculture they attributed the principal explanation of this 33% reduction in fertility, not to changes in lifestyle, but to the increasing use of agricultural chemicals.[344] This explanation of falling male fertility and other worsening problems in human reproduction is known as the Endocrine Disruptor Hypothesis. The hypothesis was first put forward in 1991 at an international conference of World Wildlife Fund scientists, who had become aware of many adverse changes taking place in birds

---

341 *Basic Information about Disinfectants in Drinking Water: Chloramine, Chlorine and Chlorine Dioxide.* U.S. Environmental Protection Agency.

342 Savitz D A et al. *Drinking Water and Pregnancy Outcome in Central North Carolina: Source, Amount, and Trihalomethane Levels.* Environmental Health Perspectives Volume 103, No. 6, June 1995.

343 Swan S H et al. *A Prospective Study of Spontaneous Abortion: Relation to Amount and Source of Drinking Water Consumed in Early Pregnancy.* Epidemiology, Volume 9, No. 2, March 1998.

344 LeMaol J et al. *Semen quality trends in French regions are consistent with a global change in environmental exposure.* Reproduction, February 2014.

and other forms of wildlife. The "Wingspread Statement" concluded, '*Many compounds introduced into the environment by human activity are capable of disrupting the endocrine system of animals, including fish, wildlife, and humans. Endocrine disruption can be profound because of the crucial role hormones play in controlling development.*'

The endocrine system is the general term for the way that the human body produces and makes use of hormones. There are many different kinds of hormone, and among other functions they regulate growth, metabolism and sexual development. Many natural and synthetic substances are able to mimic or interfere with the functioning of the human endocrine system. Substances with this property are collectively known as endocrine disrupters.

While endocrine disruptors are ubiquitous – in plastics, sun cream, face cream, shampoo, toothpaste, petrol and pesticides – one major source of concern is their possible presence in drinking water. Clearly some residue from agricultural and industrial chemicals is going to find its way into our water supplies, either through drainage from the land or else through rainfall. Hormones affect the body in incredibly tiny amounts, often in a few parts per trillion,[345] so it takes only the tiniest imaginable amount of a hormone-mimicking chemical to have an unpredictable effect. And when we consider how much water we take in compared to, say, a whiff of petrol at a filling station, the extent of the possible problem quickly becomes apparent.

Not all scientists believe there is a problem. A paper published in 2014 concluded, '*There is not enough evidence to confirm a worldwide decline in sperm counts. Also, there seems to be no scientific truth of a causative role for endocrine disruptors in the temporal decline of sperm production.*'[346] I seem to detect an inconsistency between those two statements! In a similar vein the U.K. Drinking Water Inspectorate stated in 2010, '*There is no evidence whatsoever that Endocrine Disrupting Compounds pose a risk to human health through drinking water.*'[347] In this case I wonder how objective such an organization can be when its declared purpose is '*to provide independent reassurance that water supplies in England and Wales are safe and drinking water quality is acceptable to consumers.*'

On the other side of the Atlantic, where they are generally more gung-ho about environmental issues than the British are, the endocrine disruptor hypothesis is being taken very seriously. Linda Birnbaum, the Director of the National Institute of Environmental Health Sciences at the National Institutes of Health, presented a statement to a committee of the U.S. House of Representatives, in which she expressed great concern about the

---

345 Norman A W & Litwack G. *Hormones*, Appendix A. Academic Press, San Diego, California, 1987.

346 Couzza M & Esteves S C. *Shedding Light on the Controversy Surrounding the Temporal Decline in Human Sperm Counts: A Systematic Review*. Scientific World Journal, February 2014; 365691.

347 *Endocrine disrupters and drinking water.* U.K. Drinking Water Inspectorate

whole matter. Here is a brief extract from her long and detailed statement.[348]

'Over the past fifty years, researchers have observed increases in endocrine-sensitive health outcomes. Breast and prostatic cancer incidence increased between 1969 and 1986; there was a four-fold increase in ectopic pregnancies (development of the fertilized egg outside of the uterus) in the U.S. between 1970 and 1987; the incidence of cryptorchidism (undescended testicles) doubled in the U.K. between 1960 and the mid 1980s; and there was an approximately 42% decrease in sperm count worldwide between 1940 and 1990.

These observations, set against the numerous observations of abnormalities of sexual development in amphibians and fish and the widespread detection of chemicals with endocrine disrupting properties in our bodies, have led NIEHS to increase its support for research on the effects of chemical exposures on the various endocrine systems. The detection of numerous pharmaceutical agents and chemicals with endocrine disrupting potential in surface waters around the country has raised concern about drinking water as a significant route of exposure.'

Many people are concerned that organic chemicals in drinking water are a major cause of falling fertility and increasing problems connected with pregnancy and birth. Fortunately there is a way to avoid such problems, as we shall shortly find out.

The fluorine controversy

There is similar controversy over the addition of fluorine compounds to drinking water. Fluorine itself is an element similar to chlorine, but with more powerful properties. Chemical compounds of fluorine inhibit tooth decay by strengthening the enamel of children's growing teeth, possibly because they help the body to digest calcium. In the U.S.A. the homes of some 150 million people are supplied with fluoridated water, while in Britain its use at the time of writing covers about 11% of the population. However at a typical concentration of one part per million almost half of children aged between 3 months and 8 years will suffer from dental fluorosis – permanent white blotches on their teeth – and one in eight will develop unsightly white and brown marks, or even pits in the enamel, making their teeth harder to clean.[349] A similar conclusion was reached by the U.S. National Academy of Sciences in 2006.[350]

---

348 *Endocrine Disrupting Chemicals in Drinking Water: Risks to Human Health and the Environment* Statement by Linda S. Birnbaum, Director, National Institute of Environmental Health Sciences, to the Committee on Energy and Commerce, Subcommittee on Energy and Environment, United States House of Representatives. February 25, 2010, updated 2013.

349 McDonagh M S et al. *Systematic review of water fluoridation*. British Medical Journal, October 2000.

350 *Report on Fluoride in Drinking Water: A Scientific Review of EPA's Standards.* Committee on Fluoride in Drinking Water, National Research Council. The National Academies Press, 2006.

A second problem is that while the prolonged consumption of fluorine compounds makes the bones denser, it also makes them more brittle. In 1988 Danielson reported, *'Exposure to fluoride apparently causes new bone formation of an inferior quality, especially in the femoral head where there is more cortical bone . . . .its compressive strength increases, but its tensile strength decreases.'*[351] In others words, one's bones break more easily. In support of this, three other independent studies noted an increased incidence of hip fractures in the elderly in areas with fluoridated water.[352,353,354] Although our own water is not fluoridated we have used fluoridated toothpaste for many years, and I wonder whether that is why the tops of my two central lower incisors broke off last year. A study in 1988 found that toothpaste can double the level of fluoride in the blood within 5 minutes of being used. Even when the toothpaste is not swallowed, it is absorbed into the blood directly through the skin of the tongue and cheeks.[355]

On the subject of toothpaste: don't ever buy fluoridated toothpaste for young children. They often swallow it, and taken in quantity, sodium and calcium fluorides are extremely toxic. According to an article published in the *Evening Standard*, just over 2gm of fluoride (roughly a teaspoon) is enough to kill a 70kg adult, while a mere 0.3gm, the quantity found in some tubes of toothpaste, is enough to kill a 9kg child.[356] Euthymol toothpaste and Eucryl tooth powder are commonly available tooth-cleaning products that don't contain fluorine compounds. More child-friendly kinds of fluorine-free toothpaste are available from health food stores such as Holland and Barrett and www.goodnessdirect.co.uk.

More recently fluorides in drinking water have been strongly linked to impaired mental ability. *'The prolonged ingestion of fluoride may cause significant damage to the nervous system,'* concludes a review of studies published in *Neurologia* in 2011.[357] *'It is important to be aware of this serious problem and avoid the use of toothpaste and items that contain fluoride, particularly in children as they are more susceptible to the toxic effects of fluoride.'* The authors describe studies that show fluorides induce changes in the brain's physical structure that affect neurological and mental development, including

---

351 Danielson C et al. *Hip fractures and fluoridation in Utah's elderly population.* Journal of the American Medical Association, p. 268. 1992.

352 Jacobsen S J et al. *Regional variation in the incidence of hip fracture: US white women aged 65 years and older.* Journal of the American Medical Association, 1990; 264(4):500-2.

353 Cooper C et al. *Water fluoridation and hip fracture.* Letter to Journal of the American Medical Association, 1991; 266:513-514.

354 Sowers M et al. *A prospective study of bone mineral content and fracture in communities with differential fluoride exposure.* American Journal of Epidemiology, 1991; 133:649-660.

355 Rajan B P et al. *Fluoride in toothpaste cause for concern.* Fluoride - Official journal of the International Society for Fluoride Research. October, 1988.

356 Dovey C. *Is fluoride good for our health?* Evening Standard, April 2003.

357 Valdez-Jiménez L et al. *Effects of the fluoride on the central nervous system.* Neurologia, June 2011; 297-300.

cognitive processes such as learning and memory. A different research team had earlier reported that, '*A qualitative review of the studies found a consistent and strong association between the exposure to fluoride and a low IQ*'.[358] As a result of such studies the U.S. Department of Health and Human Services at the beginning of 2011 lowered its recommended level of fluorides in drinking water to 0.7 parts per million. Yet 2 years later the Environmental Protection Agency was still reviewing its advice that anything up to four parts per million was safe!

Even the evidence that fluoridation reduces decay has been challenged. In 1999 the U.K. Department of Health commissioned a report from York University's Centre for Reviews and Dissemination to review the available evidence on the benefits and safety of fluoridation. By 2003 the University was publicly complaining that its findings had been misquoted in order to support fluoridation.[359] '*We were unable to discover any reliable good-quality evidence in the fluoridation literature world-wide,*' they reported. '*What evidence we found suggested that water fluoridation was likely to have a beneficial effect, but that the range could be anywhere from a substantial benefit to a slight disbenefit to children's teeth. Any beneficial effect comes at the expense of an increase in the prevalence of fluorosis (mottled teeth).*'

In the 5 years after Wolverhampton's water fluoridation status rose from 38% to 100% there was a 50% increase in preventative procedures and a 120% increase in spending on dental care,[360] whereas in Manchester and Liverpool, where fluorine was not used, spending on dental treatment fell during the same period.[361]

As a result of such concerns, most European governments have banned the practice of fluoridation; in Belgium the sale of fluoride tablets and fluoridated chewing gum is illegal;[362] and since 1990 more than fifty U.S. cities have withdrawn fluorine from their water supplies.

Incredibly, therefore, in 2003 the U.K. government passed a Water Act requiring water suppliers in England and Wales to comply with requests from local health authorities to fluoridate their water supply after local consultation. However, the supporting white paper stated that opponents of the practice '*should not be allowed to deprive health communities from opting for fluoridation*', and in 2009 the Southampton City Primary Care Trust decided that '*public vote could not be the deciding factor*'. So much for scientific evidence, local consultations, freedom of choice and democracy!

---

358 Tang Q et al. *Fluoride and Children's Intelligence: A Meta-analysis*. Biological Trace Elements Research, Winter 2008.

359 www.york.ac.uk/inst/crd/fluoridnew.htm

360 Holdcroft C J. *Preventative Dental Treatments and Dental Health Expenditure in Wolverhampton 1997 – 2002*. National Pure Water Association, June 2006.

361 Holdcroft C J. *The Other Side of the Coin - An appraisal of the factors influencing dental health statistics*. 6th Edition - May 2006. (May be available from www.awaywolf.com after September 2014.)

362 Dovey C. (Cited above.)

The ridiculous thing is that adding fluorine to water is expensive, and if the experience of Wolverhampton is anything to go by, fluoridation results in even greater expense to the NHS, which is supposed to be saving money. If only the government would spend our taxes on dissuading people from consuming sugar instead (or simply make the use of sucrose illegal!) then children's teeth would not decay, and fluoridation would be totally unnecessary whatever the scientific support for it may be.

It must be admitted that numerous national and international scientific committees, at least up to 2002, were firmly convinced that the case for fluoridating water was incontestable, and it is on the advice of such committees that government policy is usually based, so long as it is politically expedient. However, if you read or hear reports favouring fluoridation I would suggest that you also read the second paper by Holdcroft cited above, *The Other Side of the Coin*. This details how the scientific facts have been distorted to favour fluoridation. A much shorter article on the same theme was published in the *British Medical Journal*.[363]

One fact, which is not so welcome for tea drinkers like me, is that both black and red tea leaves contain significant amounts of naturally occurring fluorides. Dr. Gary Whitford presented a paper on this subject at the 2010 International Association of Dental Research conference in Barcelona.[364] His research was prompted by the case of four patients who had suffered from advanced skeletal fluorosis, which is caused by an excessive consumption of fluorides and is characterized by pain and damage to the bones and joints. These patients had each drunk from one to 2 gallons of tea daily for 10 to 30 years! He discovered that the actual fluoride content of tea was much higher than had been previously believed. His paper included the following statements:

- Most people (whose water is fluoridated and who use fluoridated toothpaste) ingest 2mg to 3mg of fluorides a day (mainly) from water, food and toothpaste.
- Four 250ml mugs of black tea can contain as much as 9mg of fluorides just from the tea.
- One would have to consume at least 20mg of fluoride or nine mugs of tea daily for 10 years or more before significantly compromising one's bone health.

The last statement seems rather optimistic in the light of the earlier reports that elderly patients drinking fluoridated water are more likely to suffer fractures of the hip, but it is somewhat reassuring.

On the other hand, tea is known to have some very important health benefits. It contains powerful antioxidants called polyphenols and other substances that help to

---

363 Graham, J. *Adding fluoride to water supplies.* British Medical Journal, 2007; 335:699

364 Medical College of Georgia. *Tea may contain more fluoride than once thought, research shows.* Science Daily, 14 July 2010.

combat heart disease and possibly certain cancers.[365] And what is not so widely known is that ordinary black tea relieves stress. In some carefully constructed research[366] carried out at London's University College, the cortisol levels of 37 young men who had drunk four cups of tea a day for 6 weeks and were then subjected to a stressful role-playing situation fell faster than those of a similar group who had not been drinking tea. Cortisol is a hormone produced under stress, which is associated with various mental and physical health problems if it is generated too frequently. While no one knew until afterwards who had been drinking tea and who hadn't, the tea drinkers said that they felt relaxed after the tests sooner than the non-tea drinkers did. In addition, their blood platelet levels were lower, both before and after the stress tests, indicating a lower risk of a stroke. And finally there was less C-reactive protein in their blood, indicating a reduced level of inflammation and hence a reduced risk of all kinds of disease.[367]

So I have not stopped drinking my three cups of tea a day, in spite of Dr. Whitford's research!

Types of water

(i) Bottled water

The problems with chlorine, endocrine disruptors and fluorine explain why some people buy bottled water instead of using tap water for drinking purposes, even though it is far more expensive. A more common reason may be that it tastes better than chlorinated tap water. However even bottled water may contain these chemicals: it depends on the kind you buy! There are three main kinds.

(ii) Mineral water

Water marketed as 'mineral water' must contain at least 250 parts per million of total dissolved minerals and trace elements such as calcium and magnesium at its source. The quantity of each must remain constant within specified limits and nothing must be added to it to alter or maintain these levels. Therefore each mineral water comes from a single identified source, such as Vichy in France.

---

365 Mukhtar H & Ahmad N. *Tea polyphenols: prevention of cancer and optimizing health*. The American Journal of Clinical Nutrition, 2000; 71(suppl):1698S–1702.

366 Steptoe A et al. *The effects of tea on psychophysiological stress responsivity and post-stress recovery: a randomised double-blind trial*. Psychopharmacology, January 2007: Vol. 190, Issue 1, 81-89.

367 Steptoe A et al. *The effects of chronic tea intake on platelet activation and inflammation: a double-blind placebo controlled trial*. Atherosclerosis, August 2007; 193(2):277-82.

(iii) Spring water

Water marketed as 'spring water' must be derived from an underground formation, from which water flows naturally to the surface of the earth. It will contain dissolved minerals but not necessarily in such large quantities as mineral water.

Some bottled water, such as Buxton Natural Mineral Water, can be both a mineral water and a spring water. Mineral and spring water are normally disinfected by means of ozone or ultraviolet light, so they are unlikely to contain chlorine, but they may contain very small quantities of naturally occurring fluorides. In theory they could also contain tiny amounts of agricultural chemicals unless, like Highland Spring Water, they are sourced from land certified by the Soil Association as organic.

(iv) Purified water

'Purified water' is water from which the bacteria and dissolved solids have been removed by some process. If the label does not include the words 'mineral' or 'spring' it could simply be purified tap water from the local water company, and several well-known brands of bottled water are just that. Actually, since tap water has already been purified by chlorine or possibly by some other means, 'purified water' could even be water straight out of the tap without any further processing! Research published by the U.S. National Resources Defense Council in 1999 concluded that *an estimated 25 percent or more of bottled water is really just tap water in a bottle - sometimes further treated, sometimes not.*

If purified bottled water is made from a fluoridated water supply then it will contain fluorine, unless it has been purified by means of a process called reverse osmosis or by distillation, both of which remove fluorides and other fluorine compounds. The more usual ozone treatment does not remove fluorine.

One problem with drinking bottled water is that the use of so many non-degradable plastic bottles creates environmental pollution. A more serious potential health concern relates to the presence of a hormone-like chemical called bisphenol A or BPA in the bottle plastic. There is evidence that BPA dissolved in water can adversely affect the brain, behaviour, and prostate gland development in foetuses, infants, and young children, as well as affecting the sexual development of young men and women.[368] It is very unwise to give bottled water to children, and especially unwise to make up infant formula milk with it. This subject will be covered in more detail in Chapter 18.

---

368 *Bisphenol A (BPA): Use in Food Contact Application. Update on Bisphenol A (BPA) for Use in Food Contact Applications.* U.S. Food and Drug Administration. January 2010, updated March 2013.

(v) Home treatment

A cheaper, safer and more environmentally friendly alternative to the purchase of bottled water is to treat tap water at home. This can be done using a jug filter or a unit plumbed in to a dedicated drinking-water tap in the kitchen. Jug filters are cheaper to buy and require no plumbing to install them, but plumbed in systems are more convenient to use and are cheaper in the long run.

There are various systems. Carbon-based water filters remove chlorine and its unpleasant taste. If drinking water tastes nice children are more likely to drink it instead of less healthy drinks containing sugar or artificial sweeteners and colourings. 'Activated' carbon will also remove nasty organic substances like THMs, endocrine disruptors and pharmaceuticals,[369] pesticides, herbicides and some industrial chemicals, but not nitrates or sodium.

Carbon can be in the form of granules or a solid block. A solid block will remove a higher proportion of contaminants. The only way to remove fluorides is to use a 'reverse osmosis' system or distillation, but distillation is not really practical in a home. Table 5 shows the various groups of contaminants and the most common methods of removing them at home.

Table 5: Water contaminants and treatment methods

Contaminant	Method				
	Granulated carbon	Activated granular carbon	Activated carbon block	Ion exchange	Reverse osmosis
Chlorine	✓	✓	✓		
Organic substances e.g. trihalomethanes, endocrine disruptors		✓	✓		
Pesticides e.g. lindane		✓	✓		
Herbicides e.g. atrazine		✓	✓		
Mercury		✓	✓	✓	✓
Other inorganic substances e.g. scum, scale and dissolved lead and copper				✓	✓
Radionuclides				✓	✓

---

[369] Redding A M et al. *Role of membranes and activated carbon in the removal of endocrine disruptors and pharmaceuticals.* Desalination, 2006; 202, 156-181.

Fluorides, nitrates, sodium					✓
Microbiological contaminants are bacteria, viruses and protozoa such as E. coli, cryptosporidium and hepatitis A. Water companies normally bring them to safe levels, but where there is a problem the best home treatment is to boil the water for 3 minutes or use ultraviolet light (UVC). However some types of activated carbon block will remove most microbiological contaminants.						

Since limescale is mainly calcium and magnesium carbonate, which the body uses for bones and teeth, its removal does not bestow any health benefit.

While jug filters are excellent at removing chlorine, most of them don't remove 100% of contaminants, which is why the Brita website for example simply says, '*It's all about taste*'. However the company's 'Water Report' is more specific and states that the active carbon does reduce the levels of both chlorine compounds and organic substances, and that the accompanying ion exchange resin reduces (dissolved) lead and copper, as well as scum and scale.

ZeroWater jug filters will remove very nearly 100% of the contaminants they are designed to remove, including lead and chromium. Like other jug filters they will not remove fluorides, phenols, inorganic substances like arsenic, or bacteria like cryptosporidium. A ZeroWater jug filter is relatively expensive, it's 28cm tall so it might not fit into your fridge, and it takes a long time to filter a jug of water.

Pureflo.co.uk sells an activated carbon block filter plus a three-way (hot, cold and drinking water) kitchen tap for £140. Additional filter cartridges cost £13. It can be installed by anyone who is reasonably competent in D.I.Y.

To remove fluorine you will have to use a reversed osmosis filter, or one that contains activated aluminium oxide. Most or all reversed osmosis systems include an activated carbon filter, so you will see from Table 5 that in combination they remove almost everything that can be removed.

One British company, eau-yes.co.uk, sells a five-stage under-counter reversed osmosis filter that will remove 95% to 99% of almost every harmful substance, including mercury and lead. It costs £200 including the first set of three cartridges and a separate drinking water tap to fit over the sink. A reasonably competent D.I.Y. person can install it under the guidance of a video provided. The filters cost £40 a year for a typical home, which is still less than the cost of buying the equivalent amount of bottled water. So long as you have a fairly large space under your sink, using a product like this is the best way to provide safe drinking water for you and your family. Other similar products are available both in the U.K. and abroad.

Readers in the U.S.A. can find out what various makes of filter remove by reference to the NSF website: http://nsf.org/certified/consumer/listings_results.asp.

CHAPTER 17: ALCOHOL – THE SACRED COW

What's the problem?

Towards the end of the nineteenth century there was a huge social problem in Paraguay in South America. The skin of the cassava root contains cyanide, but someone discovered that when it was dried, ground to a powder, mixed with a waterweed which was plentiful in one particular river and left in airtight pots to ferment, the resulting spongy green substance was no longer deadly but had some interesting properties. Eaten in small quantities it produced a pleasurable feeling, increased one's self-confidence, and reduced one's inhibitions. As you can imagine, it soon became popular at parties. Eaten in large quantities, however, it had terrible effects. It produced destructive behaviour in the form of violence and criminality; mental problems in the form of dizziness, headaches, hallucinations and unconsciousness; suicidal behaviour and all kinds of serious physical problems, which in some cases also led to death. The trouble was that although it tasted disgusting when people first tried it, in time their taste buds adjusted to it and before long they liked eating it so much they became addicted. So in most cases, once people started to eat it they found they couldn't imagine life without it. And because it was easily obtained and had such desirable effects, at least in small quantities, it wasn't long before pretty well everyone was addicted to the stuff and it became part of the regular diet at meal times as well as at social events. Although doctors warned about its dangers and some religious sects even forbade their followers to use it, the almost universal response was always, "I don't eat too much of it, so what's the harm?" 10 years after it first came into use it was estimated that some 70% of the adult population ate it on a regular basis.

Now you might ask, "So what?" Well, for a whole raft of reasons the government eventually decided that something had to be done about sueñera, as it was called. Social historians have analysed its effects in terms of the probable financial loss to the Paraguayan nation as a result of its use at that time:

- Although no one who started to eat it believed he would ever become so addicted that he would eat more than was safe, many people did so, and widespread life-threatening physical problems began to afflict the population. While there was no real health service as such, if similar problems occurred in the same relative numbers in our own country today they would probably cost our health service about £3.5 *billion* a year in medical care – so you can tell how serious a health

problem it was causing. It was estimated that some 9,000 deaths a year were caused by sueñera.
- The Paraguayan nation as a whole lost billions of guaranis a year in productivity due to absenteeism from work and accidents in the workplace attributed to the use of sueñera. Again, in the same relative numbers in the U.K. it would have cost our nation the equivalent of £7.3 billion.
- Worst of all, incidents of criminal behaviour attributed to sueñera were estimated to be causing the country, in terms of policing, imprisonment, etc., the equivalent of a staggering £10 billion or more every year. This did not involve any costs connected with illegal drug trafficking, because the use of sueñera remained perfectly legal.

You can imagine that if such a nasty drug were costing our country £21 billion pounds a year, not to mention the social costs of disease and death, then the government would have to act.

The action that the Paraguayan government took was both extreme and incredible. For some reason the waterweed used in the fermentation process grew in only one river, the Verde or 'Green River'. This runs parallel for much of its length with another river to the south, the Lindo or 'Nice River'. The government employed the army and teams of convicts to dig three 50-mile long canals between the two rivers. They used these canals to drain all the water from the Verde into the Lindo, but through filters that kept the waterweed from migrating to the Lindo. Thus they completely dried up the Verde and thereby stopped the weed growing. Except that they didn't. The government continued to grow it in the new canals under military guard, and they supplied it in huge quantities to licensed sueñera suppliers who then sold it to the public as a product that the government was able to tax. The logic of the government's actions was that the vast income it obtained from tax on the finished product more than compensated for the wealth the country was losing as a result of disease, absenteeism, suicides, accidents, robberies, rapes, murders and death that the drug was responsible for. They even allowed the stuff to be advertised in order to increase its sales!

All that sounds too dreadful to be true, and indeed hardly a word of my little story is true, *except* for the statistics, the effects of the sueñera, and the attitude of the government. All those, unfortunately, *are* true. Because of course what I have really been talking about is alcohol, and the statistics relate to our own country today! The figures on the cost to our nation of health care, lost productivity, crime and police work all come from official U.K. economic surveys.[370],[371] Worse still, most of the figures are several years

---

370 *Government's Alcohol Strategy - Third Report of Session 2012-2013.* Paragraph 10. House of Commons Health Committee, HC 132.

371 *Home Office Full Equality Impact Assessment.* Drugs, Alcohol and Partnerships Directorate, Alcohol Strategy Unit, November 2010.

old, and it is pretty certain that by now the total annual cost to the nation of alcohol-related problems is even greater than £21 billion.

All kowtow to the great cash cow

At one time, most people in our land saw nothing wrong with slavery; the majority of white people in South Africa saw nothing wrong with apartheid; many traditional African tribes saw nothing wrong with a man beating his wife to death if he thought she had been unfaithful to him; and when I was a child people thought there was nothing wrong with smoking. In exactly the same way today, the majority of the population sees nothing wrong with the government's allowing a deadly drug to be promoted in order to obtain tax revenues from its sale. Our thinking is so blinded that we simply cannot see that this is wrong, even though something very similar that was supposed to have happened in Paraguay sounded dreadful, or at least I hope it did when you read about it just now. Just as leaders of the Dutch Reformed Church cited the Bible to support apartheid,[372] so Christian leaders in our country today use the Bible to justify drinking alcohol (and therefore advertising it) by saying that Christ drank wine and that he turned water into wine, even though in both cases the 'wine' was more likely to have been unfermented grape juice.[373]

Years ago the European Community Economic and Social Committee issued a document that listed some fifteen reasons why cigarette advertising should be made illegal. A tiny footnote, which they did not dare to publicize more openly, said, '*Most*

---

[372] E.g. Acts 17.26: "God made from one every nation of men…having determined allotted periods and the boundaries of their habitation."

[373] The Greek word οινοσ and several Hebrew words which are translated in the Bible as 'wine' can mean either wine or grape juice. In several references they clearly do mean grape juice, while in others they clearly mean wine as we understand the word. When Jesus spoke about putting 'new wine' into new wineskins he was talking about 'wine' which had not yet fermented and would therefore have burst old wineskins as it fermented, so by 'new wine' he evidently meant *unfermented* grape juice. Therefore when he passed the cup round at the last supper and said he would not again drink of 'the fruit of the vine' (N.B. not 'wine') until he drank it 'new' at the inaugural Passover celebration in his Father's kingdom, it was almost certainly fresh grape juice he was looking forward to drinking. We have been so brainwashed by wine that most of us cannot conceive that Jesus might have preferred to drink fresh grape juice to the fermented version!
At the wedding in Cana, we are told he made 120 to 150 gallons of 'wine', once the wine provided (whatever it was) had run out. We don't know how many guests there were, but if there were 150 of them then Jesus must have made up to a gallon of 'wine' *per guest*. Even if there were 300 guests they could each have had half a gallon. Jesus would have been well aware of the various Old Testament instructions to avoid strong drink. It therefore seems unlikely that, having declared he had come to fulfil every word of the Old Testament, he would then have provided another half *gallon* or more of alcoholic wine per person to guests who had already drunk 'freely', i.e. everything in sight!

of these reasons would equally support a ban on the advertising of alcohol.' The fact is that cigarette advertising is now banned, even though smoking causes no crime, no violence, no road accidents, no absenteeism from hangovers, no mental health problems, no family breakdowns, and no suicides. Yet alcohol advertising, which contributes to all these things, continues to be supported by the government, because the government can't balance its books without its tax revenue, and the majority of the population can't imagine life without it.

In fact when it was reported that the number of NHS prescriptions for alcohol medication had increased by 73 per cent between 2003 and 2013, a Department of Health spokesman's initial response was, '*It's encouraging to see that more people are getting help for problems with alcohol.*'[374] Admittedly he did have second thoughts and go on to say, '*These figures (on hospital admissions) prove that alcohol is causing harm to the health of hundreds of thousands of people and we must continue to act. That is why we are already improving prevention by funding alcohol risk assessments at GPs and encouraging increased access to alcohol liaison nurses in hospitals.*' Drastic action indeed! Clearly the sacred cash cow itself must not be touched.

Moderate drinking

While some people think there is a case for banning advertisements for alcohol, the vast majority of people in our country still believe there to be no harm in what is termed 'moderate drinking'. This is hardly surprising considering that the drinks industry spends £600 to £800 million pounds a year in the U.K. on promotion and marketing,[375] with the whole aim of persuading us that drinking in moderation is a good thing. But let me at least try to change your mind.

If you were a strict Muslim, Hindu or Buddhist you wouldn't need me to tell you not to drink. Adherents of these religions constitute 43% of the world's population,[376] so if there is nothing wrong with moderate drinking then at least three billion people are mistaken. However, if you are at least nominally one of the world's 2.4 billion Christians, one argument you might think about is the one that persuaded me not to drink. So here are some facts. They have to be strung together like beads on a necklace to complete the argument:

- Alcohol-related diseases are increasing. According to the Health and Social Care Information Centre the number of hospital admissions due to drinking in the U.K.

---

374 *Huge rise in numbers treated for alcoholism.* Laura Donnelly, Daily Telegraph, May 2013.
375 *Advertising alcohol. Fact sheet. Summary.* www.alcoholconcern.org.uk. July 2013.
376 *The World Factbook.* CIA, July 2013. www.cia.gov/library/publications/the-world-factbook/geos/xx.html.

doubled between 2003 and 2013 to over 1.2 million a year.[377]
- About 2 in 100 women and 6 in 100 men in the U.K. are alcohol dependent.[378] This means that if they don't drink several times a day they experience unpleasant withdrawal symptoms, and in time will almost certainly arrive in hospital with some kind of serious health issue.
- Not one of these alcohol-dependent people believed that it would happen to them when they took their first drink.
- The only people who can know for certain that they will not become alcohol-dependent are those who never start to drink.
- People's behaviour is influenced by those whom they admire or respect, and most of all by their parents. If a child's youth leader, teacher or parent believes that drinking is harmless and acceptable then, generally speaking, the child will believe it is too.
- When I was a *youth leader*, the last thing I wanted to do was to encourage the young people in my care to start doing something that they would later deeply regret. That would have been deeply irresponsible. Since one in every 25 young people in my youth groups was likely to become an alcoholic even without my help, I certainly didn't want any part in turning that one into two.
- As a *parent*, if I had encouraged my own four children in any way to drink alcohol when young and one of them had later become alcohol dependent or died of alcohol poisoning, it would have been hard to live with myself.
- As a *Christian,* which you will have guessed I am, I knew that St. Paul said he wouldn't eat or drink anything that might cause an onlooking brother to stumble, and that Jesus said anyone who caused a little one to stumble would be better off thrown into the sea with a millstone round his neck than have to account for his actions at the last judgement. So could I have claimed to follow Christ and the teachings of the New Testament and at the same time ignore both of them? What about you?

Actually there is no such thing as drinking in moderation. What does drinking in moderation mean? If it means not drinking as much as other people drink, then it means drinking as much as you like, for you can always find someone who drinks more than you do. If it means that you never get drunk then you could still be drinking enough to become alcohol dependent or seriously damage your health. Neither of those definitions of moderate drinking seems a very sensible policy to base your life on.

What you probably mean by moderate drinking, if you really think about it, is not drinking enough to damage your health. However if that is what you mean then you are

---
[377] *Huge rise in numbers treated for alcoholism.* Laura Donnelly, Daily Telegraph, May 2013. (Also cited earlier.)

[378] www.patient.co.uk/health/Alcoholism-and-Problem-Drinking.htm. July 2013.

almost certainly *not* drinking moderately, because you will still be damaging your health if only to a small extent. In 2012 Dr. Melanie Nichols and some colleagues of the British Heart Foundation Health Promotion Research Group at Oxford University analysed the annual death toll from eleven conditions known to be linked to long-term alcohol consumption. Yes, eleven! These included heart disease, stroke, high blood pressure, diabetes, cirrhosis of the liver, epilepsy and five different cancers.[379]

She and her team related these conditions to the alcohol consumption of the U.K. population, as reported in the General Household Survey of 2006. Her team related the amount people drank on a regular basis to their chances of contracting each disease, taking into account the fact that regularly drinking a small amount of alcohol appears to reduce the risk of coronary heart disease, probably by reducing the blood's ability to form clots. (Not a good idea if you cut yourself on the ring pull of your beer can!) They concluded that, on average, the overall risk of an alcohol-related death is at a minimum if one drinks 5gm or half a unit of alcohol a day. This is equivalent to less than half a small glass of wine or a quarter of a pint of beer, which is far less than the government's current recommended limits. If you drink anything more than half a unit of alcohol a day, the resulting additional protection afforded against heart disease is outweighed by the even greater increase in the risk of death from one of the other causes.

Yet that is not the whole story. Drinking a tiny amount of alcohol does appear to provide a small overall benefit to people who are at average risk of contracting heart disease, but it doesn't provide even that benefit for everybody. People who are not likely to contract heart disease because they eat a genuinely healthy diet and take a healthy amount of exercise and are not leading an unduly stressful life derive zero health benefit from drinking half a unit of alcohol per day. All it does is to increase the risk of their contracting one of the other diseases that the researchers analysed.

So what is 'moderate drinking'? If it means drinking an amount that won't harm you, then for someone with an average unhealthy lifestyle it might indeed be half a unit of alcohol a day, which is very little indeed. But for someone who enjoys a healthy diet and lifestyle, 'moderation' means that you can drink any normal drink in reasonable quantities so long as it contains no alcohol.

So what about teaching your kids to drink in moderation? Would you teach them to take heroine in moderation? Would you teach them to self-harm in moderation? Should you teach them to drink alcohol in moderation? Only if by 'moderation' you mean the one sensible thing that moderation can logically mean for healthy people who want to remain as healthy as possible – to drink none at all.

Actually an alcohol-free life is not so unusual as one might imagine. In England in

---

[379] Nichols M et al. *What is the optimal level of population alcohol consumption for chronic disease prevention in England? Modelling the impact of changes in average consumption levels.* BMJ Open, 2012.

2009, 38% of the adult population drank less than one alcoholic drink a week.[380] 15% did not drink at all,[381] and this was an increase of 5% on the 1998 figure, so the proportion of teetotallers in the country is rising.

Alcohol and obesity

One thing I forgot to mention earlier is that there is a link between alcohol and obesity. Alcoholic drinks put weight on for three reasons:

- Wines, particularly sweet wines, have sugar in them, which the body stores as fat if the resulting energy is not needed immediately.
- Beers have carbohydrates in them, which the body converts to sugar and then stores as fat if it is not needed immediately.
- All alcoholic drinks have alcohol in them, which the liver converts to energy in a form that the body uses in preference to the energy it obtains from food, so the energy from food is once again stored as fat. Most of the calories in beer and wine come from the alcohol rather than their carbohydrate or sugar content. According to several websites[382] 1gm of alcohol is equivalent to 7 calories, whereas 1gm of carbohydrate or protein is equivalent to only 4 calories. Calorie books generally put the calorie count of a 142ml/5oz glass of wine and of a 284ml/half pint of beer as around 100 calories.

So drinking alcohol is a particularly bad idea for people with a weight problem.

Alcohol and diabetes

Alcohol has special health dangers for people who are diabetic, because it temporarily lowers blood sugar levels and has other upsetting effects. The term 'beer belly' suggests that the energy from beer at least is stored mainly around the belly, where excess weight is particularly associated with diabetes. Even in people who are not diabetic, alcohol can produce fatty livers and actually cause heart attacks by lowering the blood pressure and

---

[380] *Statistics on Alcohol: England 2011*. NHS Information Centre.
[381] *Smoking and drinking among adults, 2009*. Office of National Statistics, 2011.
[382] E.g. www.medicinenet.com

opening up the arteries around the heart.[383]

Finance and alcohol

When I talk about buying organically produced food and proper meat and fish I know that people on low and even average incomes may wonder how they can afford such 'luxuries'. For many families there is one easy way to find enough money to pay for good quality food, and that is simply to cut the booze. On average, households in the U.K. spend £11.70 a week on alcohol, tobacco and narcotics, with most of this going on alcohol.[384] In fact about 18% of the average family's expenditure on food and drink is spent on alcohol.[385] And if, say, a third of families buy little or no alcohol, then families who do buy it regularly must be spending at least 25% of their weekly shopping bill on alcoholic drinks. Saving that amount of money could easily cover the cost of switching to organic milk, eggs and vegetables, and buy some fresh meat and fish as well.

Health warnings on alcoholic drinks

Just before I finished writing this book, the U.K. government's All Parliamentary Party Group on Alcohol Misuse published a report recommending that a health warning should be attached to all alcoholic drinks. If this recommendation is taken up then public attitudes to alcohol will change significantly, and this chapter will no longer appear to be so radical as it probably does right now.

---

383 'Alcohol metabolism produces excess amounts of NADH (Nicotinamide Adenine Dinucleotide plus Hydrogen). This excess of NADH can lead to acidosis from lactic acid build-up and hypoglycaemia (low glucose level) from lack of glucose synthesis. It can also lead to weight gain, fatty liver, and heart attack.'
(Extract from *How to Change Your Drinking: a Harm Reduction Guide to Alcohol (2nd edition)* by K Anderson et al. The HAMS Harm Reduction Network.)

384 *Family spending, 2012. Chapter 5: Weekly household expenditure, an analysis of the regions of England and countries of the United Kingdom.* Office for National Statistics. February 2013.
(There are regional differences in alcohol and tobacco expenditure, with the smallest average amount being £10.10 a week in the London area and the greatest being £16.50 a week in Northern Ireland.)

385 Collis J et al. *Econometric Analysis of Alcohol Consumption in the U.K.* HMRC Working Paper 10, December 2010.

CHAPTER 18: INFERTILITY – ITS CAUSES AND CURE

Sadly I can't provide a cure for all causes of human infertility, but in this chapter you will find some ideas that may be helpful, especially in cases of reduced fertility on the part of a man.

What is happening to human reproduction?

The birth rates in many developed countries have declined so much that this is now more of a concern than overpopulation. An official OECD paper has reported that unless something changes the populations of several European countries will shrink to only one third of their present size within the next 100 years.[386] The number of births in England and Wales fell in 2013 by the largest amount for 40 years,[387] while birth rates in the U.S.A. are at record low levels, with National Census figures released in 2014 showing that the total number of babies born in the year ending July 2013 was the lowest for 16 years.[388] One major cause of these falling birth rates seems to be that young people are starting families later, giving them less time to have babies and at ages when their fertility levels naturally begin to fall. But there is another, more worrying, reason for decreasing birth rates.

An analysis of 61 research papers published in the *British Medical Journal* in 1992 suggested that the male sperm counts in several developed countries had fallen on average *by half* in the preceding 50 years, from 113 million per millilitre of semen to 66 million.[389] In just 16 years between 1989 and 2005 the average sperm count among a total of 26,609 Frenchmen surveyed fell by a third, and there was no sign that that

---

[386] Sleebos J. *Low Fertility Rates in OECD Countries: Facts and Policy Responses.* OECD Labour Market and Social Policy Occasional Papers, No.15. October 2003, OECD Publishing.

[387] BBC News 16 July 2014 quoting the Office of National Statistics.

[388] Reported by Josh Sanburn in *Time*, March 27, 2014.

[389] Carlsen E et al. *Evidence for decreasing quality of semen during past 50 years.* British Medical Journal, 1992; 305:609.

the decline was slowing down.[390] Commenting on the latter report in *The Telegraph* in 2012, Professor Richard Sharpe from the University of Edinburgh said: '*In the UK this issue has never been viewed as any sort of health priority, perhaps because of doubts as to whether 'falling sperm counts' was real. Now, there can be little doubt that it is real, so it is a time for action. Doing nothing will ensure that couple fertility and average family size will decline below even its present low level and place ever greater strains on society.*'

While 66 million per millilitre is still above the level of 20 million at which it becomes difficult to conceive, this was only the final *average* among thousands of men surveyed. Clearly, with such a dramatic fall in this average value, many men of childbearing age who had a low but acceptable sperm count in the middle of the last century would have been unable to inseminate successfully if they had been born 50 years later.
So what is causing this alarming drop in male fertility?

Endocrine disruptors in drinking water

Testosterone and oestrogen are two hormones involved in fertility, so if they are interfered with by substances in the water we drink then we are likely to have problems with both conception and with producing and delivering healthy babies in a normal manner. As we saw in Chapter 16 there remains some controversy as to whether or not drinking water contains harmful levels of endocrine disrupting chemicals, but the tide of evidence seems to be turning. I think that before long the remaining sandcastles built by those who maintain that there is no problem will be finally washed away.

Endocrine disturbance can be especially damaging to the formation and growth of foetuses and young babies, so if you are a potential parent it is paramount to think about where your drinking water is coming from. Spring water from remote Scottish highlands may sound like a good idea, but even that is uncertain if it is delivered in plastic bottles, as we shall see in a moment.

The solution given in Chapter 16 was to filter tap water at home using activated granular carbon, preferably in block form. So long as the filter is regularly renewed, it will remove not only endocrine disruptors but all kinds of other potentially harmful substances too.[391]

---

390 Rolland M et al. *Decline in semen concentration and morphology in a sample of 26 609 men close to general population between 1989 and 2005 in France.* Human Reproduction journal, December 2012.

391 Redding A M et al. *Role of membranes and activated carbon in the removal of endocrine disruptors and pharmaceuticals.* Desalination, 2006; 202, 156-181.

Endocrine disruptors in plastic packaging and food containers

<u>(i) BPA</u>

One serious contender for the explanation of falling sperm counts is the use of plastic food and drink containers, particularly baby feeding bottles. In the 1960s glass bottles started to be replaced by bottles made of polycarbonate plastic, but since about 2005 there has been real concern that a constituent of such plastics called bisphenol A or BPA can affect oestrogen levels which in turn can affect fertility. Although nothing seems to have been proved, there is evidence that BPA may disrupt both hormone levels and brain development in foetuses, babies and children, and that in later life it may contribute to the development of immune disorders, obesity and some cancers such as prostate cancer.[392,393] Such effects seem especially likely in small babies whose total food supply comes from such containers. The World Health Organization estimated that the intake of BPA by infants fed from polycarbonate bottles was eight times as much as for breastfed babies.[394]

As I mentioned earlier, only the tiniest imaginable amount of a hormone-mimicking chemical could wreak havoc in a youngster's developing body and mind. So mainly for reasons of public concern, the use of BPA plastic in baby bottles and children's drinking cups was banned in the European Union countries in 2008, in Canada in 2010, and in the U.S.A. in 2012.

However, it is possible that even breastfed babies may imbibe BPA from their mother's breast milk. Tests carried out in Boston on 27 new mothers and their 31 healthy infants aged from 3 to 15 months identified BPA in 75% of the mothers' breast milk samples and in 93% of the urine samples taken from their babies.[395] (Some of the babies were fed on infant formula milk, which would explain the higher percentage among the babies.) However, it is not certain that all the BPA in the babies came from their feed. Earlier research on premature babies conducted by a similar team in a neonatal unit did not detect any change in the levels of BPA in the babies after feeding. What the team did discover was that the BPA level of each baby was very dependent on the number of medical devices that had been used to keep it alive. The babies who had required the use of four or more devices in the previous 3 days had nearly three times as much total BPA

---

392 Schug T T et al. *Endocrine disrupting chemicals and disease susceptibility*. The Journal of Steroid Biochemistry and Molecular Biology. November 2011; Vol. 127, Issues 3–5, 204–215.

393 Grün F & Blomberg B. *Perturbed nuclear signaling by environmental obesogens as emerging factors in the obesity crisis*. Reviews in Endocrine and Metabolic Disorders, 2007; 8:161-171.

394 *Joint FAO/WHO expert meeting to review toxicological and health aspects of bisphenol A: summary report including report of stakeholders meeting on bisphenol A*. World Health Organization, 2010.

395 Mendonca K. *Bisphenol A concentrations in maternal breast milk and infant urine*. International Archives of Occupational and Environmental Health, January 2014; 87(1):13-20

in their urine as the babies who had required three devices or fewer.[396] This suggests that BPA from plastics and other external sources may be an even more potent source of BPA than milk or food in general.

While babies may have some protection through the banning of polycarbonate baby bottles and drinking cups, older children and adults can still be affected, because BPA plastic is not banned in other food containers such as water containers, nor in the linings of food and drink cans. In the U.S.A. the 2003-2004 National Health and Nutrition Examination Survey (NHANES III) found detectable levels of BPA in 93% of 2,517 urine samples taken from people aged 6 years and older.

Nevertheless not everyone is convinced that the current levels of BPA are harmful to humans. In 2012 Health Canada's Food Directorate concluded after extensive study that current levels of dietary exposure to BPA from food packaging was not expected to pose a health risk to the general population, including newborn babies and young children. It stated that this conclusion was consistent with those of other food regulatory agencies including the United States, the European Union and Japan.[397]

(ii) Phthalates

Not only BPA but other plastic components called phthalates have been implicated in a range of serious undesirable health effects including infertility.[398],[399] Most plastics contain phthalates, which contain xenoestrogens. Xenoestrogens mimic the effects of oestrogen and have produced a variety of undesirable effects in laboratory experiments. A mixture of three different plastic constituents, BPA and the two phthalates DEHP and DBP, produced abnormalities in rats down to the third generation, including abnormalities in puberty, diseases of the testicles and ovaries, and obesity. In addition, kidney and prostate disease occurred in the generation of rats that were dosed.[400]

(iii) Food packaging plastics in general

Pretty well all plastic materials contain chemicals that leach out into food or drink in contact with them and have oestrogenic effects. These chemicals can cause problems

---

396 Duty S M et al. *Potential Sources of Bisphenol A in the Neonatal Intensive Care Unit*. Pediatrics, March 2013; Vol. 131, No. 3.

397 *Health Canada's Updated Assessment of Bisphenol A (BPA) Exposure from Food Sources*. September 2012. Health Canada, www.hc-sc.gc.ca.

398 Schug T T et al. Cited previously.

399 Halden R U. *Plastics and Health Risks*. Annual Review of Public Health, April 2010; Vol.31:179-194.

400 Manikkam et al. *Plastics Derived Endocrine Disruptors (BPA, DEHP and DBP) Induce Epigenetic Transgenerational Inheritance of Obesity, Reproductive Disease and Sperm Epimutations*. Public Library of Science ONE, January 2013.

such as early puberty in females, altered function of the reproductive organs, obesity, increased rates of certain cancers, problems with infant and childhood development and, of course, reduced sperm counts.[401] Yang, Yaniger and others tested more than 500 different plastic products used to contain food or drink and concluded, '*Almost all commercially available plastic products we sampled—independent of the type of resin, product, or retail source—leached chemicals having reliably detectable EA (oestrogenic activity), including those advertised as BPA free. In some cases, BPA-free products released chemicals having more EA than did BPA-containing products.*'[402]

(iv) When in doubt…

Scientists continue to argue about these issues, but to be on the safe side you may want to follow the advice of the U.S. National Institute of Environmental Health Studies:

- Don't microwave polycarbonate plastic food containers, because polycarbonate may break down from repeated use at high temperatures.
- Avoid food contained in plastics with a recycle code 3 or 7.
- Reduce your use of canned foods.
- Whenever possible, opt for glass, porcelain or stainless steel containers, particularly for hot food or liquids.

(Polycarbonate plastic is tough clear, plastic, which is the kind usually made with BPA. It is sometimes identified by the recycle code 3 or 7.)

While I continue to use soft plastic containers to store frozen food, I don't use such containers to reheat it in a microwave. I use a Pyrex or earthenware bowl with a plate on top of it, or else transfer the food to a stainless steel saucepan and heat it up on a hob.

Incidentally, ever since we married we have had our milk delivered to the door in glass bottles. Besides posing no health risk they are completely recyclable.

(v) Teats, dummies, soothers, pacifiers and teethers

If you've read this far you are probably thinking twice about giving your baby any kind of plastic to suck, chew or even hold. Many products for babies to suck or chew are advertised as 'BPA-free', but as we have seen phthalates and almost any kind of plastic can be just as harmful as polycarbonate, especially in the mouth or hands of a

---

401 *Hormonally Active Agents in the Environment.* Committee on Hormonally Active Agents in the Environment, Board on Environmental Studies and Toxicology, Commission on Life Sciences, National Research Council. National Academy Press, Washington D.C., 2014.

402 Yang C Z et al. *Most Plastic Products Release Estrogenic Chemicals: A Potential Health Problem That Can Be Solved* Environmental Health Perspectives, July 2011; 119(7): 989–996.

developing baby for hours on end.

Fortunately silicone rubber appears to be safe, even for bottle teats. Although silicone contains chemicals called siloxanes that can impair reproductive processes and do other nasty things, they don't appear to leach out at normal temperatures and have been shown to be safe when used as teats in feeding bottles.[403] Wood and organic cotton soothers are becoming more widely available and are completely safe as soothers and teethers. Rubber is probably safe too, especially if you can find one made of guayule rubber.[404] And it might even be worth trying raw broccoli stalks: they are nutritious too.

Of course the cheapest and most natural solution for a comforter is a thumb. I sucked my thumb when I was a small child and it did me very little harm: it has grown back to 90% of the size of my other thumb already!

Testosterone – when the well runs dry

(i) A dramatic loss

The generation of sperm is regulated by the hormone testosterone. If a man's body stops making testosterone it will not generate sperm. So another reason for the ongoing reduction in sperm production might be a reduction in testosterone production. And that is indeed what has happened. U.S. researchers observed a 'substantial' decline in the testosterone levels of middle-aged men between 1987 and 2004.[405] So far as they could tell this was not due to increasing age, declining health, increased smoking or reduced exercise. Obesity was a factor but was only partially responsible for the decline. A survey of 991 U.S. Air Force veterans between 1982 and 2002 came to a similar conclusion,[406] as did a survey of over 3,000 Finnish men.[407] Between 1972 and 2002 the average level of testosterone of Finnish men in their sixties fell by 37%![408]

A low level of testosterone, also known as male hypogonadism, can be identified

---

403 Zhang K et al. *Determination of siloxanes in silicone products and potential migration to milk, formula and liquid simulants.* Food additives & contaminants. Part A, Chemistry, analysis, control, exposure & risk assessment, August 2012; (8):1311-21.

404 Some people are allergic to the latex in rubber; also it is thought that prolonged contact with rubber can initiate the allergy. Guayule rubber is hypoallergenic: it does not affect people who have a latex allergy.

405 Travisan T G et al. *A population-level decline in serum testosterone levels in American men.* Journal of Clinical Endocrinology and Metabolism, January 2007;92(1):196-202.

406 Mazur A. *Is Rising Obesity Causing a Secular (Age-Independent) Decline in Testosterone among American Men?* Public Library of Science ONE, October 2013, 8(10).

407 Perheentupa A et al. *A Cohort Effect on Serum Testosterone Levels in Finnish Men.* European Journal of Endocrinology (Impact Factor: 3.14), November 2012.

408 A nanomole or nmol is a measurement of the number of molecules of a chemical in a sample.

by symptoms such as low sex drive, erectile dysfunction, a paucity of body hair and tenderness in the testicles, poor concentration and memory loss.[409] High levels of testosterone are associated with sex drive, muscular strength and endurance, strong bones, body hair and aggressive behaviour.

(ii) Testosterone and the protein:fat:carbohydrate ratio

So now we must ask this: why are men in general producing less testosterone than they used to? If it is not due to age, health, smoking, exercise or even obesity, part of the explanation may well lie once again in changes to our diet.

And that is exactly what researchers at Pennsylvania State University have discovered. It was found that the testosterone levels in the blood of twelve young men at rest were closely related to the calorie ratios in their diets.[410] The more fat they ate in relation to protein and carbohydrate, the more testosterone they produced. Other papers quoted by the researchers supported this result. The conclusion is obvious: modern low-fat diets are bad news for sperm.

The researchers then analysed the kinds of fat that these men consumed. They discovered that the more *saturated and monounsaturated fat* they ate, the more testosterone they produced. The association between testosterone and saturated fat, the kind that comes mainly from animals, is easily explained. Testosterone is made from cholesterol, which the liver produces from saturated fat. So cutting down on saturated fat means starving the body of its building material for testosterone. In other words the kind of fat that is essential for testosterone production is the very kind of fat that the authorities have told all of us to avoid for the last 50 or 60 years!

And here's another point. Since testosterone is made from cholesterol, the use of cholesterol-lowering drugs is almost bound to reduce the body's ability to generate testosterone as well as other hormones, so the increasing use of statins and other cholesterol-lowering drugs may well be a further factor in the decline of human fertility.

Furthermore, the researchers discovered that the more *polyunsaturated* fat compared to saturated fat eaten by their research subjects, the *less* testosterone they produced! Polyunsaturated fat is the kind that comes from temperate seed oils and margarine, so clearly the increased use of cooking oils and margarine in place of lard and butter is another cause of the diminishing levels of male fertility.

Finally they discovered that testosterone production decreases to some extent

---

409 McNamara M. *Decreased Testosterone & Sperm Count.* Livestrong.com, 28 January 2014.
410 Volek J S et al. *Testosterone and cortisol in relationship to dietary nutrients and resistance exercise.* Journal of Applied Physiology (1985), January 1997; 82(1):49-54.

as the proportion of calories obtained from sugars and starches increases,[411] and that testosterone production decreases to a significant extent as the proportion of calories obtained from protein increases. These findings can be explained partly by the fact that a higher proportion of protein or carbohydrate calories usually means a lower proportion of the fat calories needed for testosterone production, but that doesn't fully explain the negative association between protein and testosterone. Nevertheless, any reduction in testosterone produced by the increased protein consumption that I shall be recommending in Chapter 22 will be far outweighed by the effects of the increased saturated fat consumption and the decreased consumption of polyunsaturated fat that I shall also be recommending.

So to summarize the main points:

- It is known that in various countries men's testosterone levels have been falling since 1972 or earlier.
- Testosterone is essential for the production of human sperm.
- The level of testosterone in a man's blood decreases when he adopts a low-fat diet, consumes polyunsaturated fats from seed oils and other sources rather than saturated fat, consumes more of his calories as protein or (to a lesser extent) consumes more of his calories as carbohydrates.
- A man's testosterone level increases significantly when he consumes more saturated and monounsaturated fat.
- It is very likely that the adoption of low-fat diets and the replacement of saturated fats by polyunsaturated fats have been major causes of the observed loss of male fertility during the last 40 or 50 years.

(iii) Testosterone and zinc

Insufficient dietary zinc will also reduce testosterone production. Zinc deficiency is said to be prevalent throughout the world. While it is accepted that severe and even moderate zinc deficiency is associated with hypogonadism, it was not known until 1996 that marginal zinc deficiency can also be a problem. In that year some scientists carried out two experiments.[412]

First they induced marginal zinc deficiency in the cells of four normal young men by restricting their dietary intake of zinc for 20 weeks. In consequence their serum (blood) testosterone concentrations fell from a mean of 39.9 to 10.6nmol/L, i.e. to only a quarter

---

[411] Apart from one outlier the twelve measured testosterone levels decreased only slightly as the protein/carbohydrate ratio increased. Therefore, since the measured testosterone levels decreased significantly with increasing proportions of protein calories, they must also have decreased with increasing proportions of carbohydrate, at least to some extent.

[412] Prasad A S et al. *Zinc status and serum testosterone levels of healthy adults*. Nutrition, May 1996; 12(5):344-8.

of their normal levels! That is an incredible decrease in testosterone.

Secondly they gave zinc supplements in the form of zinc gluconate for 3 to 6 months to nine elderly men who were already marginally zinc-deficient. Their mean serum testosterone concentrations increased from 8.3 to 16.0nmol/L, nearly doubling!

An even more startling experiment took place in 1981.[413] 22 married men with serum testosterone levels less than 4.8ng/ml who had been unable to produce a child for 5 years or more were treated with zinc supplements taken orally. There was a significant increase in their testosterone, dihydrotestosterone and sperm count. Six of their wives became pregnant within 3 months and three more within 2 months of a second trial! However among a further fifteen patients whose initial testosterone levels were greater than 4.8ng/ml only their dihydrotestosterone level increased and there were no conceptions. (Dihydrotestosterone is a more reactive form of testosterone but it is produced in much smaller quantities.)

As we saw in Chapters 12 and 13, the zinc content of many foods has fallen since the middle of the last century, so zinc deficiency may well be another cause of falling levels of testosterone and hence of sperm production.

According to the NHS and other agencies, the best sources of zinc are:

- shellfish
- meat (beef, pork, lamb and the dark meat of poultry)
- wheatgerm
- pumpkins
- nuts
- pulses (peas, beans, lentils, chickpeas, etc.)
- milk and dairy products
- oatmeal
- cocoa and chocolate

The very best dietary source of zinc is oysters. According to the U.S. National Institutes of Health a typical serving of cooked oysters contains more than ten times as much zinc as any other food. That might explain why oysters have the reputation of being an aphrodisiac. So instead of asking your doctor to prescribe Viagra for you, why not ask him to prescribe a bucketful of oysters?

If you think that you may be zinc deficient the simplest way to find out is to take a zinc supplement for 3 months to see if it makes a difference. Blood tests may not be reliable because most of the body's zinc, like magnesium, is stored in the tissues rather than in the blood.

---

413 Netter A et al. *Effect of zinc administration on plasma testosterone, dihydrotestosterone, and sperm count.* Systems Biology in Reproductive Medicine, January 1981, Vol. 7, No. 1: 69–73.

(iv) Testosterone and vitamin D

Vitamin D is required for testosterone production, and the main source of vitamin D is sunlight. Once again, changing lifestyles have produced a problem. Because increasing numbers of us work indoors, and because we are continually told to cover ourselves up with protective clothing or sunblock if we stay in the sun, many people are deficient in vitamin D.

In 2011, 31 men with somewhat low levels of vitamin D and testosterone were given 3,332 IU (international units) of vitamin D a day for a year, while 23 similar men were given a placebo.[414] A placebo is something that looks the same as the experimental substance but does nothing at all. It is used in scientific research for comparison purposes. The men in the supplement group experienced significant increases of around 12.5% in their levels of both free (bioavailable) testosterone and their total testosterone, but there were no changes in the testosterone levels of the placebo group.

However, there is a cheaper, faster and much more effective way to increase one's testosterone production than taking a vitamin D supplement. Many years ago Dr. Abraham Myerson of Boston University Hospital demonstrated that sunlight on the chest or back doubled the testosterone levels of his male test subjects after just 5 days of increasing exposure each day for long enough to produce a slight reddening of the skin. Furthermore, when their genitals also were exposed their testosterone levels tripled.[415] A tanning bed evidently has uses other than tanning!

(v) Testosterone and exercise

High-intensity interval training increases the level of testosterone in the blood immediately and significantly, but only for a short time.[416]

(vi) Testosterone boosts from other sources

There seems to be reliable evidence that testosterone levels can be increased by the consumption of certain other foods and dietary supplements:

- Leafy green vegetables such as broccoli, cabbage, cauliflower, Brussels sprouts and kale. On cutting them up or chewing them a phytochemical called indole-3-

---

414 Pilz S et al. *Effect of vitamin D supplementation on testosterone levels in men*. Hormone and Metabolic Research, March 2011; 43(3):223-5.

415 Myerson A & Neustadt R. *Influence of ultraviolet radiation on excretion of sex hormones in the male*. Endocrinology, 1939; 25:7-12.

416 Kraemer R R et al. *Effects of high-intensity exercise on leptin and testosterone concentrations in well-trained males* Endocrine, August 2003; 21(3):261-5.

carbinol (I3C) is produced which reduces oestrogen levels beneficially for both men and women, thereby increasing the effective availability of testosterone in men.[417],[418]

- Egg yolks contain both cholesterol and the vitamin D needed for testosterone production, as well as the protein needed to build muscles. In addition they contain calcium, which has been shown to increase free testosterone levels in athletes who were dosed with it.[419]
- Olive oil. Argentinean researchers tested the effects on rats of adding four different kinds of cooking oil to their diets – soya, grape seed, coconut and olive.[420] After 60 days the rats that were fed on olive oil and coconut oil had significantly more testosterone and heavier testes than the other rats did. The researchers explained that these oils help the Leydig cells (which produce testosterone) to absorb cholesterol better, as well as having other beneficial effects.
- Probiotic yogurt. Recent experiments on aged mice demonstrated that feeding them purified lactic acid bacteria such as those found in live yogurt restored their testosterone levels and testicular size to youthful measurements![421] It is not known whether such yogurt has the same effect on men, but before this book becomes a bestseller it might be a good idea to buy some shares in Yeo Valley or another company that sells live yogurt to supermarkets!
- Eurycoma longifolia Jack, also known as Long Jack, Malaysian ginseng and Tongkat ali. There is test evidence that this can increase testosterone levels and help men who have difficulties in achieving full sexual intercourse.[422],[423]
- L-Arginine. Among other important bodily functions L-Arginine relaxes the blood vessels, thereby facilitating penile erection. Dietary sources are similar to those for zinc, but if sufficient quantities are not obtained from one's diet then taking

---

417 http://en.wikipedia.org/wiki/Indole-3-carbinol

418 Michnovicz J J et al. *Changes in Levels of Urinary Estrogen Metabolites After Oral Indole-3-Carbinol Treatment in Humans.* Journal of the National Cancer Institute, (1997; 89 (10): 718-723.

419 Cinar V et al. Testosterone Levels in Athletes at Rest and Exhaustion: Effects of Calcium Supplementation. Biological Trace Element Research, June 2009; Vol. 129, Issue 1-3, pp 65-69.

420 Hurtado de Catalfo G E et al. *Influence of commercial dietary oils on lipid composition and testosterone production in interstitial cells isolated from rat testis.* Lipids, April 2009; 44(4):345-57.

421 Poutahidis T et al. *Probiotic Microbes Sustain Youthful Serum Testosterone Levels and Testicular Size in Aging Mice.* Public Library of Science ONE, January 2014.

422 Tambi M I et al. *Standardised water-soluble extract of Eurycoma longifolia, Tongkat ali, as testosterone booster for managing men with late-onset hypogonadism?* Andrologia, May 2012; 44 Supplement 1:226-30.

423 Udani J K et al. *Effects of a Proprietary Freeze-Dried Water Extract of Eurycoma longifolia (Physta) and Polygonum minus on Sexual Performance and Well-Being in Men: A Randomized, Double-Blind, Placebo-Controlled Study.* Evidence-Based Complementary and Alternative Medicine, 2014; Volume 2014, Article ID 179529.

L-Arginine as a supplement might be beneficial.[424],[425]

(vii) Testosterone and age

In general men's testosterone levels decline by about 1.5% per year after the age of 30 or so.[426] However researchers in Sydney found that the testosterone levels of 325 very healthy men aged 40 to 97 were all similar and they did not decline at all during the 3 months of the study.[427] Whether this is also true for men who have not grown up on a diet of kangaroo meat and Australian beer remains to be proved! Testosterone production certainly declines if one is overweight or unfit, so the Australian research is a great encouragement to all men to adopt a healthy lifestyle in order to keep their testosterone going.

Restoring fertility

It is clear that in the last 70 years human fertility has been falling at a significant rate, at least in many Western countries. In this chapter I have been able to identify a number of likely causes:

- endocrine disruptors in drinking water
- plastic packaging that releases endocrine disruptors into our food and drink
- endocrine disruptors in babies' feeding and teething equipment
- low-fat diets with too much polyunsaturated fat and too little saturated and monounsaturated fat
- excessive weight caused by eating too much sugar and other carbohydrates
- zinc deficiency resulting from eating too little zinc-rich food and a decline in the zinc content of foods that are not grown organically
- vitamin D deficiency due to insufficient exposure to the sun
- insufficient exercise to maintain full physical fitness

With a little effort and determination all these causes can be dealt with. And such effort works! Not so long ago Brett McKay, an American in his 30s who runs a website

---

424 Tapiero H et al. *L-Arginine*. Biomedicine and Pharmacotherapy, November 2002;56(9):439-45.

425 Maas R et al. The pathophysiology of erectile dysfunction related to endothelial dysfunction and mediators of vascular function. Vascular Medicine, August 2002; Vol. 7, no. 3, 213-225.

426 Vermeulen A & Oddens B J (Eds.) *Androgens and the Aging Male.* Parthenon Publishing, New York, 1996.

427 Sartorious G et al. *Serum Testosterone, Dihydrotestosterone and Estradiol Concentrations in Older Men Self-reporting Very Good Health: The Healthy Man Study*. Clinical Endocrinology, November 2012; 77(5):755-763.

called The Art of Manliness, conducted an experiment on himself. Discovering that his total and free testosterone levels were those of an average 85 to 100-year-old man he set out to improve them over a period of 90 days. Here's what he did:

- Increased his fat and cholesterol consumption. For breakfast he ate three rashers of nitrate-free bacon and three eggs.
- Increased his consumption of foods rich in zinc and magnesium. For lunch he had a salad of spinach, chuck steak, Brazil nuts and walnuts, avocados, olives, broccoli and olive oil.
- Ate a normal evening meal with his family but kept his starchy carbohydrate consumption reasonably low.
- Consumed no alcohol (he was a teetotaller anyway), and only a little sugar.
- Took supplements of vitamin D_3, omega-3 and whey protein.
- Did weight lifting and high-intensity interval training.
- Gave himself 8 to 9 hours of restful sleep each night (no late-night caffeine, etc.) instead of 4 to 5 hours as previously.
- Consciously reduced his stress levels by means of 20 minutes a day of meditation, walking, deep breathing and facing up to stressful situations.
- Avoided plastic food and drink containers.
- Ate organic foods where practical, carefully washed others to remove any traces of pesticides, etc.
- Used no grooming products containing parabens, a type of xenoestrogen

After the 90 days' trial he had his testosterone levels checked. Both his total testosterone and his free (bioavailable) testosterone measurements had doubled.

A month later, wondering what had happened to his cholesterol and triglyceride levels as a result of consuming all that fat, Brett took a blood test for lipids (fats). The results were excellent:

> HDL/Total cholesterol ratio = 0.38:1. (0.24:1 or more is ideal.) [428]
> Triglycerides/HDL ratio = 0.84:1 (2.0:1 or less is ideal.)

And what about his body fat? It went down from 18% to 12%!
You can find a more detailed description of what Brett did on his website.[429]

---

[428] Ideal values obtained from Dr Ronald Grisanti at http://www.yourmedicaldetective.com/public/523.cfm, July 2014. I have inverted Brett's Total/HDL ratio to match the more commonly quoted form.
[429] http://www.artofmanliness.com.

Now do it!

It is my sincere hope that the advice given in this chapter will help at least some couples that are having problems with conception. It is exciting that, according to the Australian research, our virility need not decline even in old age, so long as we continue to keep ourselves fit by following all the advice in this book!

Therefore once again I would encourage you to set an example of healthy living to your children. Help them to grow up naturally into a healthy way of life, so that when their turn comes to raise a family they will not have to experience the heartache suffered by increasing numbers of parents today who are unable to produce children of their own.

CHAPTER 19: HOW TO LOSE WEIGHT AND KEEP IT OFF

Cut the carbs and keep the fat

Most readers who are concerned about being overweight will have been avoiding fatty meats and full-cream dairy products, getting most of their protein from white meat and fish, and most of their carbohydrates from starchy foods like rice, bread, pasta and potatoes. They will be eating some salad and vegetables and trying not to eat too much. And they will not be losing weight.

Or, if they are losing weight, then sooner or later they will be putting it on again.

Zig Ziglar advised overweight people to stay away from cottage cheese. '*I say this*,' he wrote, '*because nobody but fat folks eat cottage cheese.*' He may have been joking, but many a true word is spoken in jest. For when you restrict your diet to low-fat foods you feel so hungry that you end up eating more and putting on weight. It's been well documented that most people who go on low-fat diets don't manage to stay on them for long, and even if they succeed in losing weight for a while, they are usually putting it on again within a year.[430] What is not so well known is that people who do the opposite, who change to a diet that is relatively rich in protein and saturated fat and who cut down on carbohydrates from starchy foods and low-fat foods, not only lose weight but find it easier to keep their weight down.

The idea of eating more fat in order to lose fat sounds ridiculous, but it's more to do with eating fewer carbohydrates than eating a lot more fat. Wing's and Phelan's 2005 study, mentioned above, showed that it's possible to lose weight without restricting one's fat intake if one cuts down on the carbohydrates. This was not news. As long ago as 1932 some very overweight British patients were divided into two groups. One group was put on a high carbohydrate, low-fat diet, and the other on a low carbohydrate, high-fat diet. In those days 'high fat' meant high in animal fats, which are mostly saturated. They didn't have huge factories processing vegetable oils and vast quantities of margarine and other low-fat spreads and shortenings. So what happened? The patients on the low-fat diet lost on average 49gm of weight per day, but the ones on the high-fat diet lost 205gm

---

[430] Wing R R & Phelan S. *Long-term weight loss maintenance*. American Journal of Clinical Nutrition 2005, 82(1 Suppl): 222S-225S.

a day.[431] The lesson from both studies is that if you want to lose weight you should reduce your intake of carbohydrates, not fat. It is carbohydrates that make people put on weight.

The same is true for children. In 2006 it was found that among healthy Swedish 4-year-olds from well-educated families, those eating a lower percentage of fat generally had a higher body mass index.[432] In particular, Table 3 of their research report showed that the children who ate less saturated fat were more likely to be obese.

Some Swiss researchers looked at five independent dietary trials and concluded that, *'Low-carbohydrate, non-energy-restricted diets appear to be at least as effective as low-fat, energy-restricted diets in inducing weight loss for up to 1 year.'*[433] In plain language, they discovered the wonderful fact that if you restrict your carbohydrate intake you can eat as much as you like of anything else and you will lose as much weight as you would on a low-fat, calorie-limited diet!

More recently, a study of 29 different weight-loss trials published in 2012 concluded that people who consume dairy products do not put on more weight than those who don't, and that, where they are making a conscious effort to lose weight by limiting their calories and taking exercise, they will lose more weight if they include butter, cheese and full-cream milk in their diets.[434]

Why is this? As I have already said, when we eat carbohydrates in the form of starchy foods like bread, potatoes, pasta or pastry, the body's digestive system starts converting them into glucose, which it needs for fuel. And if our body finds that we have kindly provided it with more fuel than it needs right now, being a prudent kind of being it stores the excess for future use by converting it into fat. Actually our digestive system can manufacture glucose out of sugars, starches, fats and even proteins. With sugars the conversion process is very fast. It starts even before the sugar reaches our stomachs. With starches it takes longer, but with fats and proteins it takes the longest of all. So when we use fat rather than starch as our main source of energy glucose is released so slowly into our bloodstreams that we can use it up for energy purposes as it becomes available, and there is no need for our bodies to store it as fat for future use.

If Jack Sprat really ate no fat he was probably fatter than his wife was!

---

431 Lyon D M & Dunlop D M. *The treatment of obesity: a comparison of the effects of diet and of thyroid extract. Quarterly Journal of Medicine* 1932; 1:331-52.

432 Garemo M et al. *Metabolic markers in relation to nutrition and growth in healthy 4-yr-old children in Sweden. American Journal of Clinical Nutrition* 2006; 84:1021-6.

433 Nordmann A J et al. *Effects of low-carbohydrate vs low-fat diets on weight loss and cardiovascular risk factors: a meta-analysis of randomized controlled trials.* Archives of Internal Medicine, February 13, 2006; 166(3):285-93.

434 Mu Chen et al. *Effects of dairy intake on body weight and fat: a meta-analysis of randomized controlled trials.* American Journal of Clinical Nutrition, October 2012; vol. 96 no. 4:735-747.

Satisfying the ghrelin goblin

A second reason why eating more fat helps you to lose weight is because, calorie for calorie, people on a fatty diet don't feel so hungry. We know this is true if you have a high-protein diet, because in 2011 Marks and Spencer paid for some research to be carried out on a range of high-protein foods they wanted to market branded as 'Simply fuller longer'. According to the *Daily Mail's* report on these trials, the subjects didn't feel particularly hungry in spite of cutting their calorie intake by 40%, because a diet containing a high proportion of protein-rich foods creates a feeling of fullness faster than one containing more carbohydrates or fat.

You may not be able to afford to feed a family regularly on Marks and Spencer's meals, but the fact is that obtaining your energy needs from protein and saturated fat rather than unsaturated fat and carbohydrates will satisfy your hunger for longer. This means you will end up eating less overall, so your food bill may be no more than it is now.

Since about 2005 there has been a lot of research into something called 'satiety', which in layman's language means 'feeling full'. It is gradually being discovered that a carbohydrate-based diet doesn't make us feel that we've had enough to eat, probably because it isn't the kind of diet our bodies have been made for. The British Egg Information Service, for example, lists five different trials that have compared the weight losses of people who eat egg-based breakfasts or lunches with those who eat typical weight-loss meals. In every case the egg eaters lost significantly more weight, because they felt full for longer. In one trial subjects who ate two eggs for breakfast every day lost 65% more weight than subjects who ate a bagel with the same number of calories![435]

There was a very interesting BBC Horizon programme in 2014 that featured two doctors who were identical twins. One was put on a high-fat diet, and the other on a high-carbohydrate (sugar and starch) diet. The high-fat doctor, Xand van Tulleken, ate sausage, bacon and scrambled egg for breakfast, while the high-carbohydrate doctor, Chris, ate cornflakes, crumpets and jam. At lunchtime they were invited to eat as much as they wanted of the foods they were each allowed. Xand had had enough after consuming 855 calories but Chris, his identical twin brother, didn't feel satisfied until he had consumed 1,250 calories. The explanation given was that protein suppresses the production of ghrelin, which is the hormone that stimulates feelings of hunger, so Xand's protein-rich food satisfied him sooner and he didn't feel the need to eat so much at lunchtime. And he lost 2.5kg more weight than his brother did.

In 2010 Weight Watchers changed their approach to dieting with a new and apparently successful 'Pro Points' plan, in which greater emphasis is given to foods high in protein and fibre rather than foods which are low in calories and saturated fat.

---

435 Van der Wal J S et al. *Egg breakfast enhances weight loss*. International Journal of Obesity, October 2008; 32(*10):1545-1551.

Foods rich in protein are therefore the best choice for keeping your weight down. In fact if you have managed to lose some weight already then you can help yourself to keep it off simply by eating more protein! In Maastricht 148 middle-aged men and women lost weight over 4 weeks on a low-energy diet.[436] After that they were encouraged to keep to the same diet for another 3 months, with regular counselling sessions to keep them going, but during this period half of them were allowed to eat an additional 48gm of protein a day. They all regained some weight, as dieters generally do after their early efforts, but the people who ate the *additional* protein gained on average only half as much weight as the others did, presumably because they didn't feel so hungry. 48gm of protein is about what you'd find in four rashers of bacon, five large eggs, two cod fillets, or a small (190gm) sirloin steak. That's an awful lot of extra food to eat every day, yet it helped them to put on less weight than the 74 people who didn't eat it.

Unless you are a vegetarian, this is wonderful news! It means that if you eat eggs and red meat and chicken skin and full-fat cheese, and drink full-cream milk, you will almost certainly lose more weight than if you stick to skinless poultry, starchy foods and low-fat dairy products. Remember again that meat, eggs and full-cream milk are the kinds of food people ate in my childhood, when hardly anyone was overweight or obese. Personally, I started eating butter and drinking full-cream milk again when I was 67, and 5 years later I weigh about 6 kilograms less.

In any case many 'low-fat' foods are loaded with carbohydrates and sugar. Most low-fat yogurts, for example, are no-no's for diabetics, because they contain far too much sugar. What is the point in buying a low-fat yogurt to lose weight if it has added sugar ready to be converted to glucose and then into body fat, and if it has lost much of the nutritional content of the full-cream milk it was made from? After all, milk, fat and butter are among the best sources of vitamins A, D, E and K, and because these vitamins have to be dissolved in fat before the body can use them they are most easily absorbed when we get them from full-cream milk rather than plants.[437] That's one reason you shouldn't feed semi-skimmed or skimmed milk to babies. Low-fat products are not a healthy option.

Farm animals like cows and sheep that feed on grass, which is a cereal crop, munch away for much of the day, whereas wild animals like lions and tigers who eat meat manage happily on one meal a day. So by obtaining more of your calories from protein-rich meat and cheese and eggs you won't feel so much need to snack between meals, and you will find it easier to lose weight and keep it off.

Food scientists are also telling us that the 'energy density' of food has a major impact

---

[436] Westerterp-Plantenga M S et al. *High protein intake sustains weight maintenance after body weight loss in humans.* International Journal of Obesity, 2004; 28(1):57-64.

[437] Fraps G S & Kemmerer A R. *The Relation of the Spectro Vitamin A and Carotene Content of Butter to its Vitamin A Potency Measured by Biological Methods. Texas Agricultural Bulletin,* February 1938; No. 560.

on satiety, and that we should choose foods that have a low energy density.[438],[439] So far as I can tell this is simply a highfaluting way of telling us to choose foods which don't have many calories in them! However, the British Nutrition Foundation has produced a chart listing the energy density of some common foods. Table 6 shows some of the best things to eat to feel full without putting on weight. You can see more in the Feed Yourself Fuller Chart on the Foundation's website, www.nutrition.org.uk.

Table 6: Some low energy-dense foods

Very low energy dense foods	Kilocalories per gram	Low energy density foods	Kilocalories per gram
Cucumber	0.10	Apples	0.47
Mixed salad	0.19	Vegetable soup	0.52
Chicken noodle soup	0.19	Low-fat yogurt	0.76
Broccoli	0.33	Baked beans	0.81
Carrots	0.35	Bananas	0.95
Oranges	0.37	Baked potatoes	1.36
Pears	0.40	Boiled eggs	1.47

Crack the snack addiction

Snacking is a major problem for most people who want to lose weight, because it is a habit difficult to break. I must say that I tend to go in search of a snack or a drink when I'm doing some work and I want a break, especially if I'm finding it hard going for some reason and I want an excuse to stop. What I do is keep a jar of pickled baby beetroots, gherkins or pitted olives in the cupboard and eat one or two of them for a snack. Or sometimes I simply drink a glass of filtered water. Water is absolutely the least energy dense substance we can consume, and most of us would benefit by drinking more of it. Actually in the light of what I was saying just now snack addicts might do even better keeping some cold chicken or salt beef or seafood in the fridge. Snacking on protein assuages hunger more effectively than crunching pickled onions.

Better still, learn to live a snack-free life. Just as we get into the habit of snacking by snacking, so we can get into the habit of not snacking by not snacking. If you can hold off snacking completely for 2 or 3 weeks then you should find that you have started to make a new non-snacking habit. The ability to form habits is really useful if you take the trouble to form good ones, because then you can live the way you want to without

---

438 Benelam B. *Satiation, satiety and their effects on eating behaviour*. Nutrition Bulletin 34: 126-173, 2009.

439 Rolls B J. *The relationship between dietary energy density and energy intake*. Physiology & Behavior 97:609-615, 2009.

thinking about it.

The habits that are hardest to change are those that are embedded into us when we are young. So if you don't want your children to grow into fattened up snackers don't give them snacks between meals. When I was small my mother told me not to eat between meals because 'it would spoil my appetite'. She thought that minced beef and cabbage would do me more good than jam sandwiches, so she wanted me to leave enough room for my dinner, disregarding the fact that a growing boy has room for both. What is clear is that she tried to keep me off snacking, and perhaps that is one reason why I've never had a weight problem.

Recently I listened to an interview with a woman whose parents split up when she was 8 years old. She comforted herself by snacking, and by the time she was 22 it had become such a habit that she weighed 21 stone. An asthma attack put her in hospital and she realized that unless she could stop eating she would not live very much longer. It is terribly important from year one to avoid comforting your children with food. Don't give them snacks when they are unhappy. Don't train them to associate eating with feeling distressed. If you do they will instinctively turn to food when they find themselves in unwelcome situations in later life, and they may do terrible damage to their health. Milk or some other healthy drink would be fine, or preferably a cuddle, song, story or some other diversion, but not a snack!

One obvious way we can all avoid snacking is simply not to buy the kind of food we are tempted to snack on. In my case it's biscuits and chocolates. A box of chocolates that survives my presence for more than 2 days can consider itself very fortunate indeed. KitKat bars, Snickers bars, Big Macs, individual pork pies and single portions of chips each contain about 500 calories. For many people that's a quarter of their daily energy requirements. It doesn't take many snacks like those to transfer a pound or two from your bank account to your waistline.

According to Professor Paul Kenny, who also made an appearance on the Horizon programme I mentioned, the snacks most likely to put weight on us are those which contains fat and sugar in equal calorific proportions, such as glazed ring doughnuts, chocolate biscuits and cheesecake. When he fed rats sugary food they didn't put much weight on, and when he fed them fatty food they didn't put much weight on, but when he fed them foods which contained both fat and sugar in equal proportions they wouldn't stop eating them. They became sedentary and overweight. Sounds familiar? For some reason foods containing fat and sugar in equal proportions act like a drug: our brain tells us to eat more and more of them. In my experience there is only one defence against such temptations: cross them off the shopping list!

Don't sugar the pill

The comedienne Victoria Wood reckoned she had discovered some effective sugar replacement therapy: it was called chocolate.[440] Unfortunately ordinary chocolate contains lots of sugar, and by now you will know that sugar is just about the worst thing to include in your diet if you want to stay slim and fit. The only thing you can do is bite the bullet and cut it out. I can still remember deciding in my teens to stop taking sugar in my tea. It took about 3 weeks before it stopped tasting disgusting, but eventually I preferred it that way. Fortunately there are now many 'no added sugar' soft drinks which taste fine, and if you can't survive without muesli and jam or marmalade for breakfast then at least you can buy reduced sugar versions of them.

If you feel you are too addicted to that sweet taste to survive without it, you could resort to using artificial sweeteners like saccharin or sucralose. Extensive research has demonstrated that they are not harmful in reasonable quantities, and they have no calorific value so they won't put any weight on you at all. Sucralose is sold in a granulated form very much like ordinary sugar, so it can be used in drinks and cooking in the same way. Stevia is a more natural option and may be cheaper. When you are looking for a sugar substitute don't buy one derived from fructose, the fruit sugar. Fructose is as bad as ordinary sugar for putting on weight, particularly around the stomach.

Small fork diet

With a name like Alan Sugar you wouldn't expect that particular business guru to be an authority on dieting, but he has one excellent piece of advice on the subject. He calls it the 'small fork diet', and it amounts to this: simply eat smaller quantities of food. I don't go all the way with that, but one thing is certain. If you are restricting your intake of carbohydrates and sugar and you are taking a reasonable amount of exercise yet are still not losing weight, there is only one solution: eat less!

Weight loss and exercise

For people who need to lose weight, the other side of the coin is exercise.

The main benefit and importance of exercise is that it improves your health. Life insurance actuaries predict that a 40 year-old who exercises at least occasionally will live about 2 years longer than someone who hardly ever exercises, and research shows that athletes who specialize in endurance sports and mixed sports live longer than average,

---

440 Victoria Wood. *Mens Sana in Thingummy Doodah.* 1990.

principally because they are less likely to suffer coronary heart disease.[441]

Most people think that exercise will help them to lose weight because any calories burnt as fuel for physical activity won't be stored as body fat. Actually, things are not quite as simple as that, as I explained earlier in the book. You may lose body fat, but you will not lose the same amount of weight because your muscles will grow larger. Nevertheless regular exercise will help you to lose weight, for the following reasons:

- Exercise requires energy. When you exercise after fasting there is little or no sugar in your blood, so your body is forced to obtain the energy it needs from stored fat. So if you exercise before breakfast you will use up body fat and hence lose some weight.
- The self-discipline required to exercise regularly will strengthen your self-control in general, and so help you to keep to a healthy diet.
- Regular exercise will make you feel better physically, mentally and psychologically, so you'll be less likely to resort to comfort eating.
- Regular exercise will increase the size of your muscles so that they can burn more energy in a given time. This means that you'll be able to burn up fat faster.

Whether or not you need to lose weight, adequate exercise is as necessary for good health as a healthy diet is, so exercise is what we shall look at in the next chapter.

---

441 Teramoto M & Bunqun T J. *Mortality and longevity of elite athletes. The Journal of Science and Medicine in Sport, July 2010.* Sports Medicine Australia.

CHAPTER 20: EXERCISE – IT'S WHAT WE WERE MADE FOR

Start young

It is so important for parents to introduce their children to sporty activities from their very early years! My father being blind, he didn't play ball games with my sisters and me, and when I went to primary school I was pretty useless at them. In fact the very first time I tried to kick a tennis ball in a playground game of football I slipped, hit my head on a wall, and was out cold for 20 minutes! I always used to say that my favourite position on a soccer field was 'Left Out'. I was terrified of swimming pools until I eventually learned to swim at the age of twelve, so you can imagine how envious I was of my grandson when I saw him happy to be underwater in a swimming pool before he was a year old.

One of the best ways to set a child up for a life of physical fitness, apart from providing a healthy diet, is to introduce him to as many different kinds of sports and physical activities as possible, and as early as possible. Everyone's mind and body is different, so different people are naturally good at different activities. Only if they try different activities will they be able to discover which ones they are good at.

The power of motivation

In my teens I discovered that my height and weight were exactly the mean height and weight of past Olympic marathon winners. Nevertheless I never once thought of running a marathon myself. One reason might have been that no one had encouraged me to try any kind of long-distance running, so running was not on my radar. Encouraging children and young people to try new things is so important! Another reason, perhaps more significant, was that no one ever told me that one can improve at a sport with practice. I used to think that boys who could run fast or were good at football or could actually hit the ball in a game of cricket were simply made that way. It never occurred to me that if I had practised long-distance running I might have become my school's champion runner. So it wasn't until I was 71 that I ran my first half-marathon, when I completed the Great North Run in a respectable time of 2½ hours.

What made me decide to train for such an event? I was motivated by the wish to experience something new and memorable, by the challenge to achieve something impressive, and most of all by the desire to raise as much money as I could through financial sponsorship for a charitable project in which I was closely involved. Those considerations were what motivated me to devote several hours each week for 6 months to train for the run.

Nobody does anything without some kind of motivation. You and your children must have adequate motivation to exercise, or you won't do it. So here are a few motivational suggestions.

(i) Play games

Having fun by playing games with your kids in the back garden or visiting the local recreation ground is a good start. If you have a back garden, create a sandpit and buy a cheap paddling pool. If you can afford it, buy or build an exciting climbing frame. Install a slide, a swing, a basketball net, a badminton net, a swingball game or a mini trampoline. If you have a big enough lawn or a long enough concrete path, buy a cheap set of boules, a set of skittles or some cricket stumps. If there is a suitable wall, draw some goalposts on it (soccer ones, not rugby ones, unless you have some very friendly neighbours!). Draw a few target crosses within the goalmouth for shooting practice. Suggest that your children invite friends round to play with them.

(ii) Encourage them to join a club or organization that includes sporty activities

This is what I was made to do – much against my will – when I was 8 years old. My mother dragged me off bawling my eyes out to join the local cub pack. I hated it, but only to start with. Then I was introduced to camping and hiking and sailing and climbing, and eventually that day when I was 8 years old changed my life.

(iii) Encourage them to join a sports team

Watching 8 and 9-year-olds going to the recreation ground in their football kit on a cold, rainy Saturday morning to practise for the local junior league shows how team membership can make you do something you would never do if you were left to your own devices. Once you are in a team the last thing you want to be is Left Out.

(iv) Encourage them to achieve something

This could be learning to fly a kite, or swim or dive, or use a skateboard or ice skates, or ride a bike or a horse, or learn archery.

Another kind of individual achievement for older children and adults alike is to reach a certain fitness level. The NHS website provides a free 5-week exercise plan called 'Strength and Flexibility'. Completing this course would be a good initial target. Why not do it with your children?

Years ago the Royal Canadian Air Force published a more comprehensive course of exercises requiring no equipment. It was called '*Physical Fitness - 5BX 11-minute-a-day plan for men - XBX 12-minute-a-day plan for women*'. Second-hand copies can still be obtained from Amazon and other second-hand bookstores, sometimes for as little as 1p plus postage. One feature of this course is that you can go as fast and as far as you like with it, so there is always a further achievement ahead if you want to fly higher. It has the additional benefit that no special equipment is required.

Currently the Royal Canadian Mounted Police publishes a free 12-week total fitness training program on its website at www.rcmp-grc.gc.ca/recruiting-recrutement/rec/pare-tape-12W-eng.htm. Anyone who manages to complete this course will be superfit by the end of it. It is suitable for anyone who is generally healthy, as the amount of effort you have to put into each exercise is related to your personal strength and endurance. You would have to buy or borrow some dumb-bells to practise it.

(v) Encourage them to aim for a public achievement

By a 'public achievement' I mean something like earning a place in a team, coming first in some athletics activity on school sports day, or completing a sponsored charity walk/swim/cycle ride/half-marathon/marshmallow eating contest, etc. The thought of achieving something special can motivate a child to make extraordinary efforts. Think of all those North African boys and girls who see themselves as world-class long-distance runners and how it motivates them to train and train and be the best in their country. For most of one term I saw a small boy jog to school every day wearing a loaded backpack. I'm sure he had some definite target in mind.

If you spot potential talent for a particular sport in any of your children, it's worth dropping a hint that it could lead to something significant if they throw themselves into it. Why should the annual world singles champion at tiddlywinks, for example, always come from the U.S.A.?

(vi) Prepare for something exciting

If you can arrange for an exciting activity holiday such as white-water rafting, climbing, skiing, sailing, youth hostelling by bike or going on a multi-activity children's adventure holiday laid on by a specialist company such as campbeaumont.co.uk or pgl.co.uk, it is reasonable to make a condition of going on it that your youngsters prepare properly beforehand. This might simply be getting themselves fit, learning a skill essential to the chosen activity such as swimming, dry skiing or rock climbing at the local sports centre, or doing some longish practice bike rides with you.

(vii) Earn some money

When your children are old enough you could pay them to do tougher physical jobs such as stripping wallpaper or painting a fence. They might be able to earn money by doing a paper round or delivering leaflets or mowing an elderly neighbour's lawn on a regular basis.

(viii) Sex

I don't intend anything immoral by this! If and when your teenagers begin to show an interest in the opposite sex, you might like to point out that although character is more important than appearance, girls are usually more attracted to boys who look fit and strong and boys are usually more attracted to girls who have a nice shape. (I wouldn't use the word 'slim' in case it prompts excessive dieting or anorexia.) Getting fit is undoubtedly one of the best ways of acquiring an attractive body, so finding a girlfriend or boyfriend generally provides a great motive for losing excess weight and for getting fit in general.

For married couples sex can provide a powerful motive to get fit, particularly for anyone who is overweight. Sex in its popular meaning is more fun if you both have lithe, strong bodies and neither of you is overweight. According to studies conducted by Philip Whitten and Elizabeth Whiteside,[442] the average world-class athlete makes love 3.4 times a week. That is exactly twice the average frequency reported by Alfred Kinsey for all men and women in their 20s and 30s.

Age is no barrier to being in trim: you don't have to be fat at 40 or flabby at 50. I am physically fitter at 70 than I was when I was 30!

(ix) Find a training partner

For adults, a regular appointment to exercise with a friend is one of the best motivations to take exercise. On 2 days every week I go out jogging with a friend. Knowing that he will be waiting for me compels me to get up early and be there for our rendezvous, even if it is raining or snowing! More energetic people might arrange a weekly game of tennis or squash with a friend, or perhaps a regular session with a friend in a gym or at the pool.

(x) Join a group

Many women and older people in particular enjoy the social interaction of a weekly visit to a keep-fit group for aerobics or other physical exercises, or for country dancing,

---

442 Whitten P & Whiteside E J. *Can exercise make you sexier?* Psychology Today, April 1989; 42-44.

ballroom dancing or even belly dancing! Regular foursomes for games such as lawn tennis, table tennis or bowls are further options.

The amazing benefits of exercise

It is strange how for many of us the word 'exercise' produces the same kind of negative response as the words 'dieting', 'abstinence' and even 'punishment'! It is strange because our bodies were made to be physically active. Most young children love to run around and dance and climb on things, but in time that natural desire seems to die down. It is almost as though we train ourselves – and our children in many cases – to prefer a lifestyle based on sitting down and avoiding physical effort. We use cars and buses and washing machines and vacuum cleaners and lifts and powered lawnmowers and car washes, and we buy ready-made meals instead of cooking food ourselves. Many of us even avoid going out to shops by buying food and clothes over the Internet and having them delivered to us.

    A lifestyle that eliminates so much physical effort is unnatural, and it is bad for us! The only way we can maintain strong hearts and lungs is to exercise them, and the only way we can develop and maintain strong muscles and bones is to use them regularly. Therefore you should encourage your children to be as active as possible, and if necessary you yourself should build some regular exercise into your weekly routine, unless of course you are a removal man, fencing contractor, bricklayer, hill farmer, miner, footballer or professional wrestler, etc. Some form of regular exercise is as vital as eating, drinking and sleeping. Don't fool yourself into thinking that you can remain healthy without it. Exercise is unpleasant only when you are unfit. Once you are fit you will not only enjoy exercising: you will also find that everything else that you do is more enjoyable.

    For simplicty we can divide exercise into four types, each with its own particular benefits.

(i) Walking

Ordinary walking is good for you. It is something that most people can do, from childhood into old age. Walking with your children gives a great opportunity to talk with them, and if you are lucky enough to have woods or footpaths nearby these can provide added interest and learning opportunities. I can still remember walking with my father in 'the bluebell woods' when I was very small; and the day when our 4-year-old walked 5 miles to the summit of Whernside in North Yorkshire, an ascent of 400m or 1,300ft, is one we shall never forget.

    Walking provides multiple benefits:

- It boosts circulation and increases oxygen supply to every cell in your body, helping you to feel more alert and alive.
- It releases stiff joints and eases muscle tension.
- It relieves stress.
- It exposes you to the sunshine so that your body can generate the all-important vitamin D.
- It helps to keep your legs and body in good shape, especially if you maintain a good posture as you walk.
- It is believed to resist osteoporosis, especially if one carries a heavy rucksack – particularly important for postmenopausal women when their oestrogen levels start to fall.
- It may stave off arthritis by helping to maintain healthy joints.
- It is very helpful to people suffering from most forms of depression, especially walking in the park or countryside. If you are depressed, start with a very short walk and try increasing it gradually. Jogging, cycling or swimming can be even more helpful if you have the energy.
- It gives you an opportunity to think, meditate or pray.

Why not head out for a walk at lunchtime instead of sitting slumped over your desk doing Sudoku or a crossword puzzle? If you are in a high-pressure job and you feel that you don't have time even for that, take a walk anyway but use it for thinking, jotting down any thoughts that come to you in a paper or electronic notebook before you forget them. Getting away from the desk frees one's mind for reflection, which can save many wasted hours and will sometimes produce some great ideas. It is even possible to read a book or a report while you are walking! I admit that while reading a comic I once walked into a lamp post and fell flat on my back, but that was when I was young. Nowadays I can walk and read simultaneously without difficulty.

Even standing up to work can be better than sitting all the time. I know a lady who lost a lot of weight when she changed her job from one in which she was sitting all day to a job in a shop where she had to stand all day.

The one thing you should never do is lie down, for there is a very strong association between lying down and dying!

Since I retired my routine has continued to include 40 minutes of brisk walking in the lunch hour each weekday, rain, shine, hail or snow.

(ii) Moderate aerobic exercise

Ordinary walking, however, does not furnish sufficient exercise to keep us in full health. We also need to engage in moderate *aerobic* exercise. Aerobic exercise is literally exercise 'with air'. It gets us at least a little out of breath but it's at a level of exertion that we could maintain for quite a while. Our muscles get enough oxygen from our lungs to keep working without feeling tired. The primary purpose of aerobic exercise is to maintain the health and strength of our heart and lungs. Even at moderate levels regular aerobic exercise:

- keeps your heart and lungs healthy
- lowers your blood pressure
- helps to control your blood sugar
- helps to keep your weight down
- helps you sleep more soundly
- makes you feel good and look good
- makes all normal physical activity easier and hence more pleasant

The NHS Livewell website says that adults should spend at least 150 minutes every week in moderate aerobic activity, or else 75 minutes a week in vigorous aerobic activity, which we shall come to in a moment.

My own moderate aerobic activity consists of jogging for half an hour three times a week before breakfast, a weekly total of 90 minutes. I spend part of each half hour warming up by brisk walking, part in slow jogging, and part in jogging as fast as I can, before I gradually slow down to a final brisk walk again. One advantage of exercising before breakfast is that one's body has to obtain its fuel from stored fat rather than sugar circulating in the bloodstream, so it is an effective way to keep one's weight down.

(iii) Vigorous aerobic exercise

An even better way to avoid heart trouble, apart from having a healthy diet of course, is to engage regularly in some form of *vigorous* exercise. People who engage in vigorous exercise have even fewer heart problems than those who exercise at only a moderate level, even if they burn the same number of calories.[443] A further advantage of vigorous exercise is that it takes up only half the time that moderate exercise does. In Tables 8 and 9 there are some examples of such exercise.

There is a special form of vigorous exercise called high-intensity interval training that takes up even less time, but I'll talk about that later.

(iv) Strength training

"*I 'ad a kettle twice the size of that 'un when I was your age, but we were stronger in*

---

[443] Swain D P & Franklin B A. *Comparison of cardioprotective benefits of vigorous versus moderate intensity aerobic exercise.* The American Journal of Cardiology. 2006; 97[1].

those days." So said Doris the cook to her struggling kitchen maid Emily back in 1914.[444] For more than a century all kinds of heavy lifting – buckets of water, hods of coal and bowls of very wet washing in the house, and outside the house the extraordinarily heavy loads carried by coalmen, dustmen, dockers, miners, farmers, builders, navvies and even milkmaids – all these loads have gradually been taken away from us by labour-saving devices and health and safety regulations. The result is that nowadays anyone who doesn't engage in deliberate strength training exercise is almost certainly weaker than his ancestors were. And that is why many of us get injured when we do have to lift something heavy; and why back pain is so commonly a reason for people having to take time off work, and why many of us suffer from excessive weight, high blood pressure, and heart trouble. In our normal daily life we are not using our bodies as they were meant to be used, and they are complaining!

Therefore all older children and adults who live in developed countries and who want to remain healthy need to engage in a completely different type of exercise, namely strength training. Strength training is sometimes called resistance exercise training. It involves the use of weights, springs, elastic bands or special machines, or simply pushing hard against the wall or floor. Whereas aerobic exercise maintains and improves the health of our heart and lungs, strength training maintains and develops the strength of our muscles and bones. Aerobic exercise is 'with air' and can be continued for extended periods of time. Strength training is anaerobic or 'without air', for in strength training our muscles simply use the energy within them. We cannot keep going for long. Lifting a heavy weight, for example, does not get us out of breath but after a few lifts our muscles tire and we have to stop and rest.

Strength training is very important indeed:

- It increases bone density, strength and size.[445],[446]
- It increases muscular strength making it easier to lift things without injury, even in older people.[447]
- It reduces back and joint pain as a result of increased muscular strength.[448]
- It improves the HDL/LDL fat ratio and other indicators of cardiovascular disease.[449]

---

444 From 'Below Stairs', a musical comedy set in 1914, written by Trevor Pilling and Alan Lewis.

445 Friedlander A L et al. *A two-year program of aerobics and weight training enhances bone mineral density of young women.* Journal of Bone and Mineral Research, 1995; 10(4), 574-585.

446 Graves J & Franklin B A. *Resistance Training for Health and Rehabilitation.* Human Kinetics, 2001.

447 Tracy B L et al. *Muscle quality. II. Effects of strength training in 65-to 75-yr-old men and women.* Journal of Applied Physiology, 1999; 86(1), 195-201.

448 Carpenter D M & Nelson B W. *Low back pain strengthening for the prevention of low back pain.* Medicine and Science in Sports and Exercise, 1999; 31:18-24.

449 Goldberg L et al. *Changes in lipid and lipoprotein levels after weight training.* Journal of the American Medical Association, 1984; 252(4), 504-506.

- It reduces blood pressure, even in older people.[450]
- It decreases body fat making you look good and feel good.
- In men it increases muscle mass and size and temporarily increases testosterone levels.[451]

Many women, it is true, think that weightlifting is something practised only by men who read 'Men's Health' magazine, or perhaps by Bulgarian women shot-putters or female weightlifters who look like something out of a 1960s sci-fi film. Never fear! When men lift weights it provides a surge of testosterone that builds up the size of their muscles, but that doesn't happen to women, or at least only to a small extent.[452] For you women it will indeed firm up and strengthen your muscles and maintain or increase your bone strength, but what it will also do is decrease your body fat and give you a bikini-shaped figure without your having to live off lettuce and zero-fat cottage cheese. What's more, weightlifting will do this as fast or faster than running on a treadmill or dodging round pedestrians while you jog along busy streets during the cold dark months of winter. And if you must know, there are even pink dumb-bells and pink ankle and wrist weights made especially for the girls.

For older women strength training is especially important to prevent osteoporosis and the risk of breaking one's hip or another bone in a fall. A group of 56 post-menopausal women undertook ten resistance exercises on a regular basis for a year, half of them doing a few repetitions under heavy loads, and half of them doing many repetitions under lighter loads. The bone densities of the first group's hips increased while the densities of the second group's decreased. Muscle strength in both groups increased significantly. This shows that the bone density of even older women, at least in their hips, can actually be increased by weight training, but only if the weights are fairly heavy.[453]

Strength training can also increase self-confidence. 16 weeks of weight training by a group of female undergraduate students increased not only their strength and cardiovascular fitness, but also their self-confidence and self-esteem.[454] Furthermore, because weightlifting produces relatively fast results, boys and girls who take it up will

---

450 Martel G F et al. *Strength training normalizes resting blood pressure in 65-to 73-year-old men and women with high normal blood pressure.* Journal of the American Geriatrics Society, 1999; 47(10), 1215-1221.

451 Fleck S J & Kraemer W J. *Designing resistance training programs, 4th edition.* Human Kinetics, 2014.

452 Mayhew J L & Gross P M. (1974). *Body composition changes in young women with high resistance weight training.* Research Quarterly, 1974; American Alliance for Health, Physical Education and Recreation, 45(4), 433-440.

453 Kerr D et al. *Exercise effects on bone mass in postmenopausal women are site-specific and load-dependent.* Journal of Bone and Mineral Research, February 1996;11(2):218-25.

454 Trujillo C M. (1983). *The effect of weight training and running exercise intervention programs on the self-esteem of college women.* International Journal of Sport Psychology.

quickly discover that they are stronger than many of their classmates in the school gym and playground, and they too will gain in self-confidence and self-esteem as a result.

Let me finish with these words from a paper that is probably the most complete scientific review of this subject.[455] *'Research demonstrates that resistance exercise training has profound* (beneficial) *effects on the musculo-skeletal system, contributes to the maintenance of functional abilities, and prevents osteoporosis, sarcopenia* (the loss of skeletal muscle mass and strength as a result of ageing), *lower back pain, and other disabilities. More recent seminal research demonstrates that resistance training may positively affect risk factors such as insulin resistance, resting metabolic rate, glucose metabolism, blood pressure, body fat, and gastro-intestinal transit time, which are associated with diabetes, heart disease, and cancer. Research also indicates that virtually all the benefits of resistance training are likely to be obtained in two 15- to 20-minute training sessions a week.'*

All exercise is worth it! At the age of 46 the inspirational American writer Zig Ziglar was told by his doctor that if he didn't want to die prematurely he must lose 37lb of weight and 7 inches off his waistline. In metric measurements that's nearly 17kg and 18cm. The thought of losing 37lb was too daunting to contemplate, but he felt he could manage 2 ounces a day, and he worked out that if he kept this up he would achieve the doctor's target in 10 months. The doctor advised him to go jogging every day before work, so in rain, snow, wind and sunshine he obeyed his doctor's orders, hating every minute of it. Whenever he found he was getting behind schedule he knew he had a choice – to get up earlier and jog further or to eat even less! Zig kept to his schedule, achieved his goal, and achieved it on time. But that isn't the whole story.

In order to maintain his weight loss Zig then continued his daily routine of jogging, press-ups and sit-ups, gritting his teeth and bearing the pain of it like a martyr. That was until one beautiful spring morning in Oregon. That morning he was jogging round a university campus, and he says that as he felt the concrete flowing beneath his feet he suddenly realized that he was having the time of his life. By then he was 50 years old and in better shape physically than he had been at the age of 25. As he ran past the students he felt confident that he could beat 98% of them in a race over 2 miles, and he knew at last that when you exercise to get fit you don't so much pay the price as enjoy the benefits. He proved this when his gall bladder ruptured and it wasn't discovered for 4 days, by which time his body was full of poison. His doctor told him that his amazingly swift recovery from the operation was due to his excellent physical condition. Zig Ziglar went on to generalize that for success in any area of life you don't pay the price: you enjoy its benefits. It is only failure that you pay the price for.[456]

So what precisely is required to enjoy the benefits of getting and staying fit?

---

455 Winett R A & Carpinelli R N. *Potential Health-Related Benefits of Resistance Training*. Preventive Medicine, 2001; 33, 503–513.

456 Ziglar Z. *See you at the top. 25th Anniversary Edition*. Chapter 13. Pelican press.

How much exercise?

The following recommendations for adults and children are compiled from the NHS and other sources including my own. The recommendations for adults apply mainly to people whose daily work is not in itself energetic. The ones for children are minimum recommendations for all children. Tables 7 to 9 suggest activities and exercises suited to each age group.

(i) Children under 5

- Youngsters need at least 3 hours of physical activity each day – a mixture of gentle and energetic activity.
- Encourage your child to be active in as many ways as possible.
- Older children in this group should spend some time out of doors. Sunlight is important.
- Minimize sitting still times – e.g. watching television, strapped into a buggy, car journeys.

Table 7: Exercises for children under 5

	Gentle activity examples	Energetic activity examples
Babies	Looking round, reaching, grasping, pulling, pushing.	Activity on tummy, crawling, swimming.
Toddlers	Walking, playing while sitting down, climbing stairs (with supervision), 'helping'.	Rolling on the floor, playing while on the feet (e.g. simple ball games, clapping, dancing), running, swimming.
Older children under 5	Walking, playing in a sandpit or paddling pool, dressing up. Standing and walking games like 'O'Grady says', 'Hunt the slipper', 'Hide and seek', 'Follow my leader'. Helping with housework and gardening.	Running, hopping, jumping, skipping, dancing, throwing, trampolining, swimming. Children's recreation ground activities such as climbing, sliding, swinging, see-sawing – in the park or garden. Energetic games and activities like tag, chasing, racing, riding a tricycle or scooter, hill climbing, rolling down hills.

(ii) Children from 5 to 18

- Children need at least 1 hour of physical activity each day – a mixture of moderate and energetic aerobic activities, and activities that strengthen the muscles and bones.
- Use the motivational ideas in the previous section to encourage your children to exercise.
- Set an example yourself. Play games and do physical exercises with them!
- Minimize their sitting still times – e.g. watching television, playing video games, travelling by car.

Table 8: Exercises for children from 5 to 18

Moderate aerobic activities	Walking to school, walking a dog, cycling on level ground. Playing in the playground or recreation ground or on the beach. Using climbing frames and slides, skateboarding, rollerblading, ice skating. Continuous stair climbing at a moderate rate. Lawn mowing, digging, sweeping up leaves. Hill walking, orienteering, bowling, table tennis, cricket, baseball, surfing, bodyboarding, canoeing, diving, gentle swimming, skiing.
Vigorous aerobic activities	Running and chasing, cycling fast or over hilly ground, mountain biking. Skipping with a rope, energetic dancing, aerobics, gymnastics, martial arts. Continuous stair climbing at a fast rate or while carrying a loaded rucksack or two heavy bags. Football, rugby, basketball, hockey, tennis, badminton, squash. Hard rowing, energetic swimming.
Muscle-strengthening activities	Swinging on bars in the playground; climbing on ropes, trees and rocks. Tugs of war, wheelbarrow races, piggybacks. Stair climbing carrying a loaded rucksack or two heavy bags. Football, basketball, netball, hockey, tennis, skiing, swimming. Field events such as long jumping and high jumping, javelin throwing, shot-putting and archery. Hiking with a loaded rucksack or cycling with loaded panniers. Sit-ups, push-ups, gymnastics, martial arts. Resistance exercises with exercise bands or weights.

Bone-strengthening activities (These are activities that stretch or compress bones.)	Walking, jogging, running. Hopping, jumping, skipping with a rope, playing hopscotch, giving piggybacks. Swinging from bars, climbing on frames and trees. Dancing, aerobics, gymnastics. Mountain biking. Football, basketball, netball, hockey, badminton, tennis. Long jumping, high jumping, javelin throwing and shot-putting. Weight training and martial arts.

(iii) Adults

- Adults over 18 years old need at least 2½ hours of moderate intensity aerobic activity a week, or 1¼ hours of vigorous intensity aerobic activity a week, or a mixture of these.
- Adults should also do some muscle-strengthening exercises at least twice a week, covering all the major muscles – another ½ hour or 1 hour a week, depending on how keen you are.

If you are unused to exercise, start gently and increase your efforts over a period of several weeks or months. Age and physical condition may limit what you can achieve. Seek a doctor's advice if you are in doubt.

Moderately intense aerobic activity will get you out of breath so that you can speak but not sing. Vigorously intense activity will get you so out of breath that you can hardly speak. One way to meet your need for 2½ hours a week of moderately intense aerobic exercise would be to put in half an hour each weekday. Perhaps you could cycle to work or go for a brisk walk in the lunch hour or choose a hilly walk home. Commuters might leave their homeward train one stop early. Or you could get up early and go jogging before work. The NHS website provides a comprehensive 9-week video guide to getting fit through jogging. It is called 'Couch to 5K'.

For guidance on muscle and bone-strengthening activities, a good start would be one of the three physical exercise courses suggested earlier in 'The power of motivation', item (iv). Encourage all your family to achieve a selected level.

If you are really keen, do a search for 'military fitness manual' in an online bookshop. You will find fitness training manuals for the army, navy, royal marines, parachutists, commandos and even the SAS! Simon Waterson's book *Commando Workout* for example, which at the time of writing could still be bought cheaply second-hand, provides a 4-week guide to total fitness based on jogging, weights and diet. I used this in preparation for the Three Peaks Challenge when I climbed Ben Nevis, Scafell Pike and Snowdon in just under 24 hours.

Table 9: Exercises for adults

Moderate aerobic activities	Walking fast, hill walking, gentle jogging, cycling on fairly level ground, rollerblading, energetic canoeing, moderately fast swimming. Playing doubles tennis, badminton, volleyball, basketball, bowling, table tennis, cricket, baseball, surfing, bodyboarding, skiing. Continuous stair climbing at a moderate rate. Using a running machine or cross trainer/elliptical trainer set at a moderate level.
Vigorous aerobic activities	Fast jogging or running, cycling fast or up hills, mountain biking, fast swimming. Playing singles tennis, football, rugby, hockey, squash. Serious aerobics, gymnastics, skipping with a rope, fast rowing, martial arts. Walking fast carrying a loaded rucksack or two heavy bags. Timed hill walking, cross-country running. Using a running machine or cross trainer/elliptical trainer set at an energetic level.
Muscle and bone-strengthening activities	Football, basketball, netball, hockey, tennis, skiing, swimming. Field events such as long jumping and high jumping, javelin throwing, shot-putting and archery. Hiking with a loaded rucksack, or cycling with loaded panniers. Carrying two loaded shopping bags, or better still continuous stair climbing carrying a loaded rucksack or two heavy bags. Sit-ups, push-ups, gymnastics, martial arts. Digging, shovelling or hard rowing. Resistance exercises with exercise bands, weights or weight-training machines.

Strength training

Weightlifting and other forms of strength training are fully useful only if they are hard! Ideally your training session should work all the major muscle groups of your legs, back and arms, with enough repetitions of each exercise and at a level of exertion such that at the end of a session you can do no more without a very long rest. Older children and everyone whose employment doesn't require the regular lifting of heavy loads should engage in strength training two or three times a week.

The fastest way to strengthen muscles and bones alike is to use weights at home.

Of course, if you can afford the time and money to visit a sports centre or gymnasium there will be weights and other equipment you can use there, and some people prefer the companionship of exercising with other people. But most parents of young children are short of time and money, and it is cheaper and less time-consuming to invest in a set of two dumb-bells and a barbell for use at home. These will be supplied with a selection of weights so that everyone can use a weight appropriate to his strength. A typical 25kg set comprises:

- six 1.25kg plates
- six 2.5kg plates
- one 1.5kg barbell bar
- two 0.5kg dumb-bell bars

A 25kg or 30kg set is adequate for most normal people. A new set will probably cost around £50, but in the long run even that is cheaper than paying for gym membership, especially for a whole family.

Alternatively, why not make your own barbell and weights, using a broomstick and bottles of water or sand? A 2-litre lemonade bottle filled with water weighs 2kg, so two or three of these on each end of a broomstick can turn it into an 8kg or 12kg barbell, good starting weights for an adult. Attach them directly to the broomstick with packaging tape. Sand weighs twice as much as the same volume of water, so a 1-litre bottle filled with sand makes a 2kg dumb-bell that is small enough for an adult to hold comfortably in one hand. Similarly a 500ml sports drink bottle is small enough for an average child to hold and weighs 1kg when filled with sand. Use silver sand or driveway jointing sand, which are fine enough to pour through a funnel.

How heavy should your weights be when you start? The weight of your barbell should be such that you can do twelve biceps curls but no more. The weight of your dumb-bells should be such that you can do twelve lateral raises but no more. These exercises are described in Table 10.

Table 10: Upper body exercises

Name	Description
Press-up	Lie on the floor face downward with your hands under your shoulders. Push yourself up, keeping your body in a straight line and your weight resting on your hands and toes, until your arms are straight. Then lower yourself to the floor. If this is too hard, keep your knees on the floor.
Bent over row	Holding the barbell down in front of you with your palms facing towards your body, stand with your feet comfortably apart, your knees bent, and your upper body bent forward from the waist at 45° to the floor. Maintaining that position, pull the barbell up to your stomach, keeping your arms close to your sides. Hold it there for 2 seconds then return to the starting position.
Shoulder press	Sit on a chair with your back well supported and your feet comfortably apart. Hold the barbell just below your chin with your palms facing forwards and your hands well apart so that your forearms are nearly vertical. Raise the barbell above your head until your arms are almost straight, and hold it there for 2 seconds before returning to the starting position.
Biceps curl	Stand with your feet comfortably apart, holding the barbell down in front of you with your palms facing away from your body. Raise the barbell slowly to your chest, keeping your elbows tucked in to your sides. Then return to the starting position.
Lateral raise	Stand with your feet comfortably apart, holding a dumb-bell in each hand with your arms at your sides and your palms facing each other. Keeping your arms fairly straight raise them outwards until they are horizontal, hold them there for 2 seconds then slowly lower them again.
Triceps dip	Standing with your back to a chair, bend your legs and place your hands on the front edge of it. Move your feet forward until your bottom just clears the front edge of the chair. This is your starting position. Lower your body until your upper arms are parallel to the floor and your bottom is nearly on the floor. Then return to the starting position by straightening your arms.

Table 11: Lower body exercises

Name	Description
Lunge	Stand with both feet together, holding a dumb-bell in each hand. Take a good pace forward with your right foot. Bend both knees until your left knee is nearly on the floor. Push yourself up again using your right heel, not your toes. Repeat this by putting your left foot forward first.
Front squat	Stand with your feet comfortably apart, knees slightly bent, holding a dumb-bell in each hand. Keeping your back straight, bend your knees until your thighs are parallel with the floor. Hold for 2 seconds then rise again until your knees are slightly bent as before.
Step-up	Stand facing a chair, holding a dumb-bell in each hand. Step up on to it with both feet, leading with one foot, then step back down again leading with the same foot. A step up and down counts as one repetition, but on each repetition you should lead off with your right or left foot alternately. Children can use a low stool or the bottom stair tread instead of a chair.
Calf raise	Stand facing a wall, about 1 foot away from it, with your hands resting flat against the wall for balance. Lift up your left foot then rise up on to the toes of your right foot, keeping your leg straight. Return to the starting position and repeat the exercise with the opposite foot.
Straight leg dead lift	Stand with your feet a comfortable distance apart, holding the barbell down in front of you with your palms facing towards your body. Bend forwards at the hips then bend your knees until your back is horizontal and the barbell nearly touches the floor. Keep your upper back straight. Return to the starting position.
Static squat	Stand with your back against a wall and your feet about 2 feet away from it. Squat down until your thighs are parallel with the floor, as though you are sitting on an invisible chair. Hold this position as long as you possibly can, but do it only once in a session. Try timing yourself to measure your increasing strength.
Note: You can make the first five of these exercises harder by wearing a backpack containing bottles of water or sand. You can then dispense with the dumb-bells.	

There are demonstrations of most of these exercises on YouTube. Raise and lower the weights slowly so that your muscles take the strain.

Before you start strength training seek a doctor's advice if you:

- are overweight
- have high blood pressure (above 140/90mmHg)
- get more breathless than other people when climbing stairs

- have an irregular heartbeat
- or if your heartbeat takes a long time to return to normal after exertion

Maintaining strong muscles is essential to reduce the risk of injury at home or at work. If you have strong back and arm muscles you are less likely to injure yourself when you have to lift a heavy suitcase or push a loaded wheelbarrow or put your shoulder to a car that is stuck in a snowdrift. And think how glad you will be that you strengthened your bones if you ever have to jump from a blazing aircraft…

Abdominal muscle exercises

Strong abdominal muscles will ward off the risk of back pain and reduce the likelihood of a hernia. Exercising them will also flatten your stomach, but unless you put in an awful lot of effort you are unlikely to acquire the 'six-pack' that bodybuilders love. Exercises to strengthen these muscles are described in Table 12.

Table 12: Abdominal muscle (ABS) exercises

Name	Description
Crunch with legs up	Lie on your back with your hands by your ears and your legs in the air. Bend your knees as far as possible then curl up by bringing your shoulders forwards and your knees towards your ribcage. Don't pull your head forward with your hands. Hold this position for 2 seconds then return to the starting position.
Crunch with feet flat	Lie on your back with your feet on the floor, your knees bent up and your hands resting on your thighs. Curl your shoulders forwards as far as possible, sliding your hands towards your knees, keeping your chin off your chest. Hold this position for 2 seconds then return to the starting position.
Leg raise	Lie on your back with your hands by your sides and your legs in the air. Tighten your lower abdominal muscles and raise your hips from the floor as far as you can. You will have to push down on the floor with your hands. Hold this position for 2 seconds then return to the starting position.
Sit-ups	Lie on your back with your hands by your sides and sit up without using your arms. If necessary hook your feet under a chair. Return to the starting position.
Note: You should breathe *out* on the exertion part of each exercise to contract your abdominal muscles fully.	

A strength-training programme

Here is my recommended programme for strength training. Each week do one session of upper body exercises, one session of lower body exercises, and one session of ABS exercises, on three different days.

A session should consist of all the exercises in turn, repeating each exercise the number of times shown in the bottom row of Table 13. Do each exercise in turn before moving on quickly to the next, and then have a short rest between each complete set. For example, for the upper body exercises at Level 1 your 5,5 training session would comprise:

- 5 press-ups, 5 bent over rows, 5 shoulder presses, 5 biceps curls, 5 lateral raises and 5 triceps dips
- 1 minute of rest
- 5 press-ups, 5 bent over rows, 5 shoulder presses, 5 biceps curls, 5 lateral raises and 5 triceps dips.

That should take about 7 minutes.

Build your strength up gradually. Start at Level 1, and when you can manage that move up to Level 2, and so on. Once you have mastered Level 5 reassess the weights of your barbell and dumb-bells, as described in the previous 'Weight training' section. Increase them as necessary.

Table 13: Strength-training programme

Upper body exercises summary (Table 10)	Press-up, bent over row, shoulder press, biceps curl, lateral raise, triceps dip.				
Lower body exercises summary (Table 11)	Lunge, front squat, calf raise, step-up, straight leg dead lift. Conclude each session with one static squat.				
ABS exercises summary (Table 12)	Crunch with legs up, crunch with feet flat, leg raise, sit-up.				
Level	1	2	3	4	5
Repetitions	5,5	5,15,5	10,15,10	10,25,10	15,25,15

High-Intensity Interval Training

In this century there has been increasing interest and research into a form of exercise called high-intensity interval training (HIT). HIT is an alternative to other forms of aerobic exercise: it is not a substitute for strength training. It has two advantages over moderate or vigorous aerobic exercise: it takes no more than 45 minutes per week, and it appears to offer increased health benefits, in particular improved aerobic capacity (the ability of the muscles to utilize oxygen efficiently), reduced fasting glucose (one is less likely to become diabetic), and a reduced likelihood of heart disease.[457,458,459] HIT is also said to promote the production of the human growth hormone (somatotropin or somatropin), a hormone that stimulates growth and cell reproduction and regeneration in humans and other animals, thereby slowing down the ageing process.[460]

In 2014 eight men and women aged 35 to 51 who had not previously engaged in any physical training did just two 11-minute sessions of HIT training a week. After 8 weeks their aerobic capacity had improved by 8%, their blood glucose levels by 6%, and their general physical abilities by around 20%.[461]

HIT involves a series of very short bursts of highly energetic exercise interspersed with short periods of rest. The exercise can be in the form of sprinting a short distance, swimming, using an exercise bike or cross trainer, or doing anything that involves a level of exertion that gets you so exhausted you couldn't continue for another second!

It has been suggested that such short bursts of effort correspond more closely to the hunting activities of our ancestors rather than to longer periods of more moderate exercise like marathon running. In fact there is some evidence that too much marathon running can damage the heart, producing arrhythmias[462] and scarring,[463] although this has been disputed more recently.[464] You probably know that the very first marathon runner, Pheidippides, collapsed and died immediately after running 26 miles from the

---

[457] Swain D P & Franklin B A. *Comparison of cardioprotective benefits of vigorous versus moderate intensity aerobic exercise.* The American Journal of Cardiology, 2006; 97(1):141-147.

[458] Gibala M et al. *Physiological adaptations to low-volume, high-intensity interval training in health and disease.* The Journal of Physiology, March 2012; 590, 1077-1084.

[459] Kessler H S et al. *The potential for high-intensity interval training to reduce cardiometabolic disease risk.* Sports Medicine, June 2012;42(6):489-509.

[460] Campbell P. *Ready, Set, Go! Synergy Fitness.* Pristine Publishers Inc, 2002.

[461] Adamson S et al. *High Intensity Training Improves Health and Physical Function in Middle Aged Adults.* Biology, May 2014; 3(2), 333-344. Each 11-minute session consisted of ten 6-second sprints at maximum speed with a minute's recovery between each sprint.

[462] Andersen K et al. *Risk of arrhythmias in 52 755 long-distance cross-country skiers: a cohort study.* European Heart Journal, 2013; Vol.34, Issue 47: 3624-3631.

[463] Wilson M. *Diverse patterns of myocardial fibrosis in lifelong, veteran endurance athletes.* Journal of Applied Physiology. June 2011;110(6):1622-6.

[464] Taylor B A et al. *Influence of chronic exercise on carotid atherosclerosis in marathon runners.* BMJ Open, 2014; 4, *e004498.*

battlefield of Marathon to Athens to announce the Greek victory over Persia. What isn't so widely known is that shortly before that the energetic fellow had run 150 miles in 2 days to summon help from Sparta. The lesson seems plain: if you enjoy long-distance running make sure you don't overdo it!

A typical 20-minute HIT session looks like this:

- Warm up for 3 minutes.
- Exercise as hard and fast as you can for 30 seconds.
- Rest for 2 minutes.
- Repeat the two cycles of exercise and rest another five times.
- Spend 2 minutes in stretching.

Total time = 20 minutes. Do this two or three times a week only, not every day! Your body will need at least 48 hours to recover and repair itself after each session.

If you have a heart rate monitor it should register your maximum heart rate during those 30 seconds of high intensity exercise. Estimates of one's maximum heart rate are shown in Table 14. If you don't have a monitor just imagine two muggers with knives are chasing you and you have 30 seconds to reach the safety of your house!

Table 14: Estimated maximum heart rates by age[465]

According to sports fitness writer Phil Campbell, for 2 hours after a HIT session you should not consume any sugar in food or drinks and preferably no starchy carbohydrates if you want to maximize your body's production of the growth hormone.[466] This is because consuming carbohydrates will generate somatostatin, otherwise known as the growth hormone-inhibiting hormone.[467] Somatostatin is involved in the regulation of digestion, and it will shut down the production of the growth hormone that you started up as a result of all that hard work.

Although it has been shown that HIT exercise is beneficial to patients recovering

---

465 One's maximum heart rate can best be estimated as HRmax = 205.8 − (0.685 × age in years), not (220-age in years) as is popularly supposed.
See Robergs R & Landwehr R. *The Surprising History of the "HRmax=220-age" Equation.* Journal of Exercise Physiology, 2002; 5 (2): 1–10.
See also http://en.wikipedia.org/wiki/Heart_rate.

466 http://fitness.mercola.com/sites/fitness/archive/2012/02/10/phil-campbell-interview.aspx. Accessed July 2014.

467 *Somatostatin.* Wikipedia, accessed August 2014.

from heart surgery,[468] it would be wise to consult your doctor before starting it if you have any doubts at all about your health. In any case it is best to begin with only one or two 30-second bouts of such high intensity exercise, and to work up to the full six bouts per session over several weeks.

Warming up, cooling down and stretching

Every session of exercise should include a warm-up and cool-down period to decrease the risk of injury. Professional tennis players spend half an hour warming up before playing a match, but for you and me 5 to 10 minutes is probably enough. The warm-up period should consist of a gradual increase in the pace and intensity of the exercise. This enables the body to increase the blood flow to the muscles. The cool-down session should last a similar time, with the pace gradually decreasing. My own regular half-hour 'jogging' sessions go like this:

- 5 minutes normal walking
- 2½ minutes fast walking
- 2½ minutes gentle jogging
- 2½ minutes normal jogging
- 2½ minutes slow running
- 2½ minutes running
- 2½ minutes slow running
- 2½ minutes normal jogging
- 2½ minutes slow jogging
- 5 minutes walking

Age in years	10	20	30	40	50	60	70
Heart rate in beats per minute	199	192	185	178	172	165	158

'Running' at my age is not very fast, but it is as fast as I can go for 2½ minutes. That is important if you want to get fitter, because it is only when you push yourself beyond what is comfortable that your heart and lungs and muscles will decide they'd better grow stronger!

Fitness trainers also recommend stretching the muscles you have used for a few minutes after exercise. This can prevent subsequent stiffness and cramp. An Internet search for 'stretching exercises' provides lots of explanations in the form of diagrams and videos. The *'Commando Workout'* book I mentioned illustrates simple stretching exercises for use following both aerobic and strength training sessions.

---

[468] Warburton D E et al. *Effectiveness of high-intensity interval training for the rehabilitation of patients with coronary artery disease.* American Journal of Cardiology, 2005; 95,1080–1084.

Don't be weak: train each week!

Here's a plan for fitting in all the recommended exercises. See if it will work for you:

(i) Don't waste the last half hour of each day doing nothing in particular: go to bed at a reasonable hour instead. (I set two alarms every day: one tells me when it's time to wake up and the other reminds me that it's the time I intended to go to bed.)

(ii) From Monday to Saturday set your alarm to give you half an hour for exercise before you shower, dress and have breakfast.

(iii) Carry out the following programme:

- Monday: Moderate/vigorous aerobic exercise, e.g. jogging and running.
- Tuesday: Upper body strength training.
- Wednesday: Moderate/vigorous aerobic exercise.
- Thursday: Lower body strength training.
- Friday: Moderate/vigorous aerobic exercise.
- Saturday: ABS training.
- Sunday: Rest.

Involve your children too!

If you want to try high-intensity interval training instead of normal aerobics, here's an alternative programme:

- Monday: Upper body strength training.
- Tuesday: HIT. (No sugar and minimal carbohydrates for breakfast.)
- Wednesday: Lower body strength training.
- Thursday: HIT. (No sugar and minimal carbohydrates for breakfast.)
- Friday: ABS training.
- Saturday/Sunday: Rest.

Stick to either of the programmes above and you will soon feel the difference. Give it a month and then look in the mirror. You will see the difference too!

Either of these programmes will keep you fit and strong enough for all normal requirements. But if you want to continue increasing in strength and muscularity do each of the three strength training sessions twice a week instead of once a week. Similarly if you want to compete in an endurance sport like cycling or cross-country running you will probably have to double the number of aerobic sessions you do each week.

Grab some excitement

Why not motivate yourselves to get fit by committing your family to something exciting? Book accommodation for a sailing holiday on the Norfolk Broads; a walking holiday in the Lake District; a long distance walk like Hadrian's Wall, the Lyke Wake Walk across the North Yorkshire Moors or the South West Coastal Path; a Youth Hostel cycling holiday; the Three Peaks Challenge or the Welsh 3,000s (aiming to accomplish them in either 1 or 3 days); a skiing holiday; a local fun run, a half-marathon or even a full marathon. The day I wrote this section Prince Harry landed in Antarctica prior to walking to the South Pole in the company of several amputee and injured service personnel. Where there's a will there's a way!

CHAPTER 21: REST – NATURE'S MEDICINE

Don't work yourself to death

In spite of regulations such as the European Union Working Hours Directive, many working people find themselves under enormous pressure to work long hours, often unpaid, in order to meet the expectations of their employers, to compete with other employees for promotion, or else to manage their own business. An extreme example of this was the case of Moritz Erhardt, a 21-year-old trainee at investment bankers Merrill Lynch in London. In August 2013 he collapsed and died after working for 72 hours without a break.

The increasing use of tablet computers and smartphones means that many people in better paid jobs find themselves at work even when they are not at work, while others in less well paid employment may have to juggle two or more part-time jobs in order to keep the bailiffs from the door. And when one has a demanding family to care for on top of earning one's daily bread, the idea of resting from work and having some good quality leisure time may seem like an impossible ideal.

Nevertheless we should not try to work all hours of day and night if we are to remain healthy, competent and happy while fulfilling our responsibilities at work and at home. As Moritz Erhardt demonstrated, all work and no play can make Jack a *dead* boy. It nearly killed John D. Rockefeller, Sr. He entered business as strong and husky as a farm lad, and by the age of 33 he had made a million dollars. By dedicating every waking moment to working he became, at the age of 53, the world's richest man and its first billionaire. Yet by then his digestion was so bad he could eat only cream crackers and milk; his hair, eyebrows and eyelashes had fallen off, probably through zinc deficiency, and it was generally agreed that he wouldn't live another year. He couldn't sleep and life no longer seemed worth living. Eventually, during his long sleepless nights, it dawned on him that he wouldn't be able to take his wealth with him when he died; that it would be better to do some good with it while he still had the chance.

So he established the Rockefeller Foundation, a charity that eventually contributed millions of dollars to universities, hospitals, missions and help for the underprivileged. It funded copious medical research, which even today is saving millions of people from death by malaria, tuberculosis, diphtheria and other diseases. John D. Rockefeller completed his earthly life, contented and satisfied, at the age of 98![469]

One study I quoted earlier found that people under the age of 40 who suffered from coronary heart disease were four times as likely to have worked 60 hours or more a week for a prolonged period than a similar group of people who had no heart trouble. An 8-year study of male employees in Japan concluded that those who put in more than 50 hours of overtime a month were 3.7 times as likely to develop type 2 diabetes during the period of study as those who put in no more than 25 hours of overtime every month.[470] A major research review carried out for the U.K. government concluded that numerous problems associated with stress appear to be associated with long hours of work, particularly work in excess of 50 hours a week. These include gastrointestinal disorders, musculoskeletal disorders, problems associated with the depression of the immune system, and psychosomatic complaints likely to reduce efficiency and increase short-term absenteeism.[471] Clearly working very long hours is likely to damage our health in a serious way.

Working shorter hours doesn't necessarily mean that one achieves less. During the last 75 years many organizations and companies in different countries have reduced working weeks of anything from 48 to 60 hours down to 40 or 45 hours, and in each case productivity has remained the same or even improved, while absenteeism has diminished.[472] According to the Wikipedia article on 'Workweek and Weekend', every reduction of the length of the working week has been accompanied by an increase in real per-capita income.[473]

If you think you may be working longer hours than are good for you, there are two things you can do to put things right:

- Take some serious thought about how you can reduce your working hours – is it *really* necessary to work such long hours; can you reduce your working hours or reduce your travel time by finding employment nearer home, even if it means a reduction in income; can you reduce your expenditure so that you don't need to work full-time; can you reduce your workload by employing someone to help; can you simplify your housework or gardening or household administration in some way; can you share childminding duties with a friend, etc.?
- Make up your mind to have 1 day a week of complete rest from work. That is what we are going to think about now.

469　Retold from "None of these diseases", by S.I. McMillen, M.D. Lakeland books, 1966.

470　Kawakami N et al. *Overtime, psychosocial working conditions, and occurrence of non-insulin dependent diabetes mellitus in Japanese men.* Journal of Epidemiological Community Health, 1999; 53:359–363 35.

471　Spurgeon A et al. *Health and safety problems associated with long working hours: a review of the current position.* Occupational and Environmental Medicine, 1997; 54:367-375.

472　Spurgeon A et al. As above.

473　Gapminder Foundation (2011) "Gapminder World" graph of working hours per week plotted against purchasing power- and inflation-adjusted GDP per capita over time gapminder.org

A weekly day of rest

'Six days you shall labour, and do all your work; but the seventh day is a Sabbath (cessation) to the Lord your God; in it you shall not do any work...'
'And God rested on the seventh day from all his work which he had done.'
'And Jesus said to them, "Come away by yourselves to a lonely place, and rest a while." For many were coming and going, and they had no leisure even to eat. And they went away in the boat to a lonely place by themselves.'
'Come to me, all who labour and are heavy laden, and I will give you rest.'[474]

Whatever you may think of the Bible, it is extraordinary how much emphasis it places on the importance of rest. In fact it contains about 136 references to the subject, and even one of the Ten Commandments tells us to rest one day in seven.

Nearly all the research into the effects of working time relates to the number of hours worked rather than the number of days per week that people work, so the benefits of taking a whole day off once a week have not been quantified objectively. However there are five pointers to the belief that a weekly day of rest is very good for us indeed:

- Employment law – throughout Europe adult workers are by law entitled to an uninterrupted rest period of not less than 24 hours in each 7-day period, or if necessary 48 hours in each 14-day period. Mexican employment law also requires workers to have a day off each week, but in addition it explains that the purpose of this is to protect the health and physical and mental integrity of employees, to allow them to rest and re-energize themselves after the working week, and to provide them with time to spend with their families. Where practical the designated rest day should be Sunday.[475]
- Physical recovery – long-distance runners are advised to take one day a week off training,[476] while professional bodybuilders recommend training only 4 or 5 days a week. Perhaps Eric Liddell's gold medal in the 1924 Olympics was actually due to his refusal to run and train on Sundays.
- Business success – Jews in general will not work on their Sabbath, yet according to the 2013 Forbes' Billionaires list, 24 out of the 100 richest men in the world are Jews – or if not Jews then (as Sammy Davis Jr. once described himself) they are at least Jew*ish*. Since Jewish men make up only 0.1% of the world's population,[477]

---
474 *The Holy Bible*, Exodus 20.9,10; Genesis 2.2; Mark 6.31,32; Matthew 11.28.
475 Sáenz P. *Employment Law – Mandatory Weekly Rest Days*. Cacheaux, Cavazos & Newton, http://www.primerus.com, accessed May 2014.
476 Eyestone E. *The Rest is Easy - Why you have to back off in order to push hard*. Runners' World, April 2009.
477 http://en.wikipedia.org/wiki/Jewish_population_by_country. Accessed June 2014.

- i.e. 0.1 out of every 100, this is impressive, to say the least.
- Enjoyment – taking 1 day a week off work reminds us that we have to work to live, not live to work. It gives us freedom to enjoy the fruits of our labour and sets us free from the stress that that comes from feeling our life will fall apart if we dare to take any time off to relax. It reminds us that there are more important things than promotion and wealth and keeping up with the Joneses, McSporrans, O'Lympics or Hatwich-Fitzbadleighs, depending on which part of Britain we live in.
- The Bible – Jesus said that the Sabbath was made for man's benefit, and the Ten Commandments include one about keeping the Sabbath, with God's promise that people who keep it will prosper.

I'm not suggesting that you should do nothing once a week. When I was young many churchgoers thought it was wrong to mow the lawn or do the washing on a Sunday because that was work. But what if our daily work involves using our brains rather than our arms and legs? In that case mowing the lawn, hanging out the washing, cooking meals or even dusting can be therapeutic, provided it is something we enjoy rather than yet another source of stress. It is always helpful to look on such mundane tasks as a part of life rather than as irritating chores that prevent us from doing more important things. That revelation can totally relieve any sense of stress that routine tasks might otherwise cause. We could also look on many such activities as opportunities for taking necessary exercise while simultaneously getting something useful done – an excellent use of our time.

Obviously if our daily work involves a lot of physical exertion then, when we are not eating and drinking, we could well spend much of our day off lounging around with our feet up, chatting to friends, driving the family to the riverside or the woods for a gentle stroll, taking a long bath or simply sunbathing! If our work is not intellectually taxing then some mental activity would also be appropriate – perhaps reading a novel or a biography, engaging in a hobby, learning a foreign language, or something even more mentally demanding such as talking to our kids!

The important thing is that we spend our special day of rest recovering from work, enjoying our family and the world God has given us, and not worrying. We have to learn to rest in the knowledge that by taking a day off we shall, over time, achieve more than if we try to work flat out every day without taking a break What we mustn't do is to spend the day worrying about the jobs that we haven't had time to finish or even start. No doubt that is where the first part of that commandment comes in – 'six days you shall labour and do *all* your work'. If we work hard enough and wisely enough during the week to complete all our most pressing tasks for that week then we won't be tempted to try to finish them off on our rest day or spend it feeling guilty about wasting time during the week before.

While taking a weekly day off work is necessary to restore our minds and bodies, its other principal purpose, of course, is to give people of faith an opportunity to worship God. Most people, I think, would agree that it is good to have some kind of spiritual refreshment as well as the mental and physical kind, even if it is only through meditation, contemplation, listening to music or writing up a personal journal. All right, I know it's hard to find the time for such things with a family of demanding youngsters, but if there are two parents and you can share the same day off then it should be possible for each of you to have a bit of time alone at some point in it. One advantage of going to church is that very often you can dispose of the brats in Sunday school for an hour!

By building a weekly day of rest into your family's routine, and by explaining to your children your reasons for doing this, you will teach them to make it a part of their lives too. You will be pointing them along a safe pathway into adult life, helping them to avoid the kind of tragic mistake that young Erhardt made.

Therefore, so far as you possibly can, make it a priority to take a weekly day off from earning your living and doing anything at all that you find stressful. Make it a day to look forward to! Spend time having fun with your kids and fun with your spouse. Go for a walk or read a book or paint a picture. Do some of those things you'd like to do when you retire! Spend time enjoying the company of your Creator and the world he has made for you. You'll have more energy, strength and health, and as a result you'll be able to do even more during the other 6 days.

A good night's sleep

(i) We need to sleep

As well as periodic rest, we need adequate sleep. If we don't get the sleep we need then we shall inevitably feel tired, function inefficiently, or feel depressed and miserable – conditions which can lead to excessive drinking or to comfort eating and a gain in weight that will make us more tired than ever! Many jobs are inevitably stressful to some extent, and this only makes adequate rest and sleep even more important. If you don't make time to maintain your car's oil and water levels and tyre pressures, or if you omit its annual service, it will eventually break down. And if you break down, through neglecting the essential maintenance of your body and mind, what use then will you be to your boss or employees or family?

(ii) How much do we need?

When I was growing up I calculated the number of hours of sleep I needed in relation to my age, on the assumption that at birth I needed 12 hours per night and at 18 I would need 8 hours per night. So at 9 years of age I tried to get 10 hours a night and at 13.5 I tried to get 9 hours a night. On the same basis a 4.5-year-old would need 11 hours.

People do differ in how much they need. I'd have thought that people who worked with their brains would need more sleep than others, but the top athletes are said to sleep on average for 8.75 hours every night, which is an hour longer than most of us. So maybe it's not only our brains that need a good night's sleep. In the end, how much we need is a matter of trial and error. But remember that if it were not for candles and light bulbs we'd all probably be sleeping for 12 hours every night.

(iii) Getting off to sleep

Going to bed early isn't much use if you can't find your way into the Land of Nod, as my grandmother called it. And even if you can get to sleep it won't do you much good if you are restless and keep waking up. Poor sleep may be due to some physical or mental problem, which I will address shortly, but if you simply find it hard to drop off or stay asleep for a reasonable time, the chances are that you have things on your mind that you can't let go. If this is a problem for you, here are some suggestions:

- Keep a journal, and either before you get ready for bed or when you are in bed write down the significant things that have happened during the day, things that you've achieved and lessons you have learned.
- Keep a day planner, and before you get ready for bed write down what you plan to do tomorrow and any things you need to remember.
- Read a few pages of a story in bed – I always read aloud to my wife before we settle down for the night, and we both look forward to this, although she does tend to fall asleep before I have finished.
- If you believe in God, thank him for the day's events, ask his forgiveness for any ways in which you have let him or yourself down, and ask him to help you to do even better tomorrow; then commit yourself, or yourselves as a couple, into his care.

One of my personal 'sleeping tablets' is Psalm 4 verse 8:

> 'In peace I will both lie down and sleep;
> for thou alone, O Lord, makest me dwell in safety.'

When I say this slowly like a prayer, my breathing immediately slows down and my body relaxes. Sometimes I am asleep even before I have repeated it a second time.

Many years ago, before China became a communist country, a Scottish missionary pitched his tent one night in an area notorious for bandits. Unable to sleep for fear of attack he started to sing to himself one of the old Scottish metrical psalms:

*'I to the hills will lift mine eyes, from whence doth come mine aid:
My safety cometh from the Lord, who heaven and earth hath made.'*

Then he sang the second verse:

*'Thy foot He'll not let slide, nor will He slumber that thee keeps:
Behold, He that keeps Israel, He slumbers not, nor sleeps.'*

At that point he stopped. "Well, Lord," he said, "if you are going to stay up a' night there's nae need for me to do the same." And with that he turned over and fell safely asleep.

These thoughts give us some important clues as to how we can help our children to settle down for a restful night's sleep. At bed time:

- Talk over the day's events with them, praising any achievements, resolving any issues that have arisen, and reinforcing any lessons learned.
- Talk about the next day, unless you think it will get them too excited. (When something exciting was going to happen next day I used to say, "The sooner you go to sleep the sooner tomorrow will come.").
- Read or tell a short story or part of a story.
- If you believe in a personal God, have a little prayer time with them, including thanks, confession and forgiveness, preferably (I would say) combined with a story from a children's Bible.
- Give them a goodnight kiss.

That may seem a lot to do, but apart from one occasion I can't remember any of our children waking us up in the night after their first year or two, so it must have helped my wife and me to have a good night's sleep too.

(iv) Waking in the night

If my sisters and I had a nightmare when we were small we would call to our mother to come and rescue us, but she never did. She would always call out, "It was only a bad dream. Turn over and go back to sleep." And that always seemed to work. Nowadays if I wake up in the night and I can't get back to sleep I do one or more of the following:

- make myself a cup of tea
- take two paracetamol tablets
- watch some television
- read a story

- write down what's on my mind for action during the following day
- pray

Why am I so tired?

Sometimes chronic tiredness or lack of energy is due, not to overwork or lack of sleep, but to some underlying mental or physical problem. Constantly feeling fatigued or tired is like the low oil level light on your car's dashboard: it is a warning signal that all is not well with you. According to the Royal College of Psychiatrists, one in ten people in the U.K. suffers from chronic fatigue, and tiredness is one of the most common complaints that GPs hear. There are lots of possible causes, many of them related to diet:

- Physical causes – anaemia, underactive thyroid, diabetes, coeliac disease (gluten intolerance), chronic fatigue syndrome or ME, sleep apnoea (pauses in breathing, often caused by bad snoring – snoring is most common in middle-aged overweight men), glandular fever, restless legs (which disturb sleep), narcolepsy (poor sleep due to a problem in the brain caused by a protein deficiency), fibromyalgia (characterized by widespread pains and an excessively painful response to pressure), heart or lung problems, insufficient vitamin D or zinc, being overweight (which makes physical activity an effort), being underweight (an inadequate diet can weaken your muscles), inadequate exercise (which results in weak muscles and can result in poor sleep), pregnancy.
- Psychological causes – anxiety (often causes insomnia and hence tiredness), stress (resulting from moving house, bereavement, relationship problems, high-pressure work, unemployment, etc.), depression.
- Lifestyle causes – too little sleep, poor diet, too much alcohol (particularly last thing at night), too much caffeine, life pattern (night-shift work, caring for babies or young children, overwork, etc.).

If you are one of those one in ten people who constantly feels tired or weary then do whatever it takes to put things right. See your doctor if you think it might be something he can cure or give advice about, change your diet or behaviour if one of them is the cause, talk to your boss or get other help if the cause is overwork or undue stress. You are not meant to feel like this! There is a reason for it. Don't let it go on dragging you down and making your life a misery. Discover what the problem is and get it put right!

Hurrah for the hols!

That may sound like the sort of thing the Famous Five would have yelled, but looking back on my childhood the times I remember with most pleasure were indeed the holidays – whether they were spent at the seaside, at cub camps, on cycling tours or even just visiting the zoo or the local lido for a day. We are told that one in three adults tries to re-enact a holiday spent in childhood. Clearly family holidays are a very important part of childhood. A holiday environment provides a unique learning experience, especially for townies who may never have seen a wave or a rock pool, a river lock or a cow. For adults, getting away from home for a family holiday is the only way to break free from work and household jobs and unwind completely, and it is by far the best way to ensure that we can spend an extended time interacting with our children.

It is true that holidays with young children may not seem to be very restful, what with packing and unpacking, squabbles in the back seat of the car, or arguments about the window seat in the plane. There may be travel sickness to contend with on the journey and pouring rain when you arrive, and always there are mountains of washing afterwards, not to mention the problem of how you can afford to pay for it all. But don't give up on holidays! They really are worth all the trouble, especially for the youngsters.

Family holidays don't have to cost a fortune. Young children will happily play on a beach all day if the weather is kind, and when they are a little older they might love a holiday on a farm. Tents are astonishingly cheap these days, seaside caravans are available all around the coast, and if you want a rest from cooking as well as housework then youth hostels provide full board and facilities for families at truly reasonable prices. Holiday camps lay on masses of entertainment for everyone, and for families with younger teenagers climbing mountains and cycling along roads and cycle paths is free (if you all own boots and bikes), while adventure holidays such as those offered by organizations like www.proadventure.org may prove to be the experience of a lifetime. The important thing, both for you and your kids, is to do something different from the normal routine. If it can involve physical activity for everyone, even better. A change really is as good as a rest. Well, almost as good!

If you possibly can, I suggest taking a fortnight's holiday in one go rather than two separate weeks. You'll have only half the total amount of packing and unpacking, and after the first week when you have wound down and you are all used to your new surroundings and routine the second week will be far more restful and refreshing.

Enjoy life!

Proverbs 17.22 says, '*A cheerful heart is a good medicine, but sorrow makes the bones rot*'.

Fear, anxiety, resentment, anger, grief and guilt all make it impossible to be cheerful, and as we discussed in the section on stress in Chapter 4, prolonged exposure to any of these emotions increases the likelihood that some illness will overtake you. It is beyond the scope of this book to address this subject in more detail, but you need to recognize that such emotions will all cause serious problems if you don't find a way to deal with them. There are strategies for doing this and there are people who can help you.

Assuming, however, that you are not unduly burdened by such things, the original version of the proverb I misquoted remains true, '*All work and no play makes Jack a dull boy*'. If we want to avoid being dull, lifeless and ill, we must take time off work to enjoy the fruits of our labour. It is pretty well impossible to work all the time and maintain a cheerful heart. So whether it is our weekly day off or our annual holiday, the most important thing is to rest and have fun, especially with our own families! We all need to build times of rest and relaxation into our lives – for they are nature's medicine.

CHAPTER 22: HOME COOKERY – MANY COOKS DON'T SPOIL THE BROTH

This chapter deals with the important subjects of home cookery and teaching your children to cook.

Why cook at home?

Contrary to popular belief, a family in which everyone takes a hand in cooking at home is going to enjoy better broth as well as better food and drink in general, and very much better health, than a family who thinks a healthy meal is a fast-food beefburger with sugar-free ketchup.

In general, food prepared at home with fresh ingredients contains more vitamins and less sugar, salt and other chemical additives than food prepared in a factory or fast-food outlet. Home-cooked food can be prepared with less polyunsaturated fat, thereby reducing the harmful inflammation produced by oxidized free radicals and providing a healthier proportion of omega-3 fatty acids. It can be prepared with free-range eggs and organic milk, which contain much more omega-3 than food from hens and cows whose diet is dependent on cereals, and which are free from possible antibiotics and growth hormones. Bread and pastries baked at home from organic flour will be free from the potentially harmful chemical additives in commercial flour, while vegetables grown at home or by small market gardeners will have higher vitamin contents than those grown on large-scale enterprises where successive crops have depleted the nutritional content of the soil.

Home-cooked food is therefore healthier than commercially prepared food, and is less likely to produce diabetes, arteriosclerosis and the many other physical problems discussed earlier in this book. So for your own sake, as well as your children's, prepare as much food as you can at home.

There is a second, equally important, reason for cooking at home, and it is this. It is the only way you can teach your children to cook. They are unlikely to learn to cook at school, so teaching them to cook at home is really important. Why? Because it:

- builds family relationships, by providing an enjoyable and useful activity in which

you and your children can engage together, whatever their age
- provides unparalleled opportunities to teach them about healthy and unhealthy diets and to supply them with convincing reasons for choosing only healthy food and drink
- builds self-confidence, giving your children opportunities to feel proud of doing something well
- encourages creativity
- introduces them to new foods and helps to overcome fussy eating, as children will generally eat something they have prepared themselves
- equips them to take over some of the food preparation fully when they are older, eventually saving you time and effort
- gives them confidence in adult life to entertain guests and practise hospitality
- makes them more eligible life partners

On the last point, what impressed my future wife and perhaps persuaded her to start going out with me was my cooking an omelette for her over a gas ring in my room at university!

Children today face enormous pressures to consume too much unhealthy food and drink. These pressures come from:

- advertisers (when did you last see a TV advertisement for broccoli or fresh fish before a children's TV programme?)
- having enough pocket money or school dinner money to buy things like sweets, crisps, chips and beefburgers
- peer pressure not to eat uncool foods like lettuce and bean sprouts
- bad family eating habits that start from a young age

Teaching your children to prepare and cook good food from their early years will give you opportunities to talk about the differences between 'good' and 'bad' food and drink, to teach them the importance of eating food from the different nutrition groups (see Annexe 3), and to encourage them to try out foods with which they are not yet familiar. These are all invaluable items in their armoury against the sticks of rock and stones of potatoes that are continually hurled at them by Giant Obesity and the Sugar Plum Duff Fairy.

I don't have time

Employment seems to leave little time to learn or practise home cookery, and the availability of ready meals and takeaways can make it all seem like unnecessary hard work. But finding time for anything is always a matter of priorities, organization and self-discipline. We always find time to eat and sleep and (if we are employed) to go to work, because these are priorities for us. However, if we have children it should be an equal priority to spend some good interactive time with them. They need this for their development, and we save ourselves many heartaches when they are older if we build good relationships with them when they are young. So why not spend some of your kids' priority time by cooking with them? And get your husband or wife to take a turn too!

Solomon wrote that there is a time for everything under the sun, and while he didn't include frying eggs among the examples he gave he did say 'everything', so he must have meant frying eggs as well. The secret of finding some time to teach your kids to cook is to set a regular time for it, perhaps once a week or once a fortnight on a Saturday morning. Have it understood by everybody involved that this time is for cookery, just as bedtime is time for bed. Education, transport, business and manufacturing wouldn't survive without having set times for different activities, so what is wrong with having some set times for our home life, where what happens is just as important as what happens in those other areas of life?

Finding time for home cookery in general is possible with determination and the sensible allocation of one's time. If you will pardon a personal memory, my mother raised my two sisters and me with relatively little assistance from our partially blind father. Somehow she managed to work full-time as a school secretary, look after the house and a very large garden, raise chickens, do all our washing and ironing, sing in a choir *and* cook our meals: a two-course breakfast every day, a cooked meal at weekends and on weekdays during the school holidays. On top of that she cooked breakfast and an evening meal every day in term time for two university students who lodged with us. And as if that wasn't enough, I can still remember the revolting smell of potato peelings, old cabbage leaves, chicken mash and eggshells she used to stew for the hens' dinner. One year she even found time to paint all six doors on the landing a different colour!

The moral seems clear. Unless your circumstances are extraordinarily difficult, you do have time to prepare your family's meals at home, if you make up your mind to do so.

I don't know how to cook

If you are one of the many people who don't know how to cook, that is a problem, but fortunately it's one that can easily be solved. If you have children, learning how to cook *with them* is a wonderful solution!

Some years ago I produced some children's cookery software for the PC. It was approved by a government body for use in U.K. schools, and a home edition of it is still available for purchase. It contains three recipe books and three simple cookery courses, one for each of three age groups ranging from 5 to 13 years. It includes 32 videos of children carrying out basic kitchen activities, a menu designer with which users can design and print out menus for parties and other special occasions, and lots of teaching material. It even has a talking parrot! Annexe 2 in this book includes eleven of the recipes provided by 'Captain Cook's Tuck Box' as it is called, and you will see that they are all very simple. Of course any of the 208 recipes in the program can be printed out for use in the kitchen or for storage in a child's personal recipe folder. If you have a PC with the Windows™ operating system on it (up to and including version 8) then I recommend buying Captain Cook's Tuck Box Home Edition from the website, www.anastasis.co.uk. Kids love watching the videos and being able to make their own private online cookery books with their personalized recipes in it.

Another way to learn is, of course, to buy a beginners' cookery book. An Internet search for 'simple cookery', 'basic cookery' or even 'student cookery' will produce a number of suitable choices. Leith's Simple Cookery, The Hungry Student Cookbook and Mary Berry's Complete Cookery Book have all received favourable customer reviews from beginners in the U.K. North American readers would want an American book of course, because their measurement systems, terminology and available foods are so different.

Also keep a look out for '*Bad Food, Good Food – How to keep your family healthy in spite of 60 years of bad advice*'. I shall be publishing this new book early in 2015. Among other things it will include 4 weeks of healthy menus (breakfasts and two-course meals) based on the findings of 'Twenty-first Century Nutrition and Family Health'.

If you'd prefer more hands-on help, how about inviting a grandparent or even an elderly neighbour with time on her hands to come in once a week to give cookery lessons to you and your children? A single elderly person who likes cooking would probably be delighted to help like this and enjoy some company. If you belong to a church or a similar organization you might discover that there is even a retired cookery teacher among your members who would be pleased to help.

Failing all else, you could pay to attend a cookery course or have lessons at home, if you can afford it.

Microwaves – good buy or goodbye?

(i) Microwaved food is safe to eat

Many articles on the popular Internet tell us that microwaved food produces long-term brain damage; free radicals; cancers of the blood, stomach and intestines; emotional instability; loss of memory, concentration and intelligence, and other awful results. Most of this is completely untrue, but it can seem so convincing that I've devoted Annexe 7 to explaining in detail my reasons for dismissing it.

There is no need to say goodbye to your microwave. Extensive tests have detected no adverse effects of eating food cooked in microwave ovens. In relation to nitrosamines, vitamins, antioxidants and free radicals, food heated or cooked in a microwave oven is as healthy or healthier than food heated or cooked by other means. All the evidence for these statements is detailed in Annex 7.

(ii) Microwave ovens are safe to use with care

Microwave oven designs have to pass safety tests to limit the escape of microwaves to what are considered to be safe levels while the door is closed. Very low levels of leakage may occur, but any damage they might do is caused simply by heating whatever they impinge upon, not by some other mysterious property. Our eyes are the organs that are most vulnerable to such damage.

In some rather unpleasant research carried out in 1997 21 rats were confined for a month in special cages containing microwave ovens with the doors closed. In one group of seven the oven was switched on for 15 minutes a day, and in a second group for 30 minutes a day. A third control group were kept in a similar cage with an oven that was not switched on. In the first two groups of rats there was some slight damage to their eyes, especially in the 30 minutes-a-day group. The researchers concluded, '*Personal exposure from microwave ovens is generally minimal because of the rapid decrease in power density with distance. Microwave oven users do not normally stand as close to the oven as the rats in our study were placed; therefore, it is difficult to suggest that microwave ovens always have cataractogenic effects on human eyes.*'[478]

Microwave ovens are probably safer now than they were in 1997. Nevertheless you have been warned. Do not stand in front of a microwave oven looking at it while is switched on!

It is equally important not to use a microwave with worn seals or a damaged door, still less with a door that doesn't switch the power off the moment it is opened. A microwave oven in operation without the protection of its door would be exceedingly dangerous.

Uncured meats such as chicken portions or pork chops rely on the heat of cooking to kill any bacteria. Microwaves don't heat food evenly, particularly meat, so if you microwave meat on a high setting it might feel very hot on the outside yet still be cool in the centre. Don't cook it too fast and make sure that it is very hot inside as well as outside before you eat it.

Never heat eggs in shells in a microwave. They may explode! Even hard-boiled eggs and Scotch eggs can burst if heated too fast.

With those caveats I know of no research demonstrating a health hazard from the proper use of a properly functioning domestic microwave oven.

---

[478] Inalöz S S. *Do microwave ovens affect the eyes?* Japanese Journal of Ophthamology. July-August 1997; 41(4):240-3.

A word about barbecues

Barbecues are the heart of many happy social occasions, and they can be a good excuse for overeating once in a while. When I was a youngster I went to a church fete wheeling an old dolls' pram I'd converted into a hot dog stall. I fried frankfurters on it over a tiny methylated spirit stove bought in Woolworths for 2s 3d; that's 10p in today's money. Then I sold them to reluctant visitors along with bread rolls and tomato ketchup. What a good thing no health and safety inspectors attended our church!

The first proper barbecue I can remember was when our own children were youngsters. It was New Year's Eve and we were all in an untidy back yard overlooking the Straits of Magellan at the southernmost tip of mainland South America. There was still some light in the sky at 11.30 pm. Our dear host was roasting half a lamb for us on a home-made spit, so at midnight we were able to celebrate the incoming New Year with Coca-Cola and more meat than was good for us, accompanied by the happy hooting of Chilean naval vessels in the port.

There are two health hazards to avoid when managing a barbecue, quite apart from setting yourself on fire or collapsing unconscious from smoke inhalation.

(i) Sodium nitrite

Bacon, most frankfurter sausages, ham and other cured meats and sausages contain a preservative called sodium nitrite to stop the growth of Clostridium botulinum during the curing process. Its presence is identified by a pink colour. While the permitted concentration of sodium nitrite is believed not to pose a healthy hazard, it may do so if it is heated to a high temperature, when it can form cancer-inducing nitrosamines. As barbecues can get very hot it is safer not to barbecue any of these foods.

Even if you fry bacon in the kitchen do it gently and take care not to burn it!

Freshly made sausages and beefburgers don't contain sodium nitrite, nor do veggie burgers, cheeseburgers, or most frozen sausages, beefburgers and hamburgers; so you can cook these safely over a barbecue grill. If you are in doubt about a particular food, check its ingredients list.

(ii) Chicken and other raw meats

Rather like microwave ovens, hot barbecues can cook or even burn the outside of chicken drumsticks or pork chops before the inside has had time to heat up. In order to kill any bacteria, either barbecue raw meat and poultry slowly, or else pre-cook it in a conventional oven and reheat it within 24 hours on a barbecue to give it an authentic smokey flavour.

Taste the difference

For many years we contented ourselves in our family with ready meals of various kinds. It wasn't until the beginning of 2013 that we began to prepare all our meals at home. When my wife went into hospital, I had to travel long distances to visit her each day. To save time I bought myself a couple of frozen roast meals, the same kind that we had previously bought as a special treat for Sunday dinners. This time I could hardly believe how tasteless and unsatisfying they were in comparison with the food we had become used to eating! So apart from all its health benefits, home-cooked food has one other great quality that is not found in many pre-cooked meals: it is truly scrumptious!

CHAPTER 23: A FAMILY HEALTH MANUAL

An ounce of common sense

To be honest we don't need the Food Standards Agency or the NHS or any scientific research to work out what is a healthy diet. It is obvious to anyone with an ounce of common sense.

Nowadays tractors and combine harvesters and flour mills make it easy and cheap to produce millions of tons of flour from vast fields of cereals, cereals which have large ears as a result of selective breeding and the use of artificial fertilizers and pesticides. Consequently we can afford to eat huge quantities of bread and cake and pastry and cereals, so much that even Windy Miller with his windmill in the children's programme of the 1960s wouldn't have been able to supply enough flour to feed the inhabitants of Camberwick Green on today's diet. Centuries ago however it was very hard to grow and harvest large quantities of cereals using scythes, flails and winnowing fans, and grinding the grain into flour by hand was a long and time-consuming process. So although bread has been eaten for at least 4,000 years it was never eaten in anything like the quantities that we eat it today. Neither was pastry. And I can't find any mention at all of cornflakes or popcorn in the Bible, the Koran or the Bhagavad Gita. There's a story that three angels once visited Abraham. To entertain them in an appropriate manner he slaughtered an entire calf and told his wife Sarah to quickly knead three large measures of flour and bake some bread for them. He presented the bread to his important guests with, presumably, a huge quantity of meat. My point is that he wanted to give them a very special meal, and freshly baked bread was something as special in those days as an entire calf.

Again, the margarine and low-fat spreads and cooking oils which we use in the kitchen and which are used for the commercial baking of pies and pastries are made from cereal crops like oilseed rape and maize and soya. Have you seen those vast fields of bright yellow rape flowers in the early summer? For most of our human existence, it was never possible to obtain and consume such quantities of oil and fat as we do now from plant crops. The vast majority of the fat consumed in man's earlier history came from meat, fish, milk, olives and nuts, and relatively little from cereals. And we certainly didn't eat any trans fats, artificially made by a rather horrid industrial process from vegetable oils to thicken them and make them last longer before they go rancid.

Or think about sugar. Although sugar was known in Britain from ad 1100, it started to be used in significant quantities only in Elizabethan times.[479] Before that sugar in our diet came from fruit and milk, and a little from root vegetables. Nowadays vast acres of East Anglia grow lorryloads of sugar beet, so that sucrose, which is deadly to the teeth and a major cause of type 2 diabetes, is added to everything from cereals, cakes and biscuits, to drinks, ready meals and baked beans.

So the diet on which most of us live today is not a natural diet at all. It is one that, relatively speaking in terms of human history, has appeared only in the last few moments. Whether one believes in creation or evolution, it is obvious that the diet most people in the Western world live on is not the one we were made for. Rabbits were made to eat grass and other plants that contain mostly unsaturated fat, so they die if they are fed on saturated fat. We were made to eat a diet that is fairly rich in saturated fat and is not augmented by added sugar, so if we feed ourselves on anything else it is unsurprising if it makes us ill, and we are lucky if it doesn't kill us.

If evolution is true then man has spent 40 million years evolving a digestive system in which cereals and sugar cane or sugar beet provided a relatively small amount of his needs for dietary fat and energy. Throughout his evolution the majority of his food came from animals, fish, seafood, fruit, nuts, and vegetables. Cereals did play a part, but a relatively small part. Then suddenly, violently, he changed his diet, giving his digestive system no time at all to evolve sufficiently to cope with the change. Is it any wonder that obesity, diabetes, cancer of the liver and colon, and coronary heart disease suddenly walked on to the stage?

If, on the other hand, the world was designed and then created in its present form by God then the truth is even more obvious. He would surely have designed our bodies to eat the kinds of food that he created and provided for us, not food that man has himself produced using unnatural chemicals, unnatural methods, and in unnatural quantities that would be unthought of without the assistance of human technology.

Keeping the lid on the truth

In the light of such common sense it is difficult to comprehend why the government and the medical establishment and the health charities persist in recommending diets and supporting the sale of foods that started all these health problems in the first place. I think the main factors, as I've said already, are the vast incomes and profits at stake in the agricultural, food manufacturing, retail, advertising and pharmaceutical industries, and even the financial interests of medical researchers and the big health charities. If the spokesmen for these bodies all told us to eat naturally grown, naturally produced, home-cooked food in reasonable quantities, and if that is all we wanted to buy then so long as we didn't smoke or drink or take drugs we would nearly all be healthy and most

---

[479] The first sugar refinery was opened in Germany in 1537.

of these businesses as currently run would go bankrupt. And that, I am convinced, is the main reason for the propaganda and misinformation we receive, and for the reluctance of Western governments to intervene.

But there may be another reason too for keeping a lid on the truth. I have a sneaking feeling that many of the food and drug manufacturers and health advisory bodies such as the BMA and the NHS continue to hold the party line on low-fat and carbohydrates being healthier than saturated fat, because if they did an about-turn and said that it was following this advice that had actually caused heart disease, diabetes and obesity, then people who had suffered as a consequence might start suing them. Dieticians and doctors must be especially concerned about this possibility. The same goes for me, as the author of this book, which is one reason I have been so careful to provide the research evidence for the various statements I have made.

A recipe for family health

Physical and mental health depends on other factors as well as food. Here is a complete list of things under the control of a family that a family needs to be healthy:

- (i) healthy food and drink
- (ii) the right quantity of food for each person's energy needs
- (iii) the right proportions of protein, fat and carbohydrate
- (iv) a healthy balance of omega-3 and omega-6 fatty acids
- (v) adequate vitamins and minerals
- (vi) adequate fluids
- (vii) adequate exercise
- (viii) adequate rest and sleep
- (ix) manageable levels of stress

And people who smoke or take drugs should stop it. GPs can provide advice and help on this.

Let's talk about each of these in turn.

<u>(i) Healthy food and drink</u>

If you've read the book up to this point, you'll know that healthy food isn't necessarily what the food and drink producers tell us or sell us. To be sure that your family's food and drink is healthy:

- prepare as much food as you can at home, and involve your children in its preparation

- use fresh, organically produced ingredients, home-grown where possible
- filter your drinking water with the best system you can afford
- eliminate alcohol and added sugar from your family's diet

The sooner you start, the better! According to Felicity Lawrence[480] even a mother's breast milk is flavoured by whatever she has been eating and drinking. Indeed my wife couldn't eat onions when she was breastfeeding one of our babies because they always gave him diarrhoea! In most cases however, if you eat a natural and healthy diet with a variety of flavours you will encourage your breastfed baby to enjoy a similar range of flavours when it is weaned. Of course, weaning children on natural foods, blended or mashed, doesn't please Heinz, Cow and Gate and the other manufacturers of the 500 or so baby foods that are sold in a typical supermarket. Lawrence writes, *'For the food business, baby cereal from a packet, and a child's palate trained on industrial tastes and textures, graduating to jars of baby food and then to yet more processed food, is the ideal path.'*

(ii) The right quantity of food for your energy needs

The quantity of food you need depends on your age, height and level of physical activity. Young children and very old people generally need less than teenagers and adults in general. Children and teenagers will need more during growth spurts than at other times.

Overall quantities of food required are measured in terms of calories consumed each day. The NHS recommends 2,500 calories a day for an average adult man in the U.K. and 2,000 calories a day for an average woman.[481] For children aged 7 to 10 it recommends 1,970 calories a day for boys and 1,740 a day for girls.

Recommendations by USDA (the United States Department of Agriculture) for the 7 to 10 age group are similar to U.K. recommendations, but include recommendations for other age groups too, as shown in Table 15. Their recommended calorie ranges are fairly wide, not only because they cover several years, but because inactive, sedentary children need far fewer calories than active ones.

---

480 Lawrence F. *Eat Your Heart Out: Why the food business is bad for the planet and your health.* Penguin Books, 2008.

481 The term 'calorie' as used here is actually short for 'kilocalorie'. A kilocalorie is 1,000 scientific calories. A scientific calorie is the amount of heat required to raise the temperature of 1ml of water by 1°C.

Table 15: Recommended daily calorie intakes for children of different ages[482]

Age range	Boys	Girls
1 – 3 years (toddlers)	1,000 – 1,300	1,000 – 1,300
4 – 6 years (pre-school/infants)	1,300 – 1,800	1,200 – 1,700
7 – 10 years (juniors)	1,500 – 2,300	1,250 – 2,000
11 – 14 years (lower secondary)	1,700 – 2,750	1,500 – 2,250
15 – 18 years (upper secondary)	2,150 – 3,250	1,800 – 2,400

In the end the quantity of food one needs each day depends on what happens to one's body:mass index (BMI) and waistline.

Although BMI is widely used in the health profession, the cut-off points at which someone's BMI is assessed as underweight, normal, overweight or obese are somewhat arbitrary. For example the 'NHS choices' calculator classifies a child as obese if his BMI puts him within the heaviest 2% of children of the same age, sex and height, whereas in the U.S.A. a child in the heaviest 3% is classed as obese.[483] Secondly the values are based simply on the average weight and overall range of weights of the sample population, so if you lived in Southern Sudan, for example, a BMI that put you in the top 2% or 3% of weight for your height would probably mean you were one of the few healthy people there! Thirdly BMIs do not distinguish between the weight of fat and muscle, so some perfectly fit rugby players, for instance, might be classified as being overweight. And finally there is no research evidence that relates any of these cut-off points to some precise measure of health or ill health.

Nevertheless, in the absence of better guidance, your children will probably be eating suitable overall quantities of food if their weights remain within the normal BMI range for their sex, height and age, as shown in Table 16. For adults a healthy BMI is considered in Britain to lie between 18.5 and 25.0.

---

[482] The values shown are derived from USDA values, assigned to age ranges more useful in the United Kingdom.

[483] *A simple guide to classifying body mass index in children.* NHS National Obesity Observatory, June 2011.

Table 16: Body Mass Index ranges for children[484]

Age in years at birthday	BOYS Under-weight if BMI is below	BOYS Over-weight if BMI is above	BOYS **Obese if BMI is above**	GIRLS Under-weight if BMI is below	GIRLS Over-weight if BMI is above	GIRLS **Obese if BMI is above**
2	13.8	17.8	**18.8**	13.3	17.7	**18.7**
3	13.3	17.3	**18.3**	13.1	17.3	**18.4**
4	13.4	17.3	**18.4**	13.1	17.6	**18.8**
5	13.5	17.4	**18.6**	13.0	17.7	**19.1**
6	13.4	17.6	**18.8**	12.9	17.9	**19.5**
7	13.3	17.8	**19.3**	12.9	18.3	**20.2**
8	13.3	18.3	**20.1**	13.0	19.0	**21.1**
9	13.4	18.8	**20.8**	13.3	19.7	**21.9**
10	13.7	19.5	**21.7**	13.6	20.4	**22.8**
11	14.0	20.2	**22.7**	14.0	21.2	**23.8**
12	14.3	20.9	**23.5**	14.5	22.0	**24.8**
13	14.8	21.7	**24.3**	15.0	22.8	**25.7**
14	15.3	22.5	**25.2**	15.5	23.6	**26.5**
15	15.8	23.2	**26.0**	15.9	24.2	**27.2**
16	16.3	23.8	**26.8**	16.3	24.7	**27.7**
17	16.8	24.5	**27.4**	16.7	25.2	**28.2**
18	17.3	25.2	**28.0**	16.9	25.5	**28.6**
19	17.7	25.7	**28.6**	17.2	25.8	**28.9**
20	18.0	26.2	**29.1**	17.4	26.2	**29.2**
Cut-offs	<2%	>95%	>98%	<2%	>95%	>98%

The Body Mass Index is assessed in the same way for both adults and children:

$$BMI = \frac{(\text{Weight in kilograms})}{(\text{Height in metres}) \times (\text{Height in metres})}$$

For example an 8-year-old boy who weighs 25kg and is 1.25 metres tall will have a BMI of

$$BMI = \frac{25}{1.25 \times 1.25} = 16.0$$

---

484 Values taken from U.K. *Growth Charts, Second Edition*, January 2013, published by the Royal College of Paediatrics and Child Health

Since 16.0 is between the values of 13.3 and 18.3 shown in Table 16 for 8-year-old boys, this particular boy is neither underweight nor overweight: his weight is about right.

Being underweight or overweight may indicate some emotional, physical or lifestyle problem and it may produce medical problems later, so if your child is underweight or overweight you might want to seek medical advice.

Some people believe that one's waistline is a more reliable guide than BMI to the possibility of weight-related health problems, or at least that one's waistline should be taken into account as well as one's height and weight. Excess weight around the midriff seems to correlate better with type 2 diabetes, for example, than excess weight in other parts of the body. One method is to measure one's waist-to-hip ratio (WHR). This is simply the circumference of your waist at your navel divided by the circumference of your hips at their widest point. (You can use centimetres or inches.) Table 17 suggests good, average and overweight values for adults.

Table 17: Guide to waist-to-hip ratios for adults[485]

	Men	Women
Good	Less than 0.8	Less than 0.7
Normal	0.81-0.94	0.71-0.85
Overweight	0.95 or more	0.86 or more

An even simpler method which has been recommended for children is just to measure their waist circumference. Table 18 suggests maximum healthy waist circumferences for boys and girls at different ages.

---

485 Waterson S. *Commando workout*. Thorsons, 2002.

Table 18: Guide to maximum healthy waist circumferences for children[486]

Age in years	Waist circumference Boys cm	Girls cm
3.5	50.3	53.1
4.5	53.3	55.6
5.5	56.3	58.0
6.5	59.2	60.4
7.5	62.0	62.9
8.5	64.7	65.3
9.5	67.3	67.7
10.5	69.6	70.1
11.5	71.8	72.4
12.5	73.8	74.7
13.5	75.6	76.9
14.5	77.0	79.0
15.5	78.3	81.1
16.5	79.1	83.1
17.5	79.8	84.9
18.5	80.1	86.7
19.5	80.1	88.4

As we have seen, the fruit sugar fructose causes weight gain around the midriff, and fructose constitutes 50% of common sucrose sugar. So if you or your children start to develop a pot belly then it really is important to reduce your family's sugar consumption in confectionery, chocolate, drinks, cakes, biscuits, many manufactured pies and pastries, fruit, fruit juice, beer and similar drinks. Abdominal fat is strongly associated with diabetes, so taking action to dispel it is essential.

If you measure your family's BMIs and waists from time to time you will know whether you and your children are eating too much or too little. If necessary you can then adjust the quantities accordingly, or perhaps encourage more exercise.

(iii) The right proportions of protein, fat and carbohydrate

Dieticians normally specify the proportions of these three major food groups, or 'macronutrients', in terms of the percentage of calories we obtain from each of them. In this context 'carbohydrate' includes both starches and sugars. According to Dr. Mary

---

[486] Taylor R W et al. *Evaluation of waist circumference, waist-to-hip ratio, and the conicity index as screening tools for high trunk fat mass, as measured by dual-energy X-ray absorptiometry, in children aged 3–19 years.* American Society for Clinical Nutrition, August 2000; Vol.72 No. 2:490-495.

Enig,[487] the approximate proportions of protein, fat and carbohydrate in many traditional, healthy diets were 20%, 40% and 40% respectively. Nevertheless in 1994 the U.K.'s Committee on Medical Aspects of Food and Nutrition Policy (COMA) recommended that 50% of energy should come from complex carbohydrates (starches) and no more than 10% from sugar – a total of 60% from all carbohydrates rather than the 40% identified by Dr. Enig's research. And the same committee recommended that no more than 35% of energy should come from fat, leaving a mere 5% from protein![488]

It is difficult to lay down a firm rule about the ideal proportions of these macronutrients, because people's needs differ, particularly people of different races and people who live in cold or hot parts of the world. African races whose bodies are designed to live near the equator need less fat, and Eskimos and other northern races need more. Asian people, who have traditionally used a lot of rice, can tolerate relatively more complex carbohydrates. More active people need more carbohydrates for immediate energy needs, and people living in colder climates need more fat for insulation purposes. In the light of everything we have talked about, and I mean everything, it seems to me that most Westerners who don't have particularly active lifestyles and who enjoy central heating in the winter need protein, fat and carbohydrate in calorific proportions of about 25%, 45% and 30% respectively, regardless of COMA's recommendations. These are the proportions I would recommend, and they are very different from the 14%, 38.5% and 47.5% proportions eaten by the average Briton,[489] North American or Australian citizen nowadays, which are producing so much obesity.

During earlier epochs of human existence eating greater quantities of meat and fish probably provided even more than 25% of a person's energy from protein and more than 45% from fat, but aiming for more than 25% from protein these days would be too expensive for many families. And while 45% of calories from fat is not that different from the 38.5% Britons typically consumed in 2011, much more of it should be obtained from saturated fat than from the seed oils that most people consume. Dr. Enig lists studies of people groups in eleven different countries around the world where the inhabitants consume up to 70% of their calories as fat, much of it saturated, yet they remain relatively free from disease and have long lifespans.[490]

So what does a 25%, 45%, 30% diet look like? I prepared a 3-day menu with proteins, fats and carbohydrates in exactly these proportions. You can see it in Annexe 1. Now I'm not suggesting that you should limit yourself to this particular menu, still less that you should try to measure the protein, fat and carbohydrate in your weekly shopping

---

487 Fallon S & Enig M G. *Americans Now and Then.* Price-Pottenger Nutrition Foundation Health Journal, 1996; 20:4:3.

488 Scientific Advisory Committee on Nutrition, SACN/02/26 03/10/02.

489 *Family Food 2011.* U.K. Government Department for the Environment, Food and Rural Affairs.

490 Fallon S with Enig M G. *Nourishing traditions: the cookbook that challenges politically correct nutrition and the diet dictocrats.* New Trends Publishing Inc. Second edition, 2001.

and keep the associated calories to the exact proportions above. My point in preparing Annexe 1 is to give you a general idea of the kinds and quantities of food we need to eat in order to achieve a healthy balance, one which won't set us or our children on the road to obesity, heart trouble, type 2 diabetes or several forms of cancer.

The recipes for the meals listed in Annexe 1 are given in Annexe 2. They include two older recipes with sugar in them, but it would be better to omit the sugar in the fruit pie recipe and replace the cooking apples with eating apples, and to use a granulated low calorie sweetener for the Floating Islands drink.

So what does Annexe 1 teach us about a healthy diet?

- A healthy diet contains only a little food that is high in starch. Although this menu plan still provides 30% of the total calories from carbohydrates, over the 3 days it includes only 4½ slices of bread per person, 25gm of flour, half a large potato, no breakfast cereals other than a small bowl of porridge, and no cakes, biscuits, rice, pasta, crisps or starchy snacks at all. Adding more of such foods would inevitably increase the percentage of calories from carbohydrates to above 30%.
- A healthy diet contains little or no added sugar or sugary foods and drinks. The suggested plan allows only a rounded teaspoonful of sugar and a level teaspoon of reduced sugar jam over the 3 days. It would be better still to omit the sugar altogether.
- Although many people on this diet would consider that they were eating well, particularly at breakfast, it provides only 1,823 kilocalories a day. This may mean that the British government's recommended daily calorie intakes of 2,000 kcals for women and 2,500 kcals for men are too high. That would help to explain why so many people in the U.K. are overweight. Alternatively it may be that with a diet richer in protein one doesn't need to consume so many calories. In the end, as I said earlier, you can discover the number of calories you need to maintain a constant weight only by trial and error, since it depends on your personal height, metabolism and lifestyle. If necessary you could always eat larger quantities than those shown, so long as you increase them all by the same proportion. Children would need smaller quantities than those shown in the table.
- In order to obtain 25% of calories from protein it may be necessary to take a protein supplement. In this menu plan, 5% of the protein calories are provided by one drink of 25gm of whey protein. Whey protein is sold as a plain or flavoured powder that makes a milky drink when mixed with water. Tubs of it are sold in health food shops at a cost of around 60p per drink, so it is fairly expensive.
- Since meat, fish and seafood are clearly the main sources of protein in food, vegetarians would have to eat plenty of fish and seafood, or huge quantities of eggs and dairy products, or gigantic quantities of nuts and mushrooms (including soya products and Quorn), in order to obtain 25% of their calories from protein.

Their only alternative, so far as I know, would be to consume substantial amounts of protein supplements such as whey protein, if that is permissible.
- The final column, headed 'Calorie Index' shows the best foods to eat to increase your protein consumption relative to your carbohydrate consumption. The higher the value the better. As you can see, the highest values, shown in white, are for cod, lamb's liver and chicken. The lowest values, shown in dark grey, are for sugar, fruit and fruit juice. The calorie indices for starchy foods such as rice, spaghetti, couscous and milk chocolate digestive biscuits, which are not included in this menu plan, are −0.8, −0.7, −0.6 and −0.5 respectively, all low values indicating that it is best not to eat too much of them.
- A healthy diet includes nourishing, cooked breakfasts. This is because eggs and other protein-rich foods delay hunger pangs longer than carbohydrate-rich foods such as breakfast cereals with the same number of calories. If you don't feel hungry you won't be tempted so much to go snack hunting.
- A healthy diet includes fruit and vegetables. Ideally, as we saw in the chapter on sugar, we should eat a fruit and five vegetables a day. Annexe 1 doesn't achieve that aim so clearly it isn't perfect.

How much would such a diet cost? The 3-day menu shown in Annexe 1 was carefully costed in 2013 mainly from Tesco's website, based on mid-range prices and normal sizes. The total cost, including all the suggested snacks, and of course the 'essential' three drinks of coffee a day, worked out at £33.72 per person per week, or nearly £68 a week for two people. (£68 is about US$110 or Aus$124.) This included the cost of minor items such as herbs, which are not shown, some rather expensive out-of-season blackberries and runner beans that found their way on to the menu, and the whey protein drink. It does not allow for possible savings on the more expensive items like meat and fish, which might be bought more cheaply in your local market or on offer in a supermarket, nor any savings that could be made on the bulk purchases of goods, home-grown produce and home-made bread and yogurt.

£33.72 is more than the average British adult spends each week on food and drink. The Office for National Statistics reports that the average household in the U.K. spent £53.40 a week on food and non-alcoholic drink in 2009-2011.[491] With an average number of 2.28 inhabitants per household, that works out at £23.40 per head per week. This includes children, who wouldn't eat so much, so the average expenditure per adult would be rather more than this, particularly in the south-east where we live and the average household expenditure was £57.80 rather than £53.40. Moreover prices have gone up since the survey was carried out, so the average weekly expenditure per adult in our area is probably over £30.00 by now and not much less than the £33.72 estimated for this

---

[491] *Family Spending, 2012. Chapter 5: Weekly household expenditure, an analysis of the regions of England and countries of the United Kingdom.* Office for National Statistics, Feb 2013.

sample healthy diet. However the same report stated that the average U.K. household spent £11.70 a week on alcoholic drinks, tobacco and narcotics, with the majority of that on alcohol. If that is representative of your family you could always switch that expenditure to pay for a healthy diet and thus be doubly better off, in both health and finances!

I'll say more about costs when I get to the end, but meanwhile, let's see if we can address some other important points.

(iv) A healthy balance of omega-3 and omega-6 fatty acids

I explained that a principal cause of 'Western' diseases is eating too many omega-6 fatty acids from seed oils in relation to omega-3 fatty acids from fish, meat and eggs, etc. Remember the red and grey squirrels? This is one matter, at least, on which all the scientists and nutritionists seem to be united. But how can you get the balance right? There are two steps you need to take:

- Follow the government's advice to eat two 140gm portions of fish or other seafood a week (two 60gm portions a week for children), one of which should be oily fish. For ecological reasons I think it is best not to eat any more.
- Reduce your omega-6 consumption to around 60gm a week. This means cutting out most of the high omega-6 foods listed near the end of Chapter 7.

Is that really practical? What would a diet with a healthy balance of omega-6 and omega-3 actually look like? It shouldn't surprise you to learn that it looks like the menu for a 25:45:30 protein:fat:carbohydrate calorie distribution that I referred to in Annexe 1. The 3 days of food and drink shown in Annexe 1 have an overall O-6-3 ratio of just under 4 to 1, which is probably the upper limit for a healthy diet. So even with such 'luxuries' as fruit pie and jam sandwich fritters, it is possible to enjoy a healthy balance of omega fatty acids, provided that you prepare such food yourself to ensure that it hasn't been made with commercial seed oils like sunflower and corn oil.

The fact that the Annexe 1 diet meets both of the requirements for a healthy diet – an overall calorie ratio of 25:45:30 and an overall O-6-3 ratio of under 4:1 – confirms to me that such a diet really is good for us, whereas a diet high in sugar, carbohydrates and omega-6 fats is the true cause of the nation's current diet-related health crisis.

In order to obtain this healthy balance of omega-3 and omega-6 fatty acids I had to include 42.5gm of crab meat and 120gm of cod per person over a 3-day period. This is equivalent to 380gm of seafood a week, which is 35% more than the minimum weekly amount of 280gm that the government recommends. As we have seen, if everybody in the country ate even the recommended amounts there would be severe problems in maintaining fish stocks without a huge increase in fish farming. I also included a little powdered flaxseed because it has a lot of omega-3 in it, although it is the ALA kind, which is not so fully utilized by our bodies.

The main 'problem' ingredients in the sample diet, the ones that produce the greatest difference in omega-6 and omega-3 fats, are the sausages, bacon, liver and salad dressing. Without these four ingredients the overall O-6-3 ratio would be a super-healthy 2.8:1, and in that case it wouldn't be necessary to eat so much fish. Omitting the salad dressing would improve everything except the taste, but if the sausages, bacon, liver were omitted then the protein level would fall too low. However it is quite likely that in the U.K. at least the three meat items have much better O-6-3 ratios than the ones I used. This is because I had to obtain the omega-3 and omega-6 contents from the American USDA database,[492] and the diet of most U.S. animals is significantly higher in omega-6 fatty acids than it should be as a result of adding maize and soya beans and other cereal products to their feedstuffs. For example, the O-6-3 ratio for eggs given by the USDA database, which I used in calculating the overall ratio for the diet, was 17:1, but as I mentioned earlier, measurements made on the eggs of naturally reared free-range hens can give a ratio as low as 1:1. So in reality, a diet like the one I have described would probably provide in the U.K. an overall O-6-3 ratio well within the healthy range even with only one portion of fish a week provided it is of the oily kind. It's a pity we have to use American data on omega contents, but that's all that seems to be available.

The 'best' ingredients in the menu, the ones that actually contain more omega-3 than omega-6, are of course the cod fillets, the crab meat and the powdered flax seed. However there are some other ingredients in this 3-day menu that provide a surplus of omega-3, albeit of the vegetable kind. These are runner beans (green beans), cabbage, red kidney beans and lettuce. All of these help in a small way to maintain a healthy balance between the red and grey squirrel populations. But although squirrels like acorns, never include acorns in your diet. Acorns have 46mg of omega-6 per gram and no omega-3 at all, so their O-6-3 ratio is infinity!

<u>(v) Adequate vitamins and minerals</u>

Chapters 11 and 12 tell you how important it is to include an adequate supply of vitamins and minerals in your family's diet. They also explain how to do this, but here is a summary of the main points:

- Make sure that your family's diet includes foods containing as many as possible of the vitamins and minerals they need. See Annexe 3: Nutrients, functions and sources.
- Buy organically grown produce, and prepare as much food as you can at home

---

[492] USDA National Nutrient Database for Standard Reference. ndb.nal.usda.gov/. (The values were obtained via the KIM-2 software - efaeducation.nih.gov/sig/kim.html.)

from fresh, organically produced ingredients, home-grown where possible.
- Vitamins B and C are gradually lost from fruit, vegetables and salads when they are stored. Fresh fruit and vegetables can lose up to 70% of their vitamin C in a week. So buy them fresh and eat them as soon as possible!
- If you live in the U.K. and you don't get out into the sunshine much take 2,000 units of vitamin D_3 a day throughout the year. If you do get out into the sunshine you probably don't need them from March 21st to September 21st.
- Consider taking a combined multivitamin and mineral supplement, or just a magnesium supplement, on a regular basis.

(vi) Adequate fluids

I've covered the subject of drinking water in Chapter 16. We saw that the widespread rule about drinking 2 litres of water a day has no scientific basis. Instead, I recommended drinking at least one cup of something at breakfast and lunchtime, preferably tea because of its antioxidant value, a full glass of water with one's evening meal, and further supplies of water or other fluids during the day as needed.

For drinking and cooking purposes it is best to use tap water filtered with at least an activated carbon block to remove chlorine, organic substances, pesticides, herbicides and mercury. Ideally combine this filter with a reverse osmosis system to remove other inorganic substances, radionuclides, nitrates, sodium and fluorides. Your local water supplier will tell you if your drinking water is fluoridated. If it is, having a reverse osmosis system is more important since nothing else can remove fluorides, protecting your children from dental fluorosis and yourself in older age from brittle bones and teeth. The only possible advantage of fluoridated water is to protect teeth from decay, and if you cut out sugary food and sugary or acidic drinks from your family's diet then tooth decay won't be a problem.

(vii) Adequate exercise

Chapter 20 explains why exercise is so important and how to motivate yourself and your family to get enough of it.

Have you ever seen a family with two young crash-helmeted kids cycling along at speed together on a summer's day, or watched a fit-looking family of four play an energetic game of volleyball on the beach, or travelled up Snowdon by the mountain railway and met two healthy-looking youngsters under 10 years old who had just climbed the same mountain by foot with both their parents? *And* via the awesome Crib Goch ridge? And did you ever wish that your family could be like that? It can be! Your kids can easily be among the fittest in their school, and you and your spouse could be two of the fittest parents. All it needs is a decision to get fit, some targets to aim at, and a mutual decision to hit those targets. All you need to know in order to do this is explained in Chapter 20. You have all the knowledge and ability that you and your family need to become very fit. So work out together what you are going to do! Involve your children in this if they are old enough. Make up your mind as a family to go for it!

(viii) Adequate rest and sleep

In Chapter 21 I wrote about the great importance of a weekly day of rest, adequate sleep, and family holidays. I listed a whole range of reasons for chronic tiredness and lack of energy, and I encouraged you, if necessary, to identify the causes and put matters right. Finally, I recommended enjoying life as the best medicine of all.

(ix) Manageable levels of stress

This final section of my 'Manual of Family Health' has to do with managing stress. As we saw in Chapter 4, constant stress is one of the three principal causes of heart trouble, and perhaps of mental illness too, as well as being a major source of tiredness and fatigue. There are various warning lights for stress on our body's dashboard:

- insomnia
- chronic tiredness
- fatigue – a feeling of weariness and a lack of energy
- irritability, bad temper and angry outbursts
- feelings of resentment
- poor concentration
- unusual clumsiness
- tearfulness
- headaches and migraines
- heart palpitations
- breathlessness
- high blood pressure

And a blood test would probably indicate higher than average levels of stress-related hormones.

If you think you may be suffering from stress then do something about it, for everyone's sake and especially for your own. Chapter 4 provides lots of suggestions on ways to manage stress, so read it again and put into practice any relevant advice you can find as soon as possible.

A personal story

For many years my wife had to take the drug metformin and strictly avoid sugar in order to control her diagnosed type 2 diabetes. Then she adopted the kind of diet recommended in this chapter. 18 months later she was told she no longer needed any medication. She stopped taking it, and her blood glucose level has remained well within normal limits ever since. Type 2 diabetes can be reversed!

CHAPTER 24: THE COST OF GOOD HEALTH

During the last 70 years the misguided advice on diet given by successive governments and other authorities, under pressure from the enormously powerful food and drink industries, has resulted in gigantic additional costs to the health service, to industry through lost working hours, and to individual human beings in terms of health and happiness. The resulting cost of alcohol alone has been estimated at £21 billion a year in the U.K., while the human cost of fatal heart attacks, diabetes damage, diet-related cancers and multiple health problems arising from obesity is incalculable.

It is true that many families will have to spend more money and time than they currently do in order to buy good quality food and prepare it at home. They may also have to assign more time to physical exercise and sleep, and less time with the TV or the latest online game to become master of the universe! So in this last chapter I need to address the important question, "Is good health affordable, in terms of money and time?"

As I wrote earlier, the 3 days of menus shown in Annexe 1 were costed in 2013 at nearly £34 per week per person, which was perhaps £5 a week more than an average adult living in the south-east of England spent on food each week. (For North American readers £34 is equivalent to US$55, although I suspect that food in general is cheaper in the U.S.A. than it is in the U.K.) There are many ways to reduce the cost of food, for example by taking advantage of special offers, bulk purchases, and end-of-week reductions; buying fruit and vegetables from market stalls; shopping at cut-price stores such as Aldi and Lidl; or simply eating smaller quantities. Sometimes the supermarket's own brand is the same as the more expensive branded product except for its labelling. Most supermarkets also sell a range of very low cost products characterized as 'Value', 'Basics', 'Savers', etc. I found that a 'Savers' tin of macaroni cheese from Morrisons contained less sugar and more protein than the most famous brand did. Similarly a 'Savers' tub of full-fat soft cheese contained more protein, less sugar and less salt than the market leader, and at a third of the price. The premium on a branded product may simply be to pay for the television commercials that promote it!

Regarding time, cooked breakfasts take about 15 minutes a day to prepare. Main meals take about 45 minutes on average, but if you make sufficient for 2 days at a time and freeze the spare food to reheat it another day then the average preparation time per meal is probably around only 30 minutes. That makes an average time of 45 minutes for preparing two cooked meals a day, assuming that older children haven't yet started to help, in their school holidays at least.

So far as exercise time goes, we've seen that children over 5 years old need at least an hour a day of energetic activity, while adults need 2½ hours a week of moderately intense aerobic exercise or 1¼ hours a week of vigorous aerobic exercise or ¾ hour a week of high-intensity interval training; plus about an hour a week of strength training.

So the final question I must answer for you is this: how can you find the money and time necessary to provide a healthy diet and lifestyle for yourself and your family?

Unless you are really hard up or exceptionally limited in time it all comes down to priorities. Many people spend a fortune on health and life insurance, even though insurance never stopped anyone from getting ill or from dying prematurely. In the U.S.A. in 2010 the amount spent on private health care was US$136 or £82 per head per week.[493] For the average American family of 2.6 people that is *£213 per week*! And a great number of the illnesses contracted in the U.S.A. are simply due to the kind of food people are spending their money on. Rather than spend their money on health insurance to pay for medical treatment when they get ill, wouldn't they be far better off spending it on a healthy diet so that they don't get ill in the first place? And wouldn't it make sense if we in the U.K. did the same?

In the U.K. most medical expenses are still covered by the NHS, which we also pay for through National Insurance, but that won't help a lot if you die of a heart attack as my brother-in-law did when he was 40, or if your children contract type 2 diabetes due to too much sugar and carbohydrate in their diet, or if you have to retire early from work due to joint problems arising from obesity. My former boss died exactly 1 week before he was due to retire at the age of 65. I wonder how much he would have been willing to pay each week into a life insurance policy that would somehow have guaranteed that he would not lose perhaps 20 years of a life of leisure as an old-age pensioner?

There isn't any such life insurance policy, but there is a way to protect ourselves from dying prematurely from the illnesses we have been talking about. That is to take out a family 'life insurance' policy by paying for good food. For make no mistake: bad diet is killing people! Poor diet was almost certainly the main factor in my brother-in-law's death. There was no history of heart trouble in his family, he kept fit through playing football and he had no job worries, but he lived on fast food, and unfortunately not for very long.

Spending money on bad food and drink is like buying ill health. The only effective way to buy good health for yourself and your family is to spend your money on healthy food and drink, and to spend your time in such a way that you all have adequate exercise, freedom from harmful stress and sufficient sleep. It is better to spend your money on good food than on lottery tickets. It is better to invest in a healthy diet than in stocks and shares. Consider the money and time that you spend in buying and preparing healthy

---

493 *Health, United States, 2012. Table 114 Personal health care expenditures, by source of funds and type of expenditure: United States, selected years 1960–2010.* U.S. Department of Health and Human Services, Centers for Disease Control and Prevention, National Center for Health Statistics.

food as an investment with a wonderful return.

Suppose that preparing healthy food at home gives you just 5 additional years of healthy life. If it costs you £5 extra per week (and you don't save that much by reducing your alcohol intake) then over 40 years you will have spent a massive £10,000 extra. But currently the government will repay you more than double that amount through an extra 5 years of state pension! And if you have a private or occupational pension you will be paid many, many times more in return. Even if you have no pension at all you might be able to pay off the extra you have spent on food by working for an extra 6 or 12 months as a result of your improved health, and still enjoy an extra 4 years or more of active retirement for the same overall cost.

On a parallel line of thought, if preparing such food takes an extra 35 minutes a day, then after 40 years you will have spent a total of one extra year in food preparation, but in return you will have gained 5 years of additional healthy life, for your family as well as yourself! A 500% personal return on your time is a good investment by any standard, not to mention eating nicer food for the rest of your life. And regard the additional time that you spend encouraging your children to grow fit and strong through physical games and exercise as a further investment for their future, as well as for your own.

In 2013 people in the U.K. spent on average an astonishing 3 hours 52 minutes every day watching live television.[494] If you spend anywhere near that amount of time it shouldn't be difficult to transfer 35 minutes of it each day into food preparation, which is surely far more important. You'll find that reducing television time isn't so hard as you might think. Three members of our family don't have a television at all in their homes.

Another way to find extra time is through delegation. That's how business bosses succeed, and in your own home you are the boss of one of the most important businesses in the world – child raising. John Wesley's mother, Susannah, gave birth to 25 children of whom sixteen survived infancy, yet she found time to converse privately with each one of them once a week, as well as educate them all at home, even when her husband had temporarily left her. How did she manage this? She did it through discipline and delegation. The children were each given duties to do according to their age, and the older ones looked after the younger ones.

In our own family, I once posted on the kitchen noticeboard a weekly rota of household jobs for our four young children to do. Each day they had a different task to carry out, suited to their abilities. It is true that within 2 days the heading had mysteriously changed from 'The Happy Helpers' Rota' into 'The *Un*happy Helpers' Rota', but so long as my wife and I persisted in our supervision of it, the helping continued.

Perhaps the most important time-saving thing you can do is to involve your children in cooking from as young an age as possible. Our grandson has enjoyed 'helping' in the kitchen since the age of 2. A little chef's hat and apron can make it more fun. As I wrote earlier, if you involve your youngsters in meal preparation they will not only learn about

---

[494] www.bbc.co.uk/news/business-26221364.

healthy eating but before many years they'll be able to take over some of the cooking for you. And even when they don't help to prepare a meal, there is no reason why Mum or Dad should have to do the washing and wiping up as well if there are younger hands capable of doing it.

It's amazing what youngsters can achieve when they are given responsibility for tough assignments. When I was 12 years old my mother decided that we needed a coal bunker. She presented me with a pile of bricks, some bags of sand and cement, a bucket, a trowel and a wheelbarrow, and told me to get on with it. The bunker housed our coal for years, and while it wasn't perfect I always felt proud of it. It even had a sliding wooden door!

A generation later, our two older children couldn't speak Spanish when we moved to Chile, but within 9 months my wife had delegated the whole of the weekly supermarket shopping to them. They were allowed to buy a hot dog each as a reward. 'Hot dog con todo' was the favourite: a frankfurter in a bread roll with avocado pear, tomato, green chillies, tomato ketchup, mustard and lots of mayonnaise!

Investments of time and money in nutritious food and an ordered family life will never lose their value through inflation or bank failures or the collapse of the stock markets. Put into practice the advice you have read in this valuable book and you will be investing in a lifetime of health for yourself and your loved ones. And not only health, but self-esteem and self-confidence, cookery skills and hospitality, better family relationships, and freedom from obesity with all its associated ills. You will be investing in a long and enjoyable life for your entire family. You are all worth it!

Keep rereading *Twenty-First Century Nutrition and Family Health* in order to maintain your motivation. When *Bad Food, Good Food – How to keep your family healthy in spite of 60 years of bad advice* is published, buy a copy for your older children to read. You and your family will then enjoy all the wonderful benefits I have just described. And if I can help you to do that then I shall die happy. But not, I trust, until at least my hundredth birthday!

Annexe 1: 3-day menu based on protein:fat:carbohydrate calorie percentages of 25:45:30

Table A.1: 3-day, 1,823 calorie per day menu for one person based on protein:fat:carbohydrate calorie percentages of 25:45:30. There is a discussion about these recipes in Chapter 23 (iii): 'The right proportions of protein, fat and carbohydrate.'

Meal	Item[1]	Details	Serving for one	Calories from Protein	Calories from Fat	Calories from Carbs	Total calories	% calories from Protein	% calories from Fat	% calories from Carbs	Calorie Index[2]
Breakfast	1 large boiled egg;	Eggs, free range	1 large	30	60	0	90	33	67	0	0.3
	1 slice of wholemeal bread with butter	Wholemeal bread	1 slice	16	10	60	86	19	11	70	-0.5
		Butter	6gm	0	44	0	44	0	99	0	0.0
Snack	Wafer thin roast Chicken on ½ slice buttered wholemeal toast.	Wholemeal toast	½ slice	8	5	30	43	19	11	70	-0.5
		Cooked chicken	7gm wafer	6	1	0	7	83	13	0	0.8
		Butter	3gm	0	22	0	22	0	99	0	0.0
Lunch	Welsh rarebit with extra cheese and tomato	Wholemeal bread	1 slice	16	10	60	86	19	11	70	-0.5
		Butter	6gm	0	44	0	44	0	99	0	0.0
		Grated Cheddar cheese, reduced fat	40gm	46	78	0	124	37	63	0	0.4
		Beaten egg	¼ egg	6	12	1	19	33	63	3	0.3
		Tomato	½ large	1	1	3	4	16	15	69	-0.5
	Floating islands (chilled milk and ice cream drink)	Sugar	4gm or small tsp	0	0	16	16	0	0	100	-1.0
		Full-cream milk	100ml	13	32	19	64	20	50	29	-0.1
		Vanilla ice cream	1 scoop	5	24	43	72	7	34	60	-0.5
Dinner	Beef curry with with extra meat	Brown onion	¼	1	0	8	10	14	5	82	-0.7
		Apple	¼	0	0	14	15	2	3	95	-0.9
		Braising steak	112.5gm	103	80	0	183	56	44	0	0.6
		Butter	4gm	0	28	0	28	0	100	0	0.0
		Sultanas	6gm	1	0	17	18	4	1	95	-0.9
		Tomato purée	4ml or small tsp	2	0	8	10	21	0	79	-0.6
		Cabbage	½ mug	4	0	20	24	17	2	81	-0.6

262

Meal	Item[1]	Details	Serving for one	Calories from Protein	Calories from Fat	Calories from Carbs	Total calories	% calories from Protein	% calories from Fat	% calories from Carbs	Calorie Index[2]
	Fruit and yogurt	Tinned apricot halves in natural tin	75gm or ¼ of small tin	2	0	30	32	6	0	94	-0.9
		Banana	½ a small one	1	1	31	33	4	3	93	-0.9
		Grapes	8	1	2	28	32	3	7	90	-0.9
		Sugar-free yogurt	50gm	7	14	9	30	22	47	30	-0.1
		Apple juice	15ml or 1 tblsp	0	0	7	7	1	0	99	-1.0
Breakfast	Fried sausages, baked beans and orange juice	Pork sausages	2	64	232	15	311	21	75	5	0.2
		Light baked beans	104gm or ¼ large tin	18	5	50	73	25	6	69	-0.4
		Fresh orange juice	150ml glass	4	0	60	64	6	0	94	-0.9
Snack	Marmite on ½ slice buttered wholemeal toast	Wholemeal toast	½ slice	8	5	30	43	19	11	70	-0.5
		Marmite	5gm or 1 level tsp	8	0	5	13	61	0	39	0.2
		Butter	3gm	0	22	0	22	0	99	0	0.0
Lunch	Fried lamb's liver, red kidney beans and lettuce; whey protein drink with full-cream milk	Lamb's liver	150gm	122	37	0	159	77	23	0	0.8
		Olive oil for frying	4ml	0	31	0	31	0	100	0	0.0
		Little Gem lettuce	¼ lettuce	1	1	2	4	23	26	51	-0.3
		Red kidney beans	65gm	18	4	46	68	27	5	68	-0.4
		Whey protein	25gm	75	12	7	94	80	13	8	0.7
		Full-cream milk	150ml	20	22	63	105	19	21	61	-0.4
Dinner	Smoked cod fillet	Cod fillets	One 120gm fillet	86	4	0	91	95	5	0	1.0
	Runner beans	Runner beans	100gm	6	4	13	23	28	16	56	-0.3
	Celery and tomato salad	Carrots	½	1	1	16	18	7	7	86	-0.8
		Cherry tomatoes	2	0	0	2	4	34	26	140	-1.0
		Celery	1 stick	0	0	0	0	0	0	0	n/a
		Salad dressing	15ml	1	37	12	50	2	74	25	-0.2
	Fruit pie and custard	Flour	25gm	10	3	71	84	12	3	84	-0.5
		Butter	12.5gm	0	92	0	92	0	100	0	0.0
		Blackberries	50gm	2	1	10	13	14	7	79	0.0

263

Meal	Item[1]	Details	Serving for one	Calories from Protein	Calories from Fat	Calories from Carbs	Total calories	% calories from Protein	% calories from Fat	% calories from Carbs	Calorie Index[2]
Breakfast		Cooking apples	125gm	2	1	45	47	3	2	94	-0.7
		Sugar	3gm or ½ tsp	0	0	12	12	0	0	100	-1.0
		Whole milk	77.5ml	10	25	14	50	40	100	58	-0.2
	Fried bacon and egg plus tomato juice	Bacon, back rasher	1 x 47gm rasher	30	78	0	108	28	72	0	0.3
		Free range eggs	1 large	30	60	0	90	33	67	0	0.3
		Olive oil for frying	4ml	0	31	0	31	0	100	0	0.0
		Tomato juice	100ml only	2	0	16	18	13	0	87	-0.7
Snack	Crab meat on buttered wholemeal toast	Toast	½ slice	8	5	30	43	19	11	70	-0.5
		Tinned crab meat	42.5gm or ¼ tin	28	0	2	31	92	1	7	0.9
		Butter	3gm	0	22	0	22	0	100	0	0.0
Lunch	**Spanish omelette**	Small onion	¼	2	1	12	15	14	5	82	-0.7
		Butter	4gm	0	28	0	28	0	100	0	0.0
		Large boiled potato	¼	5	1	43	49	11	2	87	-0.8
		Medium tomato	¼	1	1	2	4	16	15	69	-0.5
		Small green pepper	¼	1	1	3	4	20	17	64	-0.4
		Eggs	2	60	121	0	181	33	67	0	0.3
		Whole milk	½ tblsp	1	2	1	5	20	50	29	-0.1
	Courgette salad	Button mushrooms	1½	3	2	1	6	54	34	12	0.4
		Cherry tomatoes	1½	1	0	2	3	17	13	70	-0.5
		Courgettes	½	7	3	7	17	40	20	40	0.0
		Lemon juice	1ml or ¼ tsp	0	0	0	0	13	10	76	-0.6
		Olive oil	15ml or 1 tblsp	0	31	0	31	0	100	0	0.0
		Vinegar	15ml or 1 tblsp	0	0	0	0	23	17	60	-0.4
	Muesli with flaxseed	Dried apricots	2	2	1	43	46	4	1	94	-0.9
		Porridge oats	22.5gm	31	18	85	133	23	13	64	-0.4
		Chopped nuts	1 level tsp	2	23	0	26	9	90	2	0.1
		Desiccated coconut	6gm	1	35	2	38	4	92	4	0.0
		Powdered flaxseed	6gm	5	21	9	35	14	60	25	-0.1
		Plain yogurt	120ml	23	114	19	156	15	73	12	0.0

Meal	Item[1]	Details	Serving for one	Calories from			Total calories	% calories from			Calorie Index[2]
				Protein	Fat	Carbs		Protein	Fat	Carbs	
Dinner	**Meat loaf**	Minced beef	114gm	89	121	0	210	42	58	0	0.4
		Small onion	¼	1	0	5	6	14	5	82	-0.7
		Fresh breadcrumbs	1 tblsp	4	2	15	22	19	11	70	-0.5
		Large eggs	½	15	30	0	45	33	67	0	0.3
	Potato salad with peas	Small new potatoes	85gm	6	2	55	63	9	4	87	-0.8
		Sweetcorn, frozen or tinned	14gm	1	1	5	7	16	14	70	-0.5
		Olive oil	5ml or 1 tsp	0	41	0	41	0	100	0	0.0
		Vinegar	10ml or 2 tsp	0	0	0	1	23	17	60	-0.4
		Frozen peas	50gm	12	4	19	35	34	11	55	-0.2
	Jam sandwich fritters	Wholemeal bread	1 slice	16	10	60	86	19	11	70	-0.5
		Reduced sugar strawberry jam	1 level tsp	0	0	9	9	1	0	98	-1.0
		Butter	6gm	0	44	0	44	0	99	0	0.0
		Large eggs	½	15	30	0	45	33	67	0	0.3
		Whole milk	15ml or 1 tblsp	2	5	3	10	20	50	29	-0.1
DAILY	Whole milk for tea or coffee	190ml (1/3rd pint) milk		75	185	107	367	20	50	29	-0.1
	Mug of whole milk for supper	250ml	750ml total over 3 days	99	243	141	483	20	50	29	-0.1
Overall percentages of protein, fat and carbohydrate								25.0	45.0	30.0	
Average calories per person per day							1,823				

1. The recipes for meals shown in **bold type** can be found in Annexe 2.
2. In the final column Calorie Index = (P-C)/T = (Protein calories - Carbohydrate calories)/(Total calories). Higher numbers are best, especially those in the white cells.
3. Water and items such as herbs and seasoning that have negligible calorific content have been omitted from the listed ingredients. The only drinks that have been allowed for are tea and coffee with milk but no sugar, and a whey protein drink made with milk. Additional fruit drinks, fizzy drinks containing sugar and all types of alcoholic drink would increase both the total calories and the proportion of carbohydrates in the diet.
4. Some approximate measurements used are as follows: 1 teacup = 0.25 pints = 150ml. 1 small glass = 6 fl oz = 175ml. 1 mug = 1 U.S. cup = 250ml.
5. The calories for each ingredient are calculated from the weights of protein, fat and carbohydrate in each ingredient. 1gm protein or carbohydrate = 4 kcal, and 1gm fat = 9 kcal. The weight of each nutrient in any food may be found by looking it up on a website such as www.tesco.com.

6. The total of 1,823 kilocalories is calculated from the values declared by the product manufacturers or retailers, not from the values listed in the table, which total 1,748 calories. The difference is because the formulae for converting protein, fat and carbohydrate to calories are not precise and they don't include calories from bran.

Annexe 2: Recipes for the 3-day menu

Table A.2: Recipes for the 3-day menu in Annexe 1

'Total time' includes preparation and cooking, if any. Ingredient quantities are for 4 servings unless otherwise stated.

Recipe and total time	Ingredients	Method
Welsh rarebit with tomato 20 minutes	4 slices of bread 25gm butter 160gm reduced fat Cheddar cheese grated 1 egg beaten 1 teaspoon ready-made mustard 1 large tomato, sliced ½ teaspoon Worcestershire sauce Salt Pepper	1. Grate the cheese on to a plate and beat the egg in a bowl. 2. Mix the cheese, mustard, egg, Worcestershire sauce, salt and pepper together in the bowl. 3. Toast the bread on one side only under the grill. 4. While it is toasting, slice the tomato in four. 5. Butter the untoasted side of the bread, spread the cheese mixture over it and put a slice of tomato on top. 6. Replace it under the grill until the cheese bubbles up.
Floating islands 3 servings, 40 minutes	1 level tablespoon instant coffee or cocoa powder 1 level tablespoon sugar or granulated sweetener ½ teacup hot water 1 teaspoon vanilla essence 300ml cold milk 3 scoops vanilla ice cream Cocoa powder to sprinkle	1. Put the hot water into a bowl. 2. Add the coffee or cocoa powder and sweetener and stir well until dissolved. 3. Add the vanilla essence and milk and stir again. 4. Refrigerate until very cold – at least 30 minutes. 5. Take the mixture out and whisk it until it foams. 6. Put a scoop of ice cream into each of three glasses. 7. Fill each glass with the mixture and sprinkle with a little cocoa powder. 8. Pop a straw in each glass and serve!
Beef curry (Recipe for a slow cooker) 6 hours 35 minutes	1 brown onion 1 apple 2 cloves of garlic 450gm braising steak (diced by the butcher if possible)	1. Preheat the slow cooker. 2. Top, tail, peel, slice and chop the onion. 3. Cut the apple from top to bottom into four pieces and remove the core. 4. Peel the garlic cloves and crush them beneath a spatula. 5. Fry the onion and garlic with the butter in a large frying pan for 5 minutes.

	15gm butter 25gm sultanas 1 teaspoon medium strength curry powder 1 teaspoon ginger (preferably ready chopped, otherwise ground) 1 teaspoon powdered turmeric 300ml boiling water 3 teaspoons tomato purée 2 mugfuls of shredded cabbage Salt Pepper	6. If necessary use a clean knife to dice the meat on the cutting board. 7. Add the meat to the frying pan and cook it on a medium to high heat until it is browned, turning it from time to time. 8. Stir in the apple, sultanas and the three spices; cook for a further 5 minutes. 9. Empty the contents of the pan into the slow cooker, add the boiling water, tomato purée, salt and pepper to taste, and stir. 10. Cook for 6 hours on auto. 11. Serve with steamed cabbage.
Fruit and yogurt 5 minutes	1 small tin apricot halves in natural juice (e.g. apple or pear juice) 1 large banana 32 grapes 6 tablespoons yogurt – plain or Greek	1. Slice the banana and wash the grapes. 2. Divide all the fruit between four serving bowls. 3. Spoon the yogurt over the fruit. (Prepare this dessert just before eating it so that the bananas don't go brown.)
Celery and tomato salad 20 minutes	2 grated carrots 8 cherry tomatoes 4 sticks celery 60ml salad dressing	1. Chop the celery into 1cm lengths. 2. Cut four of the tomatoes into four pieces for the salad. 3. Mix all the ingredients together and add the salad dressing. 4. Cut the remaining tomatoes in two for a garnish. (If you prefer, use a small pointed knife to cut them with a zigzag pattern around the circumference, pulling the two halves apart when you have cut all the way round. Each tomato will then be in two 'water lily' shapes.)
Fruit pie and custard 60 minutes	100gm flour, plain or self-raising 50gm butter 2 tablespoons water 200gm blackberries 500gm cooking apples 1 level tablespoon sugar 2 teaspoons milk	(This is a faster method of making pastry that works well with plain flour. It is better to replace the cooking apples and sugar specified in the recipe with eating apples.) 1. Preheat the oven to 180°C. 2. Wash the blackberries in a sieve. 3. Peel, core and slice the apples. 4. Melt the butter in a saucepan and thoroughly stir in the flour. 5. Mix the water in, or at least enough to make a firm dough.

| | | 6. On a clean, lightly floured surface roll out the dough until it is the size and shape of an ovenproof pie dish. Invert the dish over the pastry and trim any excess pastry from the edges.
7. If you are using a pie funnel, place it in the centre of the dish. Place the fruit in the dish with a teaspoonful of water, and sprinkle the sugar (if used) over it.
8. Brush a little water around the edge of the dish, then carefully place the pastry on to it. (You can do this by rolling the pastry around a rolling pin to lift it up, then unrolling it over the dish.)
9. Trim off any excess, then press down the edges with the fork.
10. You can use any remaining pastry to make decorations like leaves or flowers. Brush them with milk to keep them in place on top of the pie.
11. If you are using a pie funnel, press the pastry down around it so that the top sticks through; otherwise make a small hole in the pastry to create a steam vent.
12. Brush the top of the pie with milk, place it on a baking tray and bake it in the oven for about 35 minutes until it turns a golden brown colour.
13. Serve with custard or cream. |
| Spanish omelette 25 minutes | 1 large potato
1 small onion
15gm butter
1 medium tomato
1 small green pepper
A little salt
A little pepper
8 eggs
2 tablespoons milk | 1. Peel the potato and microwave it on medium/high (750 watt) for about 8 minutes until just soft.
2. Meanwhile skin and finely chop the onion. Fry it gently with the butter in a large metal-handed frying pan for about 5 minutes, stirring occasionally.
3. Meanwhile chop the tomato into small pieces.
4. Deseed and slice the green pepper.
5. Add the tomato, green pepper, cooked potato, salt and pepper to the cooked onion and butter.
6. Lightly whisk the eggs and milk with the fork in a bowl. Add this to the vegetables and mix them together.
7. Continue to cook the omelette over a medium heat until it is just dry on top.
8. Place the pan under a hot grill and cook it until the omelette bubbles up and is golden brown in colour. |

Courgette salad 20 minutes	6 button mushrooms 2 courgettes 3 medium sprigs parsley 1 spring mint 1 teaspoon lemon juice 4 tablespoons olive oil 4 tablespoons vinegar A little salt A little pepper 6 cherry tomatoes	1. Wash the mushrooms, wiping off any dirt with a cloth. Slice them thinly and put them into the salad bowl. 2. Wash the courgettes and slice them thinly. Steam them for 3 minutes. Do not overcook them. 3. Meanwhile cut up the parsley and mint leaves, and add them to the mushrooms. 4. Put the lemon juice, oil, vinegar, salt and pepper into an empty bottle or jam jar, put the lid on, and shake it vigorously. 5. Place the courgette slices in a colander and rinse them with cold water. They should still be crunchy. Add them to the other ingredients in the bowl. 6. Cut each tomato into quarters and add them to the salad. 7. Pour the dressing over them, mix and serve. 9. Serve with a green salad and crusty bread.
Meat loaf 4 generous servings, 85 minutes	460gm minced beef 1 small onion 1 tablespoon chopped parsley ¼ teaspoon mixed herbs A pinch of salt A splash of Worcestershire sauce 4 tablespoons fresh breadcrumbs or crumbled stale bread 2 large eggs	1. Preheat the oven temperature to 180°C. 2. Brown the beef by frying it for 5 or 6 minutes in a little olive oil, turning it halfway through. 3. Skin the onion and chop it into small pieces. 4. Beat the egg in the small bowl. 5. Mix all the ingredients together in the large bowl. 6. Line a loaf tin with greaseproof paper and press the meat loaf mixture into it. 7. Bake it on a baking tray for 1 hour above the centre of the oven. 8. Turn it out on to a dish, slice it up, and serve.
Potato salad with peas 10 minutes	340gm small cooked new potatoes 55gm sweetcorn, frozen or canned 1 tablespoon olive oil 3 tablespoons vinegar ½ teaspoon mixed herbs 200gm frozen peas	1. Heat the peas with a little water in a saucepan until hot. 2. Meanwhile chop the potatoes in half. 3. Rinse the sweetcorn in cold water and put it in a salad bowl with the potatoes. 4. Put the olive oil, vinegar and herbs into a jar. Put the lid on and shake it well. 5. Pour the dressing over the salad in the bowl, mix and serve it with the peas.

Jam sandwich fritters 30 minutes	4 slices of medium sliced white bread 1 tablespoon reduced sugar strawberry jam 25gm butter 2 eggs 4 tablespoons milk	1. Butter each slice of bread and make two jam sandwiches. 2. Cut them into quarters. 3. Whisk the egg with the milk in a bowl. 4. Dip the quartered sandwiches into the egg and milk mixture. 5. Melt the butter in a large frying pan, taking care not to overheat it. 6. Fry the sandwiches for 1 or 2 minutes, then turn them over and continue to cook them until they are golden brown on both sides.

Annexe 3: Nutrients, functions and sources

Table A.3: The nature, functions, sources and effects of nutrients

Nutrient	Description	Functions	Food groups in which it is found	Effects of having too much or too little
Proteins	Proteins are complicated chemical substances. They are assembled in our bodies from a selection of much simpler chemicals called 'amino acids' in accordance with instructions from our genes. There are only 20 different amino acids, but there are probably more than a million different kinds of protein in the human body.[495] Our bodies obtain the amino acids from animal and vegetable protein, then turn these acids into the kinds of proteins that humans need. Each protein has its own particular function that is essential for bodily growth and health.	• Building and repairing bones, muscles, hair, teeth & internal organs. • Digestion and other chemical reactions. • Protection from infection. • Carrying messages around the body. • Transport and storage, e.g. building the oxygen-carrying red corpuscles in our blood.	• Meat, poultry, fish and eggs • Dairy milk products (milk, cheese, cream, butter, etc.) • Cereals, nuts (including peanut butter), seeds, lentils, beans (including products made from soya beans such as tofu and soya milk) and peas • Smaller quantities are provided by some vegetables such as sweetcorn, artichokes, potato skins, kale, broccoli & Brussels sprouts. Foods in the first two groups above contain all the amino acids that the body needs in about the right proportions. Foods in the last two groups contain most but not all of the body's requirements. However if you eat a variety of them you can obtain all that you need.	Eating *far too much* protein can produce health problems in the liver and kidneys (painful kidney stones) as these organs try to dispose of the excess, and can result in calcium being extracted from the bones producing osteoporosis (weakening of the bones). Too many meat and dairy products, just like too much starchy food and sugar, will produce weight gain, which may produce various health problems if it is excessive. If the body receives *too little protein* for its needs it starts to break down its own protein into amino acids. First the muscles grow weak and flabby, then other tissues begin to degenerate with increasingly harmful effects.

---

[495] Jensen O N. *Modification-specific proteomics: characterization of post-translational modifications by mass spectrometry.* Current Opinion in Chemical Biology, 2004; 8, 33-41.

Nutrient	Description	Functions	Food groups in which it is found	Effects of having too much or too little
Sugars	A **carbohydrate** is a chemical molecule made out of carbon, hydrogen and oxygen. Sugars are simple carbohydrates with relatively small molecules.[496] The most common kinds of sugar are sucrose, glucose, fructose, lactose and maltose. Sucrose, which is what we buy in a bag of sugar, is a slightly more complex molecule than the others. It is a combination of glucose and fructose.	• Glucose is the body's petrol.[497] The body burns glucose to produce energy, which is used for heating and working. • Our bodies can turn sucrose, fructose, lactose and maltose into glucose, so these sugars are also a source of energy. • Glucose is ready for use almost as soon as it is swallowed, but for other kinds of sugar the digestion process takes a little longer. • Sugars make food and drink taste sweet as well as providing energy.	• Glucose Pure glucose can be bought in powder or tablet form for use by athletes or people who need an urgent boost of energy. • Sucrose This is extracted mainly from sugar cane or sugar beet. It is sold as packeted sugar and icing sugar. Sugar from sugar cane is also sold as syrup and treacle. • Fructose Fructose is fruit sugar. It is found in fruit and honey, and there is a little in some vegetables. • Lactose Lactose is milk sugar. It is found in cow's and goat's milk. • Maltose Maltose is made from malted grains like barley, brown rice and millet. It can be bought as a syrup or powder for sweetening food, but it mainly occurs in drinks like beer.	Sugar in food: • causes tooth decay,[498] especially in children and teenagers • contributes to excessive weight by providing more energy than the body needs • in excess it can result in the development of type 2 diabetes If sweetening is needed then the substitution of artificial sweeteners will reduce tooth decay. It is sensible to clean your teeth immediately after eating sugary food. For the effects of being overweight, see below under starches.

---

[496] A molecule of glucose, for example, has 6 atoms each of carbon and oxygen and 12 atoms of hydrogen.

[497] Petrol is also a hydrocarbon, or rather a mixture of several different hydrocarbons.

[498] Bacteria called *Streptococcus mutans* obtain energy from all the common sugars and in the process form lactic acid which dissolves the calcium phosphate of the tooth enamel allowing cavities to form. However, these bacteria also produce plaque from sucrose. The plaque provides a home for them, and keeps the acid from being washed away by saliva, so sucrose is more destructive than other sugars.

Nutrient	Description	Functions	Food groups in which it is found	Effects of having too much or too little
Starches	Starches are complex carbohydrates, consisting of large numbers of glucose molecules chemically bonded together. The word 'starches' is also used to refer to foods rich in starch.	• Starches are a very important source of energy. The body breaks them down into glucose, but because this process takes time starchy foods provide a steady supply of energy over a long period. They do not produce excessively high levels of glucose in the blood for short periods as sugars can do.	• Root vegetables (potatoes, carrots, swedes, yams, etc.) • Pulses (peas, beans, lentils) • Grains (wheat, oats, rice, maize, etc.) • Food made from grains (bread, pasta, noodles, breakfast cereals, cakes, scones, couscous, etc.)	The body stores excess starch as fat, so eating too much increases our weight. Excessive weight is associated with various health problems,[499] such as: • type 2 diabetes • high blood pressure • heart attacks • strokes • bowel cancer • arthritis and other orthopaedic problems • asthma and sleep apnoea (when a person stops breathing while asleep) • psychological problems resulting from teasing or exclusion (which can lead to comfort eating, which makes matters worse) • medical depression Eating too few calories causes weight loss, since the body then converts stored fat into energy instead. If weight loss is taken to extremes it can produce: • dehydration • constipation • heart damage • kidney stones • medical depression

---

[499] Some of the medical problems associated with being overweight may be caused by certain foods that overweight people eat in excess, such as those containing trans fats, rather than being overweight as such.

Nutrient	Description	Functions	Food groups in which it is found	Effects of having too much or too little
Fats	Fats are various complex chemicals which involve glycerol. This makes them feel oily when they are in liquid form or greasy when they are in a solid form. There are four main kinds of fat: • 'Saturated fat' is solid at room temperature.[500] It is commonly simply called 'fat'. • 'Polyunsaturated fat' is liquid at room temperature. It is commonly called 'oil'.[501] • 'Monounsaturated fat' is intermediate between the two in its chemical properties.[502] It is also liquid at room temperature. • 'Trans fats' are unsaturated fats processed to give them a longer shelf life and, in some cases, to make them more solid. The process involves hydrogenation, so they are also called 'hydrogenated oils'.	• Fats provide the most concentrated source of energy of any nutrient. Also they enable our bodies to: • absorb vitamins A, D, E and K • assimilate calcium into our bones • saturated fats are used to manufacture sex hormones • Polyunsaturated fats from fish are known as the omega-3 polyunsaturated fatty acids. Many nutritionists believe that these protect us from heart disease. They may also help to reduce the symptoms experienced by people who suffer from arthritis, joint problems in general, and some skin diseases. • Although most governmental and mainstream medical bodies advise that unsaturated fats are more healthy than saturated fats, there is very little genuine evidence for this, whereas there is a host of research-based evidence that indicates the opposite is true.[503] The only points of agreement between the two factions seem to be that trans fats are bad and cold-pressed olive oil is good!	Saturated fat is found in animal fat (meat – particularly from animals that graze on grass, meat products, and poultry skin); dairy products (especially cream and butter); in many processed foods (cakes, biscuits, pastry, crisps); and in coconut and palm oil. Polyunsaturated fat is found in oily fish (mackerel, sardines, trout, salmon and herring); safflower, grape seed, corn and sunflower oil; and in soy/soya products. Monounsaturated fat is found in olive oil, rapeseed oil, nuts, and avocados. Trans fats (transformed fats) are still sometimes found in commercially baked foods and in fast food.	Eating too much fat leads to excessive weight, with the same problems as are listed for too much starch. Too little fat can prevent our bodies from assimilating vitamins A, D, E and K and calcium into our bones (see below under vitamins and minerals), and prevent the manufacture of essential hormones (for example preventing menstruation). In particular toddlers and young children should drink full cream milk Trans fats have been shown to increase the risk of heart disease, and the less you eat of them the better. You can identify them in the labelling of margarine and other food as 'Fats – of which trans n%'. Some manufacturers may hide them in the declared percentage of polyunsaturates, so a low declared value may be better than no declared value! On some products however it states 'No hydrogenated oils', which means that there are no trans fats present.

[500] It is called 'saturated' because all the available spaces in the molecule are filled with hydrogen atoms.
[501] It is called 'polyunsaturated' because the molecule has spaces for several more hydrogen atoms.

Nutrient	Description	Functions	Food groups in which it is found	Effects of having too much or too little
Vitamins	A vitamin is an organic compound which is necessary in tiny amounts for life. It cannot be made by the body so it must be obtained from the diet.[504] Some vitamins are fat soluble, which means that the body can store them in its fat for use when needed. Others, like vitamins B_6, B_{12} and C, are water soluble. These cannot be stored by the body so they must be replenished regularly from food that contains them. Since they are soluble in water, vegetables containing them should be steamed, grilled or eaten raw to retain their vitamin content.	Nearly all vitamins have more than one function. Vitamin A • eyesight and colour detection • immune system • growth • healthy skin Vitamins B • digestion and release of energy • making red blood cells for carrying oxygen • nerve cell functioning Vitamin C • growth and repair of bodily tissue • resistance to infection • helps body to absorb iron and calcium • contributes to brain functioning	Many vitamins are found in fruit, vegetables and whole grains (e.g. brown bread). Vitamin A • liver, cod liver oil • dark orange coloured fruits and vegetables like apricots, peaches, melons, carrots, swedes and sweet potatoes • dark green leafy vegetables like kale, broccoli and spinach Vitamins B • whole grains such as wheat, oats and brown rice • fish and seafood • poultry and meats • eggs • dairy products • leafy green vegetables • beans and peas Vitamin C • citrus fruits like oranges and grapefruit • melons • kiwi fruit • tomatoes • broccoli and cabbage • sweet peppers	Vitamin deficiencies cause various health problems: • Vitamin A: night blindness • Vitamin B_1: beriberi – a disease affecting the nervous system • Vitamin B_2: ariboflavinosis – various problems particularly in and around the mouth • Vitamin B_3: pellagra – cracking of the skin and mental disorders • Vitamin B_5: paraesthesia – burning, or itchy skin • Vitamin B_6: anaemia, nerve damage • Vitamin B_7: dermatitis and enteritis • Vitamin B_9: birth defects • Vitamin B_{12}: abnormal enlargement of red blood cells • Vitamin C: scurvy – spots on skins, soft gums, bleeding, loss of teeth

[502] It is called 'monounsaturated' because the molecule has space for one additional hydrogen atom only.
[503] For examples of such evidence, read Chapter 3: *The truth about saturated fats*, or buy *Nourishing Traditions: The Cookbook that Challenges Politically Correct Nutrition and the Diet Dictocrats* by Sally Fallon with Mary G. Enig, PhD (NewTrends Publishing, 2000). Some individuals who believe that they have become ill through the prolonged ingestion of polyunsaturated fats are considering suing the US Department of Health and Human Services (HHS) and the Department of Agriculture (USDA) for giving them bad advice.
[504] An exception is vitamin D. The body can make this, but often not in sufficient quantities.

276

Nutrient	Description	Functions	Food groups in which it is found	Effects of having too much or too little
Vitamins (cont.)	The vitamins known to be required by humans are: A B$_1$ (thiamine) B$_2$ (riboflavin) B$_3$ (niacin) B$_5$ (pantothenic acid) B$_6$ (pyridoxine) B$_7$ (biotin) B$_9$ (folic acid) B$_{12}$ (cyanocobalamin) C D E K[505]	<u>Vitamin D</u> • development of bones and teeth • helps body to absorb calcium <u>Vitamin E</u> • maintenance of eyes, skin, and liver • protection of lungs from damage by polluted air • making red blood cells • an antioxidant, which helps to prevent cell damage <u>Vitamin K</u> • clotting of blood to prevent bleeding from injuries	<u>Vitamin D</u> • fish oil • egg yolks • liver • sunlight <u>Vitamin E</u> • whole grains, such as wheat and oats • wheatgerm • leafy green vegetables • sardines and other oily fish • egg yolks • nuts and seeds <u>Vitamin K</u> • leafy green vegetables • dairy products like milk and yogurt • broccoli • soya bean oil	Excesses: It is unlikely that any health problems will occur as a result of consuming too much of a vitamin through normal eating and drinking. Various problems such as nausea, diarrhoea and vomiting may occur if the recommended dosage of vitamin supplement tablets is exceeded. Deficiencies can cause: • Vitamin D: rickets – softening and deformity of the bones, and osteomalacia – weakening of the bones • Vitamin E: mild anaemia in newborn babies • Vitamin K: bleeding

---

[505] The substances originally classified as vitamins F to J either were found not to be vitamins or were reclassified as one of the vitamin B group.

Nutrient	Description	Functions	Food groups in which it is found	Effects of having too much or too little
Minerals and trace elements	These are inorganic substances which are necessary in tiny amounts for life. The main ones are: • calcium, Ca • magnesium, Mg • sodium, Na • potassium, K • phosphorus, P • zinc, Zn • iron, Fe • copper, Cu • iodine, I Like vitamins, minerals and trace elements cannot be made by the body so they have to be obtained from one's diet.	Calcium builds strong bones and teeth. Magnesium helps the muscles and nerves to function, steadies the heart rhythm, and keeps the bones strong by enabling the body to assimilate calcium. It also helps the body to create energy and make proteins. Sodium and potassium are needed to control the fluid balance in the blood and body tissues, and for the functioning of nerves and muscles.	Calcium • dairy products • dark green leafy vegetables (spinach, broccoli, kale) • pulses (beans, peas, tofu, peanuts) • some types of fish (e.g. salmon, sardines) • certain other foods (e.g. oranges, almonds) • hard tap water Magnesium • green vegetables • some pulses (beans and peas) • some nuts and seeds • whole grains (e.g. wholemeal bread) • hard tap water Sodium Common salt (sodium chloride) is present in many foods. There is little salt in unprocessed natural foods, but a great deal in highly processed, manufactured foods, either as common salt or bicarbonate of soda or else in certain preservatives. Bacon, salami and tinned ham have more than 1% by weight. A single fast-food chicken dinner can contain more than the recommended daily amount of sodium for an adult. Potassium • bananas • avocados • nuts • leafy green vegetables • milk • orange juice • potatoes	Too much calcium can cause kidney stones. Too little calcium causes osteoporosis (thinning of the bones), which can lead to fractures and pain. Insufficient magnesium can cause irritability, nervousness and hyperactivity, depression, dizziness, muscle weakness or twitching, heart disease, arthritis, high blood pressure, brittle bones and many other conditions of body and mind. Excess sodium is believed to be a significant cause of high blood pressure in the developed world. Too little can produce dangerous results but is only likely to affect athletes competing in endurance events in hot and humid conditions. Insufficient potassium can produce muscle cramp, an increased risk of heart disease, stroke, arthritis, digestive disorders and infertility.

Minerals and trace elements (cont.)	Phosphorus helps to form healthy bones and teeth; it helps the body to turn carbohydrates and fats into energy and to make protein for the growth and repair of cells and tissues. It is also needed for the correct operation of muscles, heartbeat, kidneys and nerves. Iron is needed to transport oxygen in the blood and to turn food into energy in the muscles. Copper has multiple functions – it helps your body to utilize iron and in the formation of red blood cells; and it helps to keep your blood vessels, nerves, immune system and bones healthy. Zinc is required for normal growth, sexual development, fertility and	Phosphorus • meat • milk and milk products Iron This is found in a wide variety of foods, particularly dark green vegetables, but iron from meat, fish and poultry is absorbed more easily than from other sources. Copper • shellfish • whole grains • beans • nuts • potatoes • organ meats (kidneys and liver) • dark leafy greens • dried fruits such as prunes • cocoa Zinc • meat (beef, pork, lamb and the dark meat of poultry) • shellfish • nuts • pulses (peas, beans, lentils, chickpeas, etc.) • milk and dairy products • oatmeal	Health problems arising from too little or too much phosphorus in the diet are rare. Low levels of iron over a long period can produce anaemia, with symptoms including weakness and fatigue, headaches, irritability, light-headedness, shortness of breath, and weight loss. Excess iron is unlikely unless too many iron supplements are taken. Lack of copper may lead to anaemia or osteoporosis. In very large amounts it is poisonous. Lack of zinc can cause a range of symptoms including lethargy, poor appetite, diarrhoea and reduced resistance to infection.[506] It can retard healing of wounds, growth and sexual development; reduce fertility in men and women[507,508]; and cause problems with ovulation, pregnancy,[509] night vision and depression.[510] More severe deficiencies can cause loss of hair, loss of the senses of smell

[506] www.patient.co.uk/doctor/zinc-deficiency-excess-and-supplementation. Accessed May 2014
[507] El-Tawil A M. *Zinc deficiency in men with Crohn's disease may contribute to poor sperm function and male infertility.* Andrologia, December 2003;35(6):337-41.
[508] Prasad A S et al. *Zinc status and serum testosterone levels of healthy adults.* Nutrition, May 1996; 12(5):344-8.
[509] Sandstead H H. *Is zinc deficiency a public health problem?* Nutrition. Jan-Feb 1995;11(1 Suppl):87-92.
[510] Yary T & Aazami S. *Dietary Intake of Zinc was Inversely Associated with Depression.* Biological Trace Element Research, September 2011.

	desire, resistance to infection, wound healing, the breakdown of carbohydrates and for the senses of smell and touch. Iodine is needed make thyroid hormones, which regulate growth in the body and brain, and energy use.	Iodine • fish • seafood • kelp • some vegetables (such as the skins of potatoes grown in iodine-rich soils) • iodized salt • eggs Although iodine is present in seawater it is not a constituent of sea salt. Eating fish twice a week will generally supply sufficient iodine for the body's needs.	and touch, and damage to the brain, nerves and eyesight.[511] Iodine deficiency produces an enlarged thyroid gland (goitre), and can produce dry skin, hair loss, fatigue and slowed reflexes. It is a major cause of stunted growth and mental retardation in children in some parts of the world.

---

[511] *Risk Assessment – Zinc*. U.K. Food Standards Agency. Expert Group on Vitamins and Minerals, 2003.

Nutrient	Description	Functions	Sources of water	Effects of having too much or too little
Water	Water, H_2O, is a colourless, odourless and almost tasteless substance with a melting point of 0°C and a boiling point of 100°C at sea level.	Water comprises 50% to 70% of an adult's body weight. It is the essential medium in which many biological reactions take place. It enables the body to maintain a constant temperature by means of perspiration, and helps to remove waste products. Since it is constantly being expelled in urine and perspiration and as water vapour in the breath, it must constantly be replenished.	Tap water Comes from various sources but undergoes treatment to ensure it is pure enough to drink. It may contain chlorine to kill bacteria. In Birmingham and some other regions sodium fluoride is added to combat dental decay, and in parts of Scotland it is naturally present. These substances may affect the taste. Hard water contains higher levels of calcium and magnesium than soft water does, which is generally beneficial. There are no proven health issues with tap water, but there are concerns about the effects of low concentrations of pesticides, nitrates from fertilizers, birth control pills and HRT residues, aluminium sulphate (used to clarify the water) and even arsenic. Metals such as lead, zinc and copper are unlikely to be present in hard water, but may dissolve in soft water that flows through old pipes. Bottled water Although bottled water may have health benefits, it degrades the environment because it requires plastic bottles to be manufactured and has to be transported by road, etc. There are also concerns about endocrine disruptors leaching from the plastic. Filtered water is cheaper and does not have these disadvantages. Spring water Bottled water sold as 'spring water' is collected directly from the spring where it rises from the ground, and must be bottled at the source. U.K. spring water must meet certain hygiene standards, and may be further treated in order to comply with purity regulations. Mineral water Mineral water emerges from under the ground, then flows over rocks, resulting in a higher content of various minerals. Unlike spring water, it must not be treated except to remove grit and dirt. Table water Bottled water, which may come from more than one source, including the tap! Filtered water Filters may be used in jugs or attached in-line to a dedicated tap in the kitchen. There are various kinds of filter, and some kinds remove more contaminants than others. See Chapter 16 for further details.	Dehydration causes headaches, tiredness and loss of concentration. Chronic dehydration can contribute to a number of health problems such as heartburn, constipation, urinary tract infections, kidney stones, and autoimmune diseases such as chronic fatigue syndrome and multiple sclerosis.

Annexe 4: Glycaemic loads produced by typical servings of common carbohydrate foods

Table A.4: Glycaemic loads produced by typical servings of common carbohydrate foods

EXPLANATORY NOTES
1. Glycaemic load is the weight of available carbohydrate in a serving of food multiplied by its glycaemic index and divided by 100
2. Some of the data shown are average values derived from foods sold internationally, so they may not apply exactly to products sold in the U.K.
3. Serving sizes. 'Measure' is only an approximate guide. The values for the 'Glycaemic load' relate to the 'Quantity' such as '10gm'.
4. Meat, poultry, fish, eggs, cheese, leafy vegetables, most nuts and alcoholic drinks contain little or no carbohydrate.
6. Colour keys to Glycaemic index: Low, 55 or less | Medium, less than 70 | High, 70 or more
7. Colour keys to Glycaemic load: Low, 10 or less | Medium, less than 20 | High, 20 or more
8. Source key: see the end of the table for source keys.

Type	Food	Serving size Measure	Quantity	Carbohydrate content (gm)	Glycaemic index	Glycaemic load	Source key
Biscuits and crispbreads	Digestive biscuit	1	15gm	9.4	39	3.7	BJN1
	Morning Coffee™ biscuit	1	10gm	8.0	79±6	6.0	FP
	Oat biscuits	1	14gm	8.5	45	3.8	BJN1
	Puffed crispbread	1 slice	10gm	7.0	81	5.7	FAN
	Rice cakes	1	8gm	6.0	85	5.1	FAN
	Rich Tea biscuit	1	8gm	5.7	40	2.3	BJN1
	Ryvita™	1 slice	10gm	7.0	69	4.8	FAN
	Shortbread	1	13gm	8.0	64	5.1	FAN
Breads, rolls, scones, etc.	Bagel, white bread	1	70gm	35	69	24	FP
	Baguette, white, plain	8cm long slice	30gm	15	95±15	14.3	FP
	Bread, oatmeal batch	1 slice	50gm	25.1	62	16	BJN
	Bread, rye	1 slice	25gm	11	41	4.5	FAN
	Bread, white gluten-free	1 medium slice	30gm	15	76±5	11.4	FP
	Bread, white wheat flour	1 medium slice	46gm	20.4	59	12	BJN1
	Bread, wholemeal wheat flour	1 medium slice	30gm	13	71±2	9.2	FP
	Croissant	1	60gm	23	67	15.4	FAN
	Pitta bread	1 large	75gm	43	57	24.5	FAN
	Scone, plain	1	40gm	13	92±8	11.8	FP
	Water biscuit	1	8gm	6.0	78	4.7	FAN

Type	Food	Serving size Measure	Serving size Quantity	Carbohydrate content (gm)	Glycaemic index	Glycaemic load	Source key
Breakfast cereals	AllBran™	Small bowl	30gm	21	42±5	9.1	FP
	Bran Flakes	1 bowl	30gm	20.1	50	10	BJN
The values shown are for the cereal only, not for cereal and milk.	Cornflakes™	1 bowl	30gm	26	81±3	21.1	FP
	Fruit and fibre	1 bowl	40gm	27.6	89	18.7	BJN
	Grapenuts™	Small bowl	50gm	35	71±4	24.8	FP
	Instant hot oat cereal, made with water	Small bowl	30gm	17.2	83	14.3	BJN1
	Special K™	Small bowl	30gm	NS	69	14.5	AS
	Muesli, fruit and nut	Small bowl	50gm	30.2	59	18	BJN
	Porridge of rolled Scottish oats cooked with water	Small bowl	50gm	31.0	63	20	BJN
	Puffed wheat	1 bowl	30gm	21	74±7	15.5	FP
	Rice Krispies™	1 bowl	30gm	26	82	21.3	FP
	Shredded Wheat™	1 biscuit	22.5gm	15	83	16.6	FP
	Weetabix™	1 biscuit	22.5gm	16	75±10	12.4	FP
Cakes	Muffin	1	68gm	34	44	15.0	FAN
	Sponge cake, plain	1 slice	63gm	36	46±6	16.6	FP
Confectionery	Mars bar™	1 bar	60gm	40	65±3	26.0	FP
	Muesli bar	1 bar	33gm	20	61	12.2	FAN
	Plain milk chocolate	50gm	50gm	28	43±3	12.0	FP
	Snickers™	1 bar	60gm	35	55±14	19.3	FP
Dairy products, milk and substitutes	Custard	4 tblsp	120gm	20	43	8.6	FAN
	Milk, full fat, standardized, homogenized, pasteurized		250ml	12	46±10	5	BJN/FP
	Milk, semi-skimmed, pasteurized		250ml	12.5	25	3	BJN/FP
	Milk, whole, pasteurized, fresh, organic		250ml	12	34	4	BJN/FP
	Ice cream	1 scoop	50gm	13	61±7	7.9	FP
	Instant milk pudding	1 pot	100gm	16	44±4	7.0	FP
	Probiotic drinks	1 pot	100ml	12.2 - 13.4	30 - 60	4.0 - 8.0	BJN
	Yogurt of various kinds	1 pot	150gm	21 - 34	17 - 67	4.0 - 13.0	BJN
	Soy milk, full-fat		250gm	17	44±5	7.5	FP

Type	Food	Serving size Measure	Quantity	Carbohydrate content (gm)	Glycaemic index	Glycaemic load	Source key
Drinks – non-alcoholic	Coca-Cola®	330ml can	330ml	34	58±5	19.9	FP
	Fanta®	330ml can	330ml	45	68±6	30.5	FP
	Lucozade®	330ml can	330ml	55	95±10	52.7	FP
	Milo™ with full-fat cow's milk	250ml mug	250ml	25	35±2	8.8	FP
	Milo™ dissolved in water	251ml mug	250ml	16	55±3	8.8	FP
	Squash (diluted)	250ml glass	250ml	14	66	9.2	FAN
	Yakult®, fermented milk drink		65ml	12	46±6	5.5	FP
Fruit – tinned	Fruit cocktail, drained	1 large cup	214gm	NS	55	19.8	AS
	Peaches, tinned, light syrup	Small tin drained	120gm	18	52	9.4	FP
	Peaches, tinned, natural juice	Small tin drained	120gm	11	38±8	4.2	FP
	Pear halves, tinned, natural juice	Small tin drained	120gm	13	43±15	5.6	FP
Fruit – dried	Dried apricots	6 – 8	60gm	21·6	31	7	BJN
	Sultanas	2 tblsp	60gm	41·6	58	24	BJN
	Mixed fruit	2 tblsp	60gm	40·7	60	6	BJN
Fruit – fresh	Apple	1	120gm	15	38±2	5.7	FP
	Apricots	3	120gm	9	57	5.1	FP
	Banana	1	120gm	24	52±4	12.5	FP
	Grapefruit	1/2	120gm	11	25	2.8	FP
	Grapes	small bunch	120gm	18	46±3	8.3	FP
	Mango	1	120gm	17	51±5	8.7	FP
	Orange	1 small	120gm	11	42±3	4.6	FP
	Peach	1	120gm	11	42±14	4.6	FP
	Pear	1	120gm	11	38±2	4.2	FP
	Pineapple	1 large slice	120gm	13	59±8	7.7	FP
	Plums	2	120gm	12	39±15	4.7	FP
	Prunes	1	60gm	33	29±4	9.6	FP
	Raisins	3 tblsp	60gm	44	64±11	28.2	FP
	Rock melon/cantaloupe	1 small slice	120gm	6	65±9	3.9	FP
	Strawberries	10	120gm	3	40±7	1.2	FP
	Watermelon	1 small slice	120gm	6	72±13	4.3	FP

Type	Food	Serving size Measure	Serving size Quantity	Carbohydrate content (gm)	Glycaemic index	Glycaemic load	Source key
Fruit – juice	Apple juice, unsweetened	4 glass	160ml	18	40±1	7.2	FP
	Cranberry juice drink	1 glass	160ml	19	56±4	10.4	FP
	Grapefruit juice, unsweetened	5 glass	160ml	13	48	6.1	FP
	Orange juice	2 glass	160ml	15	52±3	7.7	FP
	Pineapple juice, unsweetened	6 glass	160ml	22	46	10.0	FP
	Tomato juice, no added sugar	3 glass	160ml	6	38±4	2.2	FP
Jam	Strawberry jam	1 tblsp	30gm	20	51±10	10.2	FP
Meals – home-made	Corn tortilla, fried, with mashed potato, fresh tomato and lettuce.		100gm	15	78	11.7	FP
	Corn tortilla, served with refried mashed pinto beans and tomato sauce		100gm	23	39	9.0	FP
	Ravioli, durum wheat flour, meat filled, boiled		180gm	38	39±1	14.8	FP
	Sirloin chop with mixed vegetables and mashed potato		360gm	53	66±12	35.0	FP
	Spaghetti bolognaise		360gm	48	52±9	25.0	FP
	Stir fried vegetables with chicken and boiled white rice		360gm	75	73±17	54.8	FP
	White boiled rice, grilled beefburger, cheese and butter		440gm	50	25±2	12.5	FP
Meals – ready meals	Cannelloni, spinach and ricotta		400gm	71·6	15	11	BJN
	Chicken korma with rice		450gm	71·6	45	32	BJN
These are a few examples of ready meals that can be bought in the U.K. The values for brands not tested will differ. For a more comprehensive list with more detailed information see BJN cited below.	Chow mein, chicken		475gm	60·0	47	28	BJN
	Cottage pie		500gm	56·0	65	36	BJN
	Cumberland fish pie		250gm	26·0	40	10	BJN
	Cumberland pie		500gm	62·0	29	18	BJN
	Lasagne		400gm	40·4	25	10	BJN
	Lasagne, vegetarian		430gm	68·8	20	14	BJN
	Pasta bake, tomato and mozzarella		340gm	48·3	23	11	BJN
	Sausage and mash		500gm	67·0	61	41	BJN
	Shepherd's pie		500gm	73·5	66	49	BJN
	Sweet and sour chicken with noodles		475gm	81·7	41	33	BJN
	Tandoori chicken masala and rice		550gm	111·7	45	50	BJN

285

Type	Food	Serving size Measure	Serving size Quantity	Carbohydrate content (gm)	Glycaemic index	Glycaemic load	Source
Miscellaneous	Chicken nuggets		100gm	16	46±4	7.4	FP
	Fish fingers		100gm	19	38±6	7.2	FP
	White bread with butter	2 medium slices	100gm	48	59	28.3	FP
	White/wholemeal wheat bread with peanut butter	2 medium slices	100gm	44	59±8	26.0	FP
Nuts	Cashew nuts, salted		50gm	13	22±5	2.9	FP
	Peanuts		50gm	6	14±8	0.8	FP
Pasta, dry	Fusilli pasta twists		50gm	36.3	54	20	BJN
	Lasagne, egg		50gm	33.1	53	18	BJN
	Tagliatelle, egg		50gm	33.2	46	15	BJN
Pasta, noodles, rice & grains, cooked	Chapatti, wheat, boiled (very variable)		200gm	50	63±19	31.5	FP
	Couscous, boiled 5 minutes	5 tblsp	150gm	35	65±4	22.8	FP
	Linguine, durum wheat		180gm	45	52±3	23.4	FP
	Macaroni, plain, boiled	3 tblsp	180gm	48	47±2	22.6	FP
	Noodles, cooked	4 tblsp	230gm	30	46	13.8	FAN
	Pearl barley		150gm	42	25±1	10.5	FP
	Rice, brown, boiled	5 tblsp	150gm	33	55±5	18.2	FP
	Rice, white, basmati, boiled	5 tblsp	150gm	38	57±4	22.0	FP
	Rice, white, long grain, boiled	5 tblsp	150gm	41	56±2	23.0	FP
	Rice, white, short grain, boiled	5 tblsp	150gm	36	64±7	23.0	FP
	Semolina		150gm	11	55±1	6.1	FP
	Spaghetti, white, boiled	3 tblsp	180gm	47	42±3	19.7	FP
	Sweetcorn		150gm	32	53±4	17.0	FP
	Vermicelli, white, boiled	3 tblsp	180gm	44	35±7	15.4	FP
Pies, pizzas and sausages	Beef pie		100gm	27	45±6	12.2	FP
	Pizza	1 slice	100gm	25	70	13.1	FP
	Sausages	2	100gm	3	28±6	0.8	FP
Snacks	Popcorn	2.5 cups	20gm	11	72±17	7.9	FP
	Potato crisps	1 packet	25gm	10	54±3	5.6	FP

Type	Food	Serving size Measure	Quantity	Carbohydrate content (gm)	Glycaemic index	Glycaemic load	Source key
Soups, tinned	Green pea		250ml	41	66	27.1	FP
	Minestrone		250ml	18	39±3	7.0	FP
	Noodle soup		250ml	9	1	0.1	FP
	Tomato soup		250ml	17	38±9	6.5	FP
Sugars and sweeteners	Fructose	2 tsps	10gm	10	19±2	1.9	FP
	Glucose	2 tsps	10gm	10	99±3	9.9	FP
	Honey	1 tblsp	25gm	18	55±5	9.9	FP
	Lactose	2 tsps	10gm	10	46±2	4.6	FP
	Maltose	2 tsps	10gm	10	105±12	10.5	FP
	Sucrose (table sugar)	2 tsps	10gm	10	68±5	6.8	FP
Vegetables – legumes	Baked beans	1 small tin	200gm	20	48±8	9.6	FP
	Black-eyed beans	Small serving	150gm	30	42±9	12.6	FP
	Broad beans	2 tblsp	120gm	7	79	5.5	FAN
	Butter beans	Small serving	150gm	20	31±3	6.2	FP
	Chickpeas	Small serving	150gm	30	28±6	8.4	FP
	Green lentils	Small serving	150gm	17	30±4	5.1	FP
	Kidney beans	Small serving	150gm	25	28±4	7.0	FP
	Marrowfat peas	Small serving	150gm	19	39±8	7.4	FP
	Peas	2 tblsp	80gm	7	48±5	3.4	FP
	Pumpkin	2 tblsp	80gm	4	75±9	3.0	FP
	Sweetcorn	2 tblsp	80gm	17	54±4	9.2	FP
Vegetables – root	Beetroot		80gm	7	64±16	4.5	FP
	Carrots	2.5 tblsp	80gm	6	47±16	2.8	FP
	Cassava, boiled, with salt	Small portion	100gm	27	46	12.4	FP
	Mashed potato	4 tblsp	150gm	20	74±5	14.8	FP
	Parsnips	1	100gm	15	97±19	14.5	FP
	Potato boiled	2 medium	175gm	33	50±9	16.3	FP
	Potato chips	Average portion	165gm	59	75	44.3	FAN
	Potato, white, baked in skin	1 large	300gm	60	60	36.0	FP
	Potatoes, new, boiled	2 small	150gm	21	57±7	12.0	FP
	Swede	4 tblsp	150gm	10	72±8	7.2	FP

Type	Food	Serving size		Carbohydrate content (gm)	Glycaemic index	Glycaemic load	Source key
		Measure	Quantity				
	Sweet potato	1 medium	150gm	28	61±7	17.1	FP
	Yam	1 medium	150gm	36	37±8	13.3	FP

Source keys:
BJN: *Glycaemic index and glycaemic load values of commercially available products in the U.K.*
    Jeya C et al. British Journal of Nutrition/Volume 94/Issue 06/December 2005, pp 922 – 930.
BJN1:*Glycaemic index and glycaemic load values of cereal products and weight management meals available in the U.K.*
    Jeya C et al. British Journal of Nutrition/Volume 98/Issue 01/July 2007, pp 147 – 153.
FP: Based on data from *International table of glycemic index and glycemic load values: 2002.*
    Foster-Powell K. Holt S.H.A.. Brand-Miller J.C. American Journal of Clinical Nutrition. July 2002; 76(1):5-56.
FAN: Quantities and glycaemic index from www.findanutritionist.com/resources/tables/glycaemic_carbohydrate.html. 2013.
AS: Dr Al Sears at www.alsearsmd.com/glycemic-index/. 2013.

Annexe 5: Omega-3 content of marine foods

Nearly all the omega-3 in marine foods consists of EPA[512] and DHA,[513] two extremely important fatty acids which can be obtained only in our diet. The total weight of EPA and DHA contained in each 140gm serving of fish or seafood is shown in the following tables.

The values are derived from three different sources: seafish.org (a U.K. source), labbio.net (a French source), and USDA (the United States Department of Agriculture[514]). The differences between them are partly explained by the different places where the fish consumed in each country is caught. For any particular species of fish the omega-3 content can vary considerably depending on its exact species, where the fish is caught, its age, the time of year, and whether it is wild or farmed. Farmed fish such as farmed trout and salmon are generally fed with cereal products, so their omega-3 content will be less than that of fish caught in the wild, which feed on krill and other organisms.

---

512 Eicosapentaenoic acid.
513 Docosahexaenoic acid.
514 www.health.gov/dietaryguidelines/dga2005/report/HTML/table_g2_adda2.htm

Table A.5.1: Omega-3 content of marine foods, best sources, in mg per 140gm serving

Species	Combined	Seafish.org UK	Labbio.net France	USDA 2005 USA
Caviar, black and red, granular	9157			9157
Roe, mixed species, cooked, dry heat	4210			4210
Mackerel	3080		3080	
Salmon, Atlantic, farmed, cooked, dry heat	3006			3006
Herring, Pacific, cooked, dry heat (mean of 3 values)	2934			2934
Anchovy, European, canned in oil, drained solids	2877			2877
Herring cooked	2817	2817		
Mackerel cooked	2804	2804		
Spiny dogfish	2800		2800	
Sardines	2660	2660		
Mackerel, Pacific and jack, mixed species, cooked, dry heat	2587			2587
Salmon, Atlantic, wild, cooked, dry heat	2576			2576
Salmon, Atlantic	2380	2380		
Herrings	2380		2380	
Sardines	2380		2380	
Pilchards (large sardines)	2380		2380	
Tuna (bluefin)	2240		2240	
Trout (lake)	2240		2240	
Anchovy	2232	2232		
Tuna, fresh, bluefin, cooked, dry heat	2106			2106
Sturgeon (Atlantic)	2100		2100	
Anchovy, European, raw	2029			2029
Salmon	1960		1960	
Anchovies	1960		1960	
Oyster, Pacific, cooked, moist heat	1926			1926
Crab white meat & brown meat	1892	1892		
Sprats	1820		1820	
Oysters, Pacific	1804	1804		
Salmon, pink, cooked, dry heat	1803			1803
Mackerel, Spanish, cooked, dry heat	1744			1744
Salmon, Pacific	1705	1705		
Mackerel, Atlantic, cooked, dry heat	1684			1684
Bluefish	1680		1680	

Halibut, Greenland, cooked, dry heat	1649			1649
Oysters native	1648	1648		
Mullet	1540		1540	

Table A.5.2: Omega-3 content of marine foods, excellent sources, in mg per 140gm serving

Species	Combined	Seafish.org UK	Labbio.net France	USDA 2005 USA
Trout, rainbow, wild, cooked, dry heat (mean of 3 values)	1436			1436
Sardine, Atlantic, canned in oil, drained solids with bone	1375			1375
Bass, striped, cooked, dry heat	1354			1354
Halibut	1260		1260	
Hake	1218	1218		
Tuna, white, canned in water, drained solids	1207			1207
Bass (striped)	1120		1120	
Mussel, blue, cooked, moist heat	1095			1095
Sea bass, mixed species, cooked, dry heat	1067			1067
Whitebait	1036			1036
Mussels cooked	956	956		
Squid prepared meat	890	890		
Trout (rainbow)	840		840	
Trout (Arctic char)	840		840	
Mullet (striped)	840		840	
Oysters	840		840	
Carp	840		840	
Squid (short-finned)	840		840	
Oyster, eastern, wild, cooked, dry heat	771			771
Pollock, Atlantic	757	757		
Sea Bream	728	728		
Shrimps brown, as eaten	720	720		
Octopus	718	718		
Flatfish (flounder and sole species), cooked, dry heat	701			701
Sea Bass	700	700		
Tuna (skipjack)	700		700	
Mussels (blue)	700		700	
Periwinkles	700		700	
Shark	700		700	
Pollock	700		700	
Sea trout, mixed species, cooked, dry heat	666			666
Halibut, Atlantic and Pacific, cooked, dry heat	651			651
Halibut	651	651		

Sole cooked	644	644		
Rockfish, Pacific, mixed species, cooked, dry heat	620			620
Oyster, eastern, farmed, cooked, dry heat	616			616
Crustaceans, crab, queen, cooked, moist heat (mean of 4 values)	615			615
Lobster	580	580		
Mackerel, king, cooked, dry heat	561			561
Hake (Pacific)	560		560	
Prawns, cold water	546	546		

Table A.5.3: Omega-3 content of marine foods, good sources, in mg per 140gm serving

Species	Combined	Seafish.org UK	Labbio.net France	USDA 2005 USA
Scallops Queen (+ roe)	487	487		
Cockles, cooked meat	487	487		
Tuna, skipjack, fresh, cooked, dry heat	459			459
Crustaceans, shrimp, mixed species, cooked, moist	441			441
Shrimp, mixed species, cooked, moist heat	441			441
Hoki or Blue Grenadier	420	420		
Cod, Pacific, cooked, dry heat	386			386
Tuna, light, canned in water, drained solids	378			378
Whelks	352	352		
Coley	343	343		
Cod	342	342		
Plaice, cooked	336	336		
Haddock, cooked, dry heat	333			333
Pollock, Alaskan	322	322		
Scampi tails	302	302		
Fish portions and sticks, frozen, preheated	300			300
Haddock	280	280		
Prawns warm water, cooked, farmed	270	270		
Barramundi	266	266		
Tuna	223	223		
Cod, Atlantic, cooked, dry heat	221			221
Scallops, king (without roe)	207	207		
Tuna, light, canned in oil, drained solids	179			179
Monkfish	140	140		
Sole, lemon	140	140		

Annexe 6: Derivation of recommended fish oil consumption

This Annexe explains the derivation of the recommendations for fish consumption shown in Chapter 7, Table 2. They are derived from a range of widely differing recommendations, as shown below, which are all intended to prevent cardiac and other types of disease in people who live on an otherwise typical Western diet.

Table A.6: Derivation of recommended fish oil consumptions

Source	Recommended number of 140gm portions of mixed fish per week	Comments
UK Food Standards Agency	2 at least	With limitations on maximum consumption.
UK Scientific Advisory Committee on Nutrition	2 or 3	To reduce the risk of heart trouble, various sources.
	4	For people over 65 or those who have survived some form of heart attack.
	6 at least	To reduce significantly the risk of heart trouble.
American Heart Association	2	'Especially oily fish'.
	4 at least	People who have had a heart attack.
	9 to 18	Equivalent in capsule form under medical supervision for people who have to lower their triglyceride level.
Holland & Barrett	Up to 7 portions of fish, or the equivalent in fish oil.	From various cited research sources, for cardiac and other types of health.
US National Institutes of Health	9	For someone on a 2,000 Kcal a day diet, or proportionately.

The U.K. Food Standards Agency (FSA) advises everyone to eat at least two 140gm portions of fish per week, one of which should be oily.[515] This is particularly important for pregnant and nursing women, because the omega-3 fatty acids in fish are needed for the proper development of a baby's brain. However, women who are likely to have a child, and pregnant and nursing women, should eat no more than two portions a week of oily fish, and other people should eat no more than four. This is because of concerns about harmful contaminants in sea water such as mercury and dioxin, which may get into some fish.[516]

The U.K. Scientific Advisory Committee on Nutrition (SACN), which advises the FSA, makes the same recommendations, but adds that everyone should consume a minimum of 450mg per day or 3150mg per week of long-chain omega-3 fatty acids.[517] The two most important long-chain omega-3 fatty acids so far as our diet is concerned are EPA and DHA,[518] and those are the two kinds of omega-3 which are found in fish.

In terms of fish, a 140gm portion of the oily fish salmon contains about 2800mg of EPA and DHA and a similar portion of the non-oily fish plaice contains about 350mg, so together these would provide the 3150mg weekly ration recommended by SACN. A 120gm tin of Tesco's sardines in brine contains 2800mg of omega-3 in the drained fish, the same as a portion of fresh salmon, while a 155gm tin of Glenryck pilchards in tomato sauce contains 2660mg of EPA + DHA. So roughly speaking 450mg a day of EPA + DHA = two portions of fresh or canned fish a week.

The American Heart Association (AHA) in its Diet and Lifestyle Recommendations 2006 recommended that people with no history of coronary heart disease or heart attack should consume fish, especially oily fish, at least twice a week. People who have had a heart attack should consume a total of 1000mg of EPA + DHA per day from oily fish or supplements,[519] which is over twice the amount recommended by SACN for the general population and is equivalent to more than *four* portions of fish a week. The same paper says that people whose triglyceride levels need to be lowered should take 2000 to 4000mg of EPA + DHA per day as capsules under a physician's care. People without documented heart disease are also recommended to include in their diet oils and foods rich in α-linolenic acid (ALA), for example flaxseed/linseed, canola/rapeseed and soybean oils, and flaxseeds and walnuts.

---

515 *Oily fish advice: your questions answered*. Food Standards Agency, 2004. www.food.gov.uk/multimedia/faq/oilyfishfaq/?version=1. Accessed April 2014.

516 *Advice on fish consumption: benefits and risks*. Scientific Advisory Committee on Nutrition: Committee on Toxicity. Food Standards Agency and the Department of Health, 2004.

517 Scientific Advisory Committee on Nutrition. FICS/04/02, dated 14/04/04.

518 EPA = eicosapentaenoic acid; DHA = docosahexaenoic acid. The human body can create these from ALA, or linolenic acid, which is found in seed oils, but the process is not very efficient so it is better to obtain them from dietary sources, of which oily marine sources are best.

519 Kris-Etherton P M et al. *Fish consumption, fish oil, omega-3 acids and cardiovascular disease*. Circulation, 2002; 106 (21): 2747–2757.

In 2004 SACN reviewed the existing research findings on this subject,[520] and they made the following discoveries:

- Various studies showed that up to 40gm to 60gm per day, the more fish (of all types) eaten by people in high-risk populations such as the U.K. and the U.S.A., the less likely they are to suffer from coronary heart disease (CHD). This means that in order to reduce your risk of heart trouble to a minimum you should eat two or three 140gm portions of fish a week. (It was on this that they based their advice of '*at least* two portions of fish a week'.)
- In people aged 65 years and in people of all ages who have survived some form of heart attack, deaths from CHD progressively decrease with increasing doses of omega-3 up to 900mg a day, corresponding to *four* portions of mixed fish per week, similar to the AHA recommendations.
- But to make a significant reduction in cardiovascular risk factors[521] at least 1500mg a day of omega-3 (EPA + DHA) is required, i.e. more than *six* portions of fish per week.

They also found that it might take from 2 to 6 months for the benefits of increasing one's intake of fish oil to be measurable.

The British Holland and Barrett website lists a number of health problems that can be alleviated by taking fish oil or other omega-3 supplements.[522] The website describes the supporting scientific trials and the corresponding quantities of fish oil taken by the subjects of the experiments. The most common dosage to produce a measurable improvement in health seems to have been around 3000mg of omega-3 a day, or nearly *seven* portions of fish a week.

And in 1999 the US National Institutes of Health recommended a daily target of 4,000mg of omega-3 a day for someone on a 2,000 calorie diet,[523] or *nine* portions of fish a week! In my view such a recommendation is totally irresponsible. While it may have some scientific support, if everyone took this advice I would guess there would be no fish left in the oceans within a month.

---

520 www.sacn.gov.uk/pdfs/fics_sacn_04_02.pdf. Accessed March 2013.

521 The cardio-vascular risk factors quoted in the SACN paper are plasma triacylglycerol levels, blood pressure, platelet aggregation and the inflammatory response.

522 www.hollandandbarrett.com. Search for 'fish-oil-and-cod-liver-oil-epa-and-dha'. The conditions listed, which omega-3 supplements have been proved to alleviate, are cardiovascular problems, high blood pressure, high triglyceride levels (which can lead to heart disease), lupus (a breakdown of the body's immune system which can produce all kinds of nasty results) and rheumatoid arthritis.

523 *Workshop on the Essentiality of and Recommended Dietary Intakes (RDI) for Omega-6 and Omega-3 Fatty Acids*, sponsored by the U.S. National Institutes of Health (NIH), 1999.

Annexe 7: Microwaved food – noxious or nutritious?

The case against microwaving

Although microwave ovens are fast, convenient and energy efficient, many people wonder if food heated or cooked in a microwave is safe to eat. The Internet is full of articles informing us about the dangers of eating microwaved food, but few of these articles reference properly traceable research. Wading through oceans of anti-microwave rhetoric (I never was much good at surfing) I found only four referenced scientific papers relating to the dangers of microwaved food.

<u>(i) Dr. Hans U. Hertel</u>

The first and most serious of the anti-microwave sources was a research paper written by the Swiss food scientist Dr. Hans Hertel and Professor Bernard Blanc, a biochemical engineer.[524] It concluded, '*The measurable effects on human beings of food treated with microwaves, as opposed to food not so treated, include changes in the blood which appear to indicate the initial stage of a pathological process such as occurs at the start of a cancerous condition.*'

This is the paper which describes the effects of microwaved food on eight volunteers (one of whom was Dr. Hertel himself), and which is said to have been published by Raum and Zelt.

Hertel submitted the paper to the Journal Franz Weber for publication in issue no. 19 dated January to March 1992. Its editor wrote an alarmist article headed, '*The danger of microwaves: scientific proof*', complete with a picture on the front cover of the Grim Reaper pointing to a microwave oven. The article was followed by the research paper.

The Swiss Association of Manufacturers and Suppliers of Household Electrical Appliances took the editor and Dr. Hertel to court in Switzerland, seeking an injunction forbidding either of them to state that scientific research proves that food which has been exposed to radiation in a microwave oven is a hazard to health. The court approved the injunction, but Dr. Hertel eventually took the matter to the European Court of Human

---

[524] Blanc B H & Hertel H U. *Vergleichende Untersuchungen über die Beeinflussung des Menschen durch konventionell und im Mikrowellenofen aufbereitete Nahrung* ('Comparative study of the effects on human beings of food prepared by conventional means and in microwave ovens') June 1991.

Rights, on the grounds that it unjustly violated his right to freedom of expression. Here the judges decided in favour of Dr. Hertel by a split decision of six to three. They did not make any judgement as to whether microwaved food was hazardous to health.

What the popular websites don't report is that during the court proceedings Dr. Hertel's fellow researcher Professor Blanc stated, '*I totally dissociate myself from the presentation and interpretation of the preliminary exploratory experiment carried out in 1989, which was published without my consent by the co-author of the study in the journal cited above. The results obtained do not in any circumstances justify drawing any conclusions as to the harmful effects of food treated with microwaves or a predisposition to the appearance of a given pathological condition.*'

Professor M. Teuber of the Food Research Institute of the Zürich Federal Institute of Technology provided an independent opinion on behalf of the appliance manufacturers. This was the only peer review that Blanc and Hertel's paper ever received. Teuber concluded, '*Blanc and Hertel's experiments ...were not conducted and described according to scientifically recognized criteria. They are of no scientific value; the conclusions drawn from them as to the alleged harmfulness of food cooked by microwaves have no verifiable basis and are unsustainable.*'

Finally, one reason that the Court of Human Rights finally found in favour of Dr. Hertel was that his research paper did *not* claim that microwaved food was harmful. The judgement read, '*Although it is stated that the results "show changes which bear witness to pathogenic disorders"...there is no assertion that the consumption of irradiated food is harmful for man...but merely a suggestion that it "might" be.*' It was the editor of the Journal Franz Weber who asserted that microwaved food was harmful. He was not a scientist, neither was his journal a scientific journal.

Therefore it is completely false to claim that Dr. Hertel proved that eating microwaved food is harmful.

All these facts were fully recorded by the European Court of Human Rights, and at the time of writing they were available online.[525]

(ii) Lubec's paper in The Lancet

A second oft-quoted source is a research paper called *Aminoacid Isomerisation and Microwave Exposure*.[526] It was published in *The Lancet* in 1989, and it is the paper that is widely but incorrectly attributed to a Dr. Lita Lee. It reported that proteins in microwave-heated infant milk formula were altered into forms that could theoretically lead to structural, functional and immunological changes and have a toxic effect on the brain.

---

525 http://hudoc.echr.coe.int/sites/eng/pages/search.aspx?i=001-59366#{%22item id%22:[%22001-59366%22]}

526 Lubec G et al. *Aminoacid Isomerisation and Microwave Exposure*. The Lancet, December 1989; Vol. 334, Issue 8676:1392–1393.

Just 2 months later these conclusions were publicly rebutted,[527] and in 1991 they were overturned by a research group in Lausanne, Switzerland. The Swiss researchers heated UHT milk and three different infant formula milks in a microwave under two sets of conditions: 3 minutes at 600 Watts and 20 minutes at 70 Watts. They reported, *"No significant differences could be found between treated and untreated samples...heating of milk or infant formula in a microwave oven under conditions corresponding to those normally applied for heating food does not induce significant inversion of protein-bound amino acids."*[528]

A similar result was reported a few years later from Florida, U.S.A. There the researchers heated ordinary whole and skimmed pasteurized milk in a microwave for 10 minutes on medium power and compared it with milk heated over a hot water bath at 80°C. They concluded, *'Within experimental error, there is no significant difference in the levels of these D-amino acids between the conventionally heated and microwave heated milks, thus having no significant effect on the nutritional value of the milk proteins.'*[529]

As you can guess, neither of those two papers is referred to by the microwave doom-mongers.

(iii) Norma Levitt's death following a blood transfusion

The third negative source frequently mentioned is not a research paper but a court case. It concerns a hip surgery patient in Oklahoma, Norma Levitt, who died in 1989 immediately after receiving a transfusion of blood that had been warmed in a microwave oven. A report of the proceedings was available at the time of writing on the website of the Wyoming State Law Library.[530]

By some contorted logic this unhappy accident is presented as evidence that somehow eating microwaved food will produce fatal alterations in our blood. That would be something quite different. Even if microwaving blood did render it poisonous this would be of real concern only to a vampire who had first microwaved his victim.

The first thing to state is that in the initial court case it was determined that Mrs. Levitt's death was *not* the result of heating her blood in a microwave. The report states, *'The defendants argued that Levitt died from a blood clot, rather than the hemolyzed blood. A defendants' verdict was returned.'* This means that after hearing the medical evidence the court decided Mrs. Levitt's death was simply due to the formation of a

---

527 Segal W. *Microwave heating of milk*. The Lancet, February 1990; Vol. 335, Issue 8687:470.

528 Fay L et el. *Evidence for the absence of amino acid isomerization in microwave-heated milk and infant formulas*. Journal of Agricultural and Food Chemistry, October 1991; 39 (10):1857–1859.

529 Petrucelli L. & Fisher G H. *D-aspartate and D-glutamate in microwaved versus conventionally heated milk*. Journal of the American College of Nutrition. April 1994; 13(2):209-10.

530 http://wyomcases.courts.state.wy.us/applications/oscn/DeliverDocument.asp?citeID=4387#marker0fn1

blood clot, not to the microwaved blood. Whatever the microwave oven did or did not do, it was not responsible for Mrs. Levitt's death, so the case should never be cited as proof that microwaving food is dangerous. It is true that there were many subsequent legal challenges but these did not relate to the cause of her death.

A footnote to the court's report explained the reference to 'hemolyzed blood' as follows. '*Heating blood in a microwave destroys the red blood cells, resulting in "gross hemolysis" of the blood, releasing large amounts of potassium. Excessive potassium, when introduced into the body, is often fatal.*' While this statement is true it is misleading as it stands. Microwaves are not some mysterious force that can somehow target red cells in our bodies or have other unknown effects. All that they do is heat things up. They do it in the same way as the radiant heat from a grill heats food up, except that they are more powerful. It is true that heating blood in a microwave can destroy red blood cells, but only if it makes the blood too hot, and any other way of overheating blood would destroy the blood cells equally well.

This was investigated in 1997 by Herron and others.[531] They heated refrigerated red blood cells in microwave blood warmers to settings ranging from 0°C to 60°C. They measured seven or eight resulting factors, including potassium levels, and found no changes in the size of the red cells or in their structure or function up to temperatures of around 52°C. They concluded, '*An inline microwave blood warmer may be used to heat blood safely to 49 degrees C.*' So long as the staff at Hillcrest Medical Center in Tulsa didn't warm Mrs. Levitt's blood above that temperature it would have been fine.

What is particularly interesting is that Herron's team used standard microwave blood warmers, meaning that by 1997 the medical profession had decided that heating blood with a microwave was no more dangerous than heating it by any other means.

(iv) Anti-infective elements in human breast milk

The fourth paper was about an investigation into the effect of thawing frozen human breast milk in a microwave.[532] These researchers found that microwaving the milk reduced the effectiveness of the antibacterial chemicals in it, with the result that when E. coli bacteria were then introduced and incubated at blood temperature for 3½ hours the bacteria multiplied much more rapidly than in similar milk which had not been heated in a microwave.

Evidently microwaving does affect some chemical properties of human milk. However there was no mention, in the abstract at least, that any comparison was made with milk heated by another means. It may be that it was simply heating human milk that

---

531 Herron D M et al. *The limits of bloodwarming: maximally heating blood with an inline microwave bloodwarmer.* Journal of Trauma, August 1997;43(2):219-26.
532 Quan R. *Effects of microwave radiation on anti-infective factors in human milk.* Pediatrics, April 1992; 89 (4 Pt 1):667-9.

reduced its bacteria-resistant properties. In any case microwaving the milk didn't make it more harmful, so nothing was discovered akin to the doomsday plagues prophesied on the popular websites.

The case for microwaving

After looking at those somewhat negative papers I did the obvious thing and looked for research on the effects of heating food in a microwave oven in general. Here is what I unearthed.

(i) Nitrosamines

In this first study the researchers compared the effects of cooking bacon by frying it in a pan and cooking it in a microwave. The reason they did this was that bacon and other cured meats contain a preservative called sodium nitrite, which can be converted to carcinogenic substances called nitrosamines on heating.

Half the test rashers were fried at either 171°C or 206°C. In both cases 11ng/g of nitrosamines were measured after cooking.[533] The remaining rashers were microwaved at 700w for 45 seconds or 75 seconds. The 45-second microwaved rashers had *no detectable nitrosamines* after cooking, while the 75-second rashers had approaching 5ng/g, less than half the quantity in the fried bacon.[534]

Conclusion: bacon cooked in a microwave is healthier than fried bacon.

(ii) Vitamins

In an investigation into the effects of microwaving infant formula milk the researchers concluded, *'There was no significant loss of either riboflavin or vitamin C.'*[535]

In a similar vein, a review of various studies made prior to 1985 concluded, *'Studies showed equal or better retention of nutrients for microwave, as compared with conventionally reheated foods, for thiamin, riboflavin, pyridoxine, folacin and ascorbic acid.'*[536]

---

533 ng/g means nanograms per gram. 1ng/g means 1 gram of nitrosamines in every 1,000,000,000 grams of bacon! If strips of bacon were laid end to end from Land's End to John o'Groats then the total length of bacon occupied by nitrosamines would be 1.4mm!

534 Miller B J. et al. *Formation of N-nitrosamines in microwaved versus skillet-fried bacon containing nitrite*. Food and Chemical Toxicology, May 1989; 27(5):295-9.

535 Sigman-Grant M et al. *Microwave heating of infant formula: a dilemma resolved*. Pediatrics, September 1992; 90(3):412-5.

536 Hoffman C J & Zabik M E. *Effects of microwave cooking/reheating on nutrients and food systems: a review of recent studies*. Journal of the American Dietetic Association, August 1985; 85(8):922-6.

In other words, microwaving preserves several important vitamins as well or better than other methods of heating food.

(iii) Antioxidants

What about antioxidants? In a comprehensive study the effects of boiling, microwaving, pressure-cooking, griddling, frying, and baking on the antioxidant activity of twenty different vegetables were evaluated and compared. The researchers concluded, *'Griddling, microwave cooking, and baking produce the lowest losses, while pressure-cooking and boiling lead to the greatest losses. Frying occupies an intermediate position. In short, water is not the cook's best friend when it comes to preparing vegetables.'*[537]

Microwaving came in joint first on the subject of antioxidant preservation!

(iv) Free radicals

And what about those 'harmful free radicals' we read about? Peanuts are a source of polyunsaturated fat, which on heating can oxidize and produce damaging free radicals. Nevertheless peanuts are usually roasted to improve their colour and flavour and to destroy any salmonella bacteria that are sometimes present.

Research was carried out in 2014 to compare the effects of roasting peanuts in a conventional oven and in a microwave.[538] Some oxidation did occur, but it *'was not significantly different between the roasting methods'*. Both methods killed previously inserted salmonella bacteria to a similar extent, and in both cases the peanuts looked and tasted just as nice!

Microwaving produces no more free radicals than cooking food in an oven does.

(v) Body chemistry

Finally, what about the effects of microwaved food on our bodies – the changes in our blood, tissues and body chemistry that it is supposed to induce? To assess these effects, diets containing beef, potatoes and vegetables were fed to ten male and ten female rats. The diet ingredients were cooked either in a microwave or by conventional methods, and were then freeze-dried, ground and mixed with supplements of vitamins and minerals to meet the rats' requirements. A second control group was fed a cereal-based rodent diet.

After 13 weeks almost everything possible was examined in the rats except their

---

537 Jiménez-Monreal A M et al. *Influence of cooking methods on antioxidant activity of vegetables.* Journal of Food Science, April 2009; 74(3):H97-H103.

538 Smith A L et al. *Oven, Microwave, and Combination Roasting of Peanuts: Comparison of Inactivation of Salmonella Surrogate Enterococcus faecium, Color, Volatiles, Flavor, and Lipid Oxidation.* Journal of Food Science, August 2014; 79(8):S1584-94.

memory, intelligence, emotional well-being... and the length of their whiskers.[539] The conclusion? *'The results indicated no adverse effects of the diets cooked by microwave compared with those cooked conventionally.'*[540]

Summary

I could find no evidence that heating food in a microwave oven renders it any more harmful than other methods of heating food. On the contrary there are some respects in which microwaved food is healthier than food heated or cooked by other means.

Whether there is a health risk in standing close to a microwave oven in operation is another question, which has been addressed in the main text.

---

539 Criteria to assess toxicity included clinical observations, ophthalmoscopy, growth, food and water intake, haematology, clinical chemistry, urinalysis, organ weights, micronucleated erythrocytes in bone marrow, gross examination at autopsy and microscopic examination of a wide range of organs.

540 Jonker D & Til H P. *Human diets cooked by microwave or conventionally: Comparative sub-chronic (13-wk) toxicity study in rats.* Food and Chemical Toxicology, April 1995; Issue 4:245-256.

Index

1

180degreehealth.com 77
1940s 4
    Diet 44
    Rickets controlled 116
1950s 4, 45

2

25-45-30 diet 251

3

3 day healthy menu 261A

Abdominal muscles
    Benefits of exercise 218
    Exercises 218
Abel and Cole
    Organic food deliveries 157
ABS. *See* Abdominal muscles
Advisory bodies
    Not always impartial 13
Aerobic exercise 206
    Benefits 206
    Moderate 206
    Vigorous 207
ALA. *See* Alpha-linolenic acid
Alcohol 171
    And diabetes 177
    And obesity 177
    Annual cost to NHS 34
    Annual cost to U.K. 172, 258
    Did Jesus Christ drink wine? 173
    Does red wine protect against heart disease?. 175
    Health warnings on labels 178
    Hospital admissions doubled in 10 years 174
    Household weekly expenditure 178, 252
    Moderate drinking 174
    U.K. advertizing expenditure 174

Alcohol dependency
    Prevalence in the U.K. 175
Allergenic foods
    Identification of 144
    List of 143
Allergies 140
    Definition 140
Allergy UK 140
Alpha-linolenic acid 64, 74
Alzheimer's disease
    Associated with nitrates 156
American Academy of Pediatrics
    Support for meat and dairy products 46
American Cancer Society
    Smoking 27
American Heart Association 19
    Financial support 13
    Fish/fish oil consumption recommendations.... 66
    Fish/fish oil recommendations 65
American Institute of Medicine
    Vitamin D requirements 115
Anaphylaxis 142
Anitschkov, Dr. N.
    Fed cholesterol to rabbits 7
Antibiotics
    In livestock rearing 154
Antioxidants 53
Appleton, Dr. N.
    Effects of sugar on health 90
Arterial plaque
    Cause of 25
Art of Manliness 190
A sick nation 34
Associations
    Are not proofs 9
    Between CHD and fat 8

B

Babyfood manufacturers

Cultivate taste for unnatural foods 245
Barbecues
    Health hazards 240
Barnett, Dr. L.
    Magnesium deficiency causes brittle bones .. 134
Basketball
    Calories 5
BBC
    Facts distorted to make headline 18
BBC Horizon programme
    High fat / high carbohydrate diets compared . 195
Bed time
    Routine with children 231
Beef
    Grass fed v. grain fed 75
    Omega ratio 75
Bentover row (upper body exercise) 216
Bergstrom, Samuelsson & Vane
    Nobel Prize for omega-3 research 57
Bible teaching about a rest day 227
Bicep curl (upper body exercise) 216
Big Mac. *See* Calories
Birnbaum, L.
    Endocrine disruptors in drinking water. 162
Birth rates
    Declining 179
Bisphenol A 181
    Absorbed by babies from neonatal equipment
        181
    Advice to avoid 183
    Effects on health 168
    In baby feeding bottles and cups 181
    In bottled water 168
    In breast milk... 181
    Prevalence in humans 182
BMI. *See* Body Mass Index
Body Mass Index
    Definition... 246
    Healthy and unhealthy ranges 246
Bottled water 167
    And BPA 168
Bowel cancer
    No association with red meat 18
    Prevalence and trends, Great Britain 38, 43
BPA
    See Bisphenol A 168
BPA-free
    May not be phthalate-free 183
Bread

Chorleywood process 6
Breast cancer
    Increase in 20th century 162
Breast milk
    Flavoured by mother's diet 245
Brita jug filters 170
British Dietetic Association 17
British Egg Information Service, The
    Egg-based breakfasts avert hunger 195
British Heart Foundation 19
    Health Promotion Research Group
        Research into moderate drinking 175
British Journal of Nutrition
    Caerphilly Project 25
British Medical Association 17
British Medical Journal 99
    Facts distorted in favour of fluoridation 166
    Salt and health 123
    Study of fluid intake requirements 159
British Medical Research Council
    Common Cold Unit closed 132
British Nutrition Foundation 13
    Energy density of common foods 196
Butter
    Consumption in U.S.A. 12
    Safer than margarine. 12
Buxton Natural Mineral Water 168

C

Cadmium in food 154
Caerphilly Project 25
Calf raise (lower body exercise) 217
Calories
    Big Mac 4
    Cross-trainer 5
    Deep pan pizza 4
    Recommended daily quantities 245
    Sponge pudding 4
    Used by exercise 5
Cancer
    Liver and bowel, prevalence and trends 38
Canola oil. *See* Rapeseed oil
Captain Cook's Tuck Box 237
Carbohydrates 93
    And heart disease 94
    And satiety 93
    And weight gain 93
    Dietary sources 93

    Effects on health 97
    Functions and sources 261
    Increase triglycerides 47
    Low carbohydrate diets reduce weight 193
CD. *See* Coeliac disease
CHD. *See* Coronary heart disease
Cheerfulness
    And health 233
Children learning to cook
    Benefits 235
Chlorinated water
    Associated with miscarriages 160
Cholecalciferol. *See* Vitamin D
Cholesterol 48, 99
    And eggs 101
    Blood level independent of fat intake 101
    Does not cause heart disease 99
    Functions 102
    High levels can be healthier 15
    In elderly people 99
    In women 100
    Kills rabbits 7
    Little in arterial plaque 14
    Needed for testosterone production 185
    Not established as cause of heart disease 20
    No trials on cardiovascular health 14
    Suppressed by statins 20
Cholesterol lowering spreads 14
Chorleywood process 6
Cochrane Reviews 123
    Salt and health 123
Coconut oil
    And testosterone 189
Coeliac disease 140, 146
Colds
    A zinc-based cure? 131
Colic 142
COMA. *See* Committee on Medical Aspects of Food and Nutrition Policy
Comfort eating 198
Commando Workout
    4 week guide to total fitness 213
Committee on Medical Aspects of Food and Nutrition Policy
    Recommended proportions of macronutrients 249
Common Cold Unit 132
Cookery. *See* Home cookery
Cookery books for beginners 238
Cooking oils

    Effects of burnt oils on health 51
Cooling down 222
Corineus and Gogmagog 78
Coronary heart disease
    And cholesterol 99
    And diet 23
    And glycaemic load 95
    And stress 29
    Causes 27
    Coronary Prevention Study 24
    Cost to NHS 34
    Deaths
        6 countries 8
        22 countries 11
        Trends 8
        U.S.A. 7, 11
    Deaths and trends
        England and Wales 38
        U.S.A. 38
    Diet related 33
    Helsinki study of low fat diets 24
    Incidence
        France 10
        India 10
    Linked to fat consumption 8
    Linked to overwork 226
    Multiple Risk Factor Intervention Trial 23
    Prevalence and trends
        England and Wales 38, 41
        U.S.A. 38, 40
    Prudent Diet 23
    Risk factors 33
Coronary Prevention Study 24
Cost
    Of alcohol to U.K. 34, 172, 258
    Of diabetes and obesity in Scotland 137
    Of obesity to NHS 34
Cost of a healthy diet 252
Cottonseed oil 75
Couch to 5K
    NHS 9 week exercise video 213
C-reactive protein 166
Cross-trainer
    Calories 5
Crunch with feet flat (ABS exercise) 218
Crunch with legs up (ABS exercise) 218
Cryptorchidism
    Increase in 20th century 162
Cryptosporidium 169

307

Curly hair stories 87
CVD. *See* Coronary heart disease
Cycling
    Calories 5

D

Dancing
    Calories 5
Daniel, prophet 2
Danone
    Water products 158
DBP. *See* Phthalates
Deans, Dr. E.
    Magnesium and mental health 135
Deep pan pizza. *See* Calories
DEHP. *See* Phthalates
Dehydration
    Effects 158
    Symptoms 158
Delegation
    In the family 261
Dental fluorosis 163
Depression
    A modern illness 135
    And walking 206
    Can be caused by magnesium deficiency 135
    Prevalence in England and U.S.A. 135
Derriford Hospital
    Overweight children 35
DHA. *See* Docosahexaenoic acid
Diabetes 87
    And alcohol 177
    Associated with nitrates 156
    Cost to NHS in Scotland 137
    Deaths, England 38
    In children 1
    Prevalence and trends, England and U.S.A. 38, 41
    Type 2 reversed 257
Diabetes UK 20
Diarrhoea 148
Diet
    25-45-30 diet described 251
    1950s 5
    And coronary heart disease 33
    Changes in 20th century 44
    COMA recommendations for proportions of macronutrients 249
    Healthy proportions of protein, fat and carbohydrates 249
    High fat / high carbohydrate diets compared . 195
    Historical 242
    Inuits 60
    Israel 60
    Macronutrients in traditional diets 249
    Recommendations in 20th century 45
    Recommendations in 21st century 46
    Traditional Japanese 60
    U.S.A. 60
Dietary Cohort Consortium
    No association between red meat and bowel cancer 18
Dietary deficiencies 126
    Discovering the source of 137
Dietary supplements
    Example 122
Dihydrotestosterone 187
Disease
    And stress 29
Docosahexaenoic acid 63
Docosapentaenoic acid 64
DPA. *See* Docosapentaenoic acid
Drinks
    And tooth decay 80, 83
Drinks industry
    U.K. advertizing expenditure 174
Dummies and teethers 183

E

Eat Well, Live Well
    Dietary recommendations 45
Eau-yes.co.uk
    Home water filtration system 170
Eby, G.
    Depression caused by magnesium deficiency 135
    Zinc-based cold cure? 131
E.coli 169
Ectopic pregnancies
    Increase in 20th century 162
Eggs
    And cholesterol 101
    Boost testosterone production 188
    Egg-based breakfasts avert hunger 195
Eicosapentaenoic acid 63
Endocrine disruptors 162
    Advice to avoid 183

Detected in surface waters 162
In drinking water 180
In most plastic food packaging 182
In plastic packaging and food containers 181
Not cause of falling sperm count claim.......... 162
Safety of drinking water................................. 162
Endocrine Society
Vitamin D advice.. 115
Endocrine system 162
Energy density of common foods 196
Enig, Dr. M.
Macronutrients in traditional diets 249
Omega-3 76
Environmental Protection Agency
Permitted levels of fluorides in drinking water
.... 164
Environmental Working Group
Report on tap water purity in the U.S.A......... 160
EPA. *See* Eicosapentaenoic acid
Erhardt, M.
Died after working for 72 hours..................... 225
Eskimos. *See* Inuits
European Food Safety Authority
Fluid intake recommendations 158
European Heart Journal
Cholesterol and CHD 20
Eurycoma longifolia Jack
And testosterone 189
Exercise 201
Aerobic 206
And life expectancy.. 199
And weight loss.. 199
A weekly programme 223
Benefits.. 200, 205
For abdominal muscles 218
For adults.. 213
For children 211
For lower body 217
For upper body 216
Recommended amounts 211
Start young 201
Ten motivational suggestions......................... 202
Expenditure on alcohol 252
Expenditure on food and drink 252

F

Facts distorted to make headline
BBC 18

Independent Newspaper 18
Family health 242
FAO
See UN Food and Agriculture Organization 97
Fat
Campaign of misinformation 7
Fatigue... 232
Causes 232
Remedies 232
Fats .... 48. *See* also Saturated, Monounsatured, Polyunsaturated & Trans fats
Choice of for cooking....................................... 51
Cleaning 51
Cooking with lard and dripping 51
Dietary sources... 48
Functions and sources 261
Fertility. *See* also Infertility, Sperm counts falling, Testosterone
And testosterone... 184
Fibre
Bad for IBS 148
Film about saturated fat 13, 25
Financial power and influence. *See* Supermarkets, Food industry, Pharmaceutical manufacturers
Fish
Omega-3 contents.................................... 64, 261
Fish/fish oil
Consumption recommendations................. 65, 66
Fish oil
Effectiveness compared with fish..................... 67
Fish oil consumption
Derivation of recommendations..................... 261
Five A Day
Not generally practised 120
Suggested amendment..................................... 86
Flax oil
Omega ratio.. 74
Flaxseed oil
Effectiveness compared with fish..................... 67
Flora
Change of spread formula 55
Pro.activ and cholesterol 14
Flour
Refining removes minerals............................ 120
Fluid intake
Daily requirements... 159
NHS recommendations 158
No evidence for NHS recommendations........ 158

309

Fluoridated toothpaste
- Doubles level of fluoride in blood 164
- Not for young children 164
- Toxicity 164

Fluoridated water
- Increases dental problems 165
- No overall benefit 165
- Prevalence in U.S.A. and U.K. 163

Fluoridation
- Facts distorted to promote it 166

Fluoride-free toothpastes 164

Fluorides and fluorine
- Home removal 170

Fluorine compounds
- In tea 166
- Linked to impaired mental ability 164
- Make brittle bones 164

Fluorine controversy 163

Food
- Advertizing 236
- Home cooked is healthier 235
- Quantities required 245
- Reducing the cost 258

Food allergies
- Causes of increasing prevalence 141
- Distinguished from food intolerance 140
- Prevalence 140
- Symptoms 141

Food and drink
- Weekly expenditure 252

Food and symptom diary 144

Food and Water Watch
- U.S. government promotion of GM food 16

Food consumption
- Fruit and vegetables 120

Food industry
- Financial power and influence 16

Food intolerance 140
- Causes of increasing prevalence 141
- Distinguished from food allergy 140
- Prevalence 141
- Symptoms 142

Food packaging
- Most plastics contain endocrine disruptors 182

Food Standards Agency
- Comparison between organic and non-organic food 150
- Dietary recommendations 46
- Film about saturated fat 13

Fish/fish oil recommendations 65
Recommendations for fish consumption 63

Football matches
- Food suggestions 97

Forbes' Billionaires list 227

Framingham Heart Study 100

Free radicals 52
- Effects on health 53

Front squat (lower body exercise) 217

Fructose
- And type 2 diabetes 88
- And waist circumference 249
- Effects on Health 85

Fruit and vegetables
- Average consumption in U.K. 120

Fruit juice
- And health 84

Fuerteventura 159

G

Gardening
- Calories 5

Garland, Dr. C. F.
- Vitamin D requirements 114

Genetically modified food
- Promoted by U.S. government 16

GI. *See* Glycaemic index

Glutathione 53

Gluten 146
- Intolerance 145
- Sensitivity 147

Gluten free food
- Not healthier for normal people 147

Glycaemic index
- Definition 97

Glycaemic load
- And diabetes 98
- And heart disease 95
- Definition 97
- Of common foods 261

GM food. *See* Genetically modified food

Good and bad cholesterol 103

Granulated carbon 169

Grapeseed oil
- And testosterone 189

Grehlin
- Hunger-stimulating hormone 195

Groves, B.

Fats 50
Growth hormones
    In livestock rearing 154
Guyanet, S.
    Vitamin D requirements 115

H

HDL. *See* High density lipoprotein
HDL/Total cholesterol ratio 191
Health
    And cheerfulness 233
    And stress 29
    Complete recipe for 244
Health Canada Food Directorate
    No health risk from BPA 182
Health care
    Cost of private in the U.S.A. 259
Health charities
    Motivation 19
    Not scientific institutions 20
Healthy diet
    25-45-30 diet described 251
    Cost of 252
    Proportions of protein, fat and carbohydrates 249
Healthy food and drink 244
Healthy menu for 3 days 261
Heart attacks
    Cause of 25
Heart disease. *See* Coronary heart disease
Heart rate, maximum 221
Heart UK 20
Helicobacter pylori 130
Helsinki Study
    Low fat diets 24
Hepatitis A 169
High density lipoprotein 103
High fat diets
    Can reduce weight 193
High fructose corn syrup 80, 89
High-intensity Interval Training 219
    Benefits 219
    Health warning 221
    In a weekly exercise programme 223
    Typical session 221
Highland Spring Water 168
Highly unsaturated fatty acids
    Associated with CHD death rates 60, 61
High oleic sunflower oil 75

HIT. *See* High-intensity Interval Training
Holdcroft, C. J.
    Facts distorted in favour of fluoridation 166
Holick, Dr. M. F.
    Vitamin D requirements 114
Holidays
    Ideas for family holidays 233
    Importance for children 233
    Suggestions for exercise 224
Holland & Barrett
    Fish/fish oil recommendations 65
Home cookery 235
    Benefits 235
    Finding time 236
    How to learn to cook 237
Honey
    And teeth 80
H. pylori. *See* Helicobacter pylori
HUFA. *See* Highly unsaturated fatty acids.
Hydration For Health
    Financial sponsors 158
    Fluid intake recommendations 158
Hypogonadism, male
    Associated with zinc deficiency 186
    Definition and symptoms 184
Hyponatremia 159

I

IBS. *See* Irritable bowel syndrome
IBS Network 147
IgE. *See* Immunoglobulin E
IHerb 116
Immunoglobulin E 140
Independent Newspaper
    Facts distorted to make headline 18
Indole-3-carbinol 188
Infertility 179
    Solved by zinc supplementation 187
    Summary of causes for decline 190
Insulin 87
International Cod Liver Omega-3 Foundation
    Recommendations for omega-3 intake 63
Intolerable foods
    Identification of 144
    List of 143
Inuits
    Diet 60
Ion exchange 169

311

Irritable bowel syndrome 147
Israel
    Diet 60
    Ill health 60

J

Japan
    Traditional diet 60
Jews
    Among world's wealthiest men 227
Jogging
    Calories. *See* also Running
Johnson, Dr. D.
    Tooth-decaying drinks 80
Journal of Alzheimer's Disease
    Nitrates and human health 156
Journal of Epidemiology 99
Journal of Evaluation of Clinical Practice
    Cholesterol and CVD 100
Jug water filters 170

K

Kenny, Prof. P.
    Addictive snacks 198
Keys, Dr. A. 7
    6 countries 8
    22 countries 11
Kinsey, A.
    Frequency of sexual intercourse 204
Krill oil
    Effectiveness compared with fish 67

L

Lancet, The
    Arterial plaque 14
Lands, Dr. B.
    Omega fatty acids and CHD 61
Lard
    Omega ratio 75
L-Arginine
    Penile erection 189
Lateral raise (upper body exercise) 216
Lawrence, F.
    Breast milk flavoured by mother's diet 245
LDL. *See* Low density lipoprotein
Leg raise (ABS exercise) 218
Leydig cells 189
Life Expectancy
    Linked to exercise 199
Linseed oil. *See* Flax oil
Lipid peroxidation 52
Lipoproteins ..103. *See* also Low and High density lipoprotein
Liver
    Cholesterol production 103
    Functions 103
Liver cancer
    Prevalence and trends, Great Britain 38, 42
LongJack. *See* Eurycoma longifolia Jack
Loperamide 148
Low density lipoprotein 103
Low fat diets. *See* also Diet
    And heart disease 94
    And older women 94
    And triglycerides 47
    Caerphilly Project 25
    Coronary Prevention Study 24
    Helsinki Study 24
    Multiple Risk Factor Intervention Trial 23
    Prudent Diet 23
Low fat yogurt
    Not so healthy 196
Lunge (lower body exercise) 217

M

Macronutrients
    Definition and recommended proportions 249
Macular degeneration
    Associated with excessive carbohydrates 97
Magnesium 132
    And depression 135
    Daily intake recommendations 136
    Deficiency causes brittle bones 134
    Deficiency widespread 133
    Dietary sources 120, 132, 136
    Effects of deficiency 133
    Functions 133
    In eggs 119
Malaysian ginseng. *See* Eurycoma longifolia Jack
Mann, Prof. G. 10
    Masai diet and heart disease 10
Marathon running
    May strain the heart 220
Margarine
    Consumption in U.S.A. 11
Masai tribe 10

McCance & Widdowson
  The Composition of Foods 118
McKay, B.
  Experiment to raise testosterone level 190
Medical Research Council
  Caerphilly Project 25
Melatonin 53
Menu for 3 days 261
Mercola, Dr.
  Effects of dehydration 158
Metchnikoff, E.
  Yogurt may alleviate IBS symptoms 149
Microwaved food
  Noxious or nutritious? 261
Microwave ovens 238
  Alleged dangers 238
  Benefits 238
  Danger to eyes 239
  Safe use 239
Milled flaxseed 69
Minerals 118
  Declining food content 118
  Definition 118
  Dietary sources 120
  Functions and sources 261
  How to obtain sufficient 122, 254
Mineral water 167
Moderate drinking 174, 175
Monounsaturated fats 48
Moritz Erhardt
  Died after working for 72 hours 225
Motivation
  Holiday suggestions for exercise 224
  Needed by children to exercise 201
  Ten suggestions to encourage exercise 202
Multiple Risk Factor Intervention Trial 23
Myerson, Dr. A.
  Sunlight can triple testosterone levels 188

N

National Foundation for Celiac Awareness 147
National Health and Nutrition Examination Survey, U.S.A.
  Prevalence of BPA in humans 182
National Health Service. *See* also Cost
  5 week exercise plan 203
  A sickness service 54
  BMI ranges 246
  Costs 34
  Couch to 5K exercise video 213
  Dietary recommendations 46
  Fluid intake recommendations 158
  Magnesium intake recommendations 136
  Recommended daily calories 245
National Institute for Health and Care Excellence
  Advice on sterols and stanols 14
National Institute of Environmental Health Sciences
  Endocrine disruptors in drinking water. 162
National Institutes of Health
  Fish/fish oil recommendations 65
  Vitamin D research 115
  Zinc deficiency statistics 128
Natural Hydration Council
  Fluid intake recommendations 158
  Sponsors 158
NHS. *See* National Health Service
NICE. *See* National Institute for Health and Care Excellence
Nichols, Dr. M.
  Research into moderate drinking 175
Nitrates
  Common dietary sources 156
  Effects on health 156
Nitrosamines
  In cured meats 240
Non steroidal anti inflammatory drugs 58
Norwegian Heart Study
  Cholesterol and CVD 100
NSAIDS. *See* Non steroidal anti inflammatory drugs
Nurses' Study
  Glycaemic load and carbohydrates 95
  Glycaemic load and heart attacks 95
  Sugar and diabetes 88
  Sugar and heart attacks 90
  Trans fats a disaster 56
  Trans fats and heart disease 45
Nutrients. *See* also also Vitamins and Minerals
  Causes of deficiencies 126
  Functions and sources 261
  Mineral content of food declining 118, 119
Nuts
  Source of protein 76

313

O

O-6-3 ratio. *See* also Omega ratio
   Definition 60
Obesity 34, 84
   And alcohol 177
   And triglycerides 47
   And vitamin D deficiency 113
   Consequences 34, 37
   Cost to NHS 34
   Cost to NHS in Scotland 137
   Definition 34
   In children 34
   Not recognized or acknowledged 35
   Obese children eat less saturated fat 194
   Prevalence 35
   Projected costs 37
   Statistics 1
   Trends 35
   Worst snacks 198
Oestrogen 180
Office for National Statistics
   Weekly food expenditure 252
Oils for cooking 75
Olive oil
   And testosterone 189
Omega-3
   Added to spreads, etc. 57
   Amounts of different supplements required 69
   Behaviour problems caused by deficiency 58
   Contents of marine foods 261
   Cost of different supplements 69
   Dietary sources 62
   Health problems caused by deficiency 57, 58
   In canned fish 62
   Supplements 66
   Too little causes inflammation 57
Omega-3 fatty acids
   Types 63
Omega-6
   Associated with CHD death rates 60
   Foods high in Omega-6 77
   Health problems caused by surplus 58
   How to reduce consumption 76
   Too much causes inflammation 57
Omega fatty acids 57
   Build signalling molecules 57
   Compete for enzymes 57
Omega ratio
   How to achieve a healthy level 253
   Importance 57
   In organic food 76
   Ways to achieve healthy levels 62
   Ways to correct imbalance 62
Ondansetron 148
ONS. *See* Office for National Statistics
Organic food
   Comparison between organic and non-organic food 150
   Fewer pesticides 153
   Magnesium content of eggs 119
   Mineral content not declined 119
   Omega ratios 76, 151
Overweight
   Not recognized or acknowledged 35
Overwork 225
   Linked to heart disease 226
   Linked to stress-related illnesses 226
Oxidative stress
   Effects on health 53
Oysters 187
Ozone gas
   As drinking water disinfectant 161

P

Pacifiers. *See* Dummies and teethers
Palm oil 76
Parabens 191
Parkinson's disease
   Associated with nitrates 156
Parks, E. J.
   Low fat and triglycerides 47
Partially hydrogenated vegetable oil. *See* Trans fats
Peanut butter 77
Peanut oil 75
Penile erection
   L-Arginine. *See* also Testosterone
Pennsylvania State University
   Testosterone dependent on dietary fat 185
Pesticides
   Health effects 153
   Less in organic food 153
Pesticides Residues Committee 154
Pharmaceutical manufacturers
   Advertising literature 18
   Financial power and influence 17

Questionable research	17
Pheidippides	220
Phthalates	182
Advice to avoid	183
Produce abnormalities in rats	182
pH value	
Common drinks	80
Plaque. *See* Arterial plaque	
Polycarbonate plastic	183
Polyphenols	166
Polyunsaturated fats	48
Effects on health	53
In arterial plaque	14
Oxidation	52
Pork	
Grass fed v. grain fed	75
Press-ups (upper body exercise)	216
Pro.active. *See* Flora	
Probiotic yogurt	
And testosterone	189
May alleviate IBS symptoms	149
Prostatic cancer	
Increase in 20th century	162
Protein	
Assuages hunger longer	195
For vegetarians	251
Functions and sources	261
Helps to sustain weight loss	196
Suppresses grehlin production	195
Suppresses hunger	195
Prudent Diet	23
Pureflo.co.uk	170
Purified water	168

R

Rabbit food stories	87
Rabbits	
And cholesterol	7
Rapeseed oil	
Omega ratio	75
Ravnskov, Dr. U.	
A hypothesis out of date	99
Egg diet experiment	101
Vitamin D requirements	114
Recipe for family health	244
Recipes for 3 day menu	261
Red meat	
No association with bowel cancer	18

Red wine	
Does it protect against heart disease?	175
Refining	
Minerals removed	120
Research	
Not always impartial	17
Rest	225
Rest day	227
Benefits	227
Bible teaching	227
Reverse osmosis	169
Filters	170
Rhode Island Hospital	
Nitrates and health	156
Rickets	
A contemporary problem	113
Controlled in 1940s	116
Rockefeller Foundation, The	225
Rockefeller, J.D.	
Outline of life	225
Rodale, J. I.	
Magnesium content of eggs	119
Royal Canadian Air Force	
5BX/XBX daily exercises	203
Royal Canadian Mounted Police	
Free on-line 12 week fitness programme	203
Rubber, guayule	
For Dummies and teethers	184
Rubber, natural	
For Dummies and teethers	184

S

Sabbath. *See* Rest day	
Saccharin	199
SACN. *See* Scientific Advisory Committee on Nutrition	
Salt	122
Advice summary	125
Content of ready meals	125
Effects on health reviewed	123
Functions	123
In home cooked food	124
Recommended intake	124
Research shortcomings	124
Too little can be harmful	124
Satiety	195
Saturated fat	48
Assists weight loss.	193

Assuages hunger longer 195
Campaign of misinformation 7
Dietary sources.. 50
Essential functions 50
Needed for cholesterol production 185
Needed for testosterone production 185
Not associated with CHD......................... 23, 25
Obese children eat less saturated fat 194
The truth 23
Scientific Advisory Committee on Nutrition
Fish/fish oil recommendations 65
Recommendations for omega-3 intake............ 63
Sugar 91
Seafood
Omega-3 contents... 261
Senna.. 148
Sexual intercourse
Frequency survey 204
Sharma, Dr. H.
Free radicals and disease 53
Sharpe, Prof. R
Comment on falling sperm counts 179
Shoulder press (upper body exercise)............... 216
Silicone rubber... 184
Sit ups (ABS exercise).................................... 218
Sleep
Getting to sleep 230
How much is needed? 229
Importance...229
Waking in the night 231
Smoking 27
Snacking.. 197
Snacks
For Kids.. 82
Healthy 98
Sodium nitrite
And nitrosamines 240
Soil Association, The 157
Somatostatin.. 221
Soothers. See Dummies and teethers
Soya oil
And testosterone.. 189
Sperm counts falling
33% decrease in France in only 16 years 161
42% decrease worldwide................................ 162
50% decrease in developed countries 179
Due to agricultural chemicals......................... 161
Not confirmed... 162
Sponge pudding. See Calories

Spring water.. 168
Stairs
Calories 5
Starch, starches. See Carbohydates
Static squat (lower body exercise)..................... 217
Statins
And cholesterol 20
Functionality 20
May reduce testosterone production 185
Step-up (lower body exercise) 217
Sterols and stanols
Health warnings 14
Straight dead lift (lower body exercise)............ 217
Strength and Flexibility
NHS 5 week exercise plan 203
Strength training................................. 207, 208, 214
Benefits... 218
For older women 209
For younger women 209
Health warning 217
Programme 219
Stress 29
And coronary heart disease 29
And disease 29
And health 29
Consequences 29
In family life.. 30
Reduced by drinking tea................................ 166
Reduction strategies 30
Warning signs 256
Stretching after exercise.................................... 222
Sucralose 199
Sugar 79
And children 79
And heart disease 89
And obesity 84
And teeth 80
And Type 2 diabetes 87
Functions and sources 261
Health effects on children 90
Historical use.. 242
In foods and drinks.. 84
Sunflower oil... 75
Supermarkets
Encourage over-eating...................................... 5
Financial power and influence 14
Sweets
Strategies to limit tooth decay......................... 83
Swimming

Calories 5

T

Tea
   And skeletal fluorosis 166
   Health benefits 166
Teaching children to cook
   Benefits 235
Teats. *See* Dummies and teethers
Teeth
   Preventing decay 82
Teetotalism
   Prevalence in the U.K. 176
Tegaserod 148
Testosterone 180, 184
   And ageing 190
   Beneficial foods 188
   Dependent on proportions of dietary fats 185
   How to increase levels 190
   Increases immediately after exercise 188
   Production depends on adequate vitamin D ... 188
   Production depends on adequate zinc 186
   Reduced by eating polyunsaturated fat 185
   Significant decline in men since 1972 184
   Symptoms of deficiency and excess 184
The Endocrine Disruptor Hypothesis 161
The World's Healthiest Foods website 144
THMs. *See* Trihalomethanes
Thomas, D.
   Mineral content of food 118
Three Peaks Challenge 213
Time
   Finding time for home cookery 260
   Finding time through delegation 260
Tiredness. *See* Fatigue
Tongkat ali. *See* Eurycoma longifolia Jack
Tooth decay
   Cause of 80
   Prevention in toddlers 82
Tooth-decaying drinks 80
Towton, Battle of 80
Trans fats 10, 48, 55
Tree of knowledge 1
Tricep dip (upper body exercise) 216
Triglycerides 103
   And low fat diets 47
   And obesity 47
   Definition 33
   Increased by carbohydrate consumption 47
Triglycerides/HDL ratio 191
Trihalomethanes
   In impure chlorinated water 160
   Permitted limits in drinking water 160
Type 2 diabetes. *See* Diabetes
Types of water 167

U

U.K. Drinking Water Inspectorate
   \ 162
Ultraviolet C 169
Ultraviolet light 113
UN Food and Agriculture Organization
   Glycaemic index 97
United States Department of Agriculture
   Recommended daily calories 245
University of Newcastle
   Comparison between organic and non-organic food 151
   Overweight children 35
University of Oxford
   Research into moderate drinking 175
University of Stanford
   Comparison between organic and non-organic food 150
University of York Centre for Reviews and Dissemination
   No overall benefit in drinking water fluoridation 165
Unsaturated fats 48, 51
   Dietary sources 10, 51
   Oxidation 51
Uric acid 53
U.S.A.
   Diet 60
USDA. *See* United States Department of Agriculture
U.S.Department of Health and Human Services
   Reduction in permitted fluorides in drinking water 164
U.S.National Academy of Sciences
   Dental fluorosis 163
U.S. National Institutes of Health. *See* National Institutes of Health
UVB. *See* Ultraviolet light

V

van Tulleken, X. & C.
    High fat / high carbohydrate diets compared . 195
Vegetable oil. *See* Rapeseed oil
Vegetables
    And testosterone 188
    Health benefits 86
    How to cook 121
Vegetarians 74
    Protein requirements 251
VITAL vitamin D research project 115
Vitamin C 53
Vitamin D 114
    And mineral absorption 121
    And obesity 113
    And testosterone 188
    Dementia risk not proved 18
    People at risk of deficiency 115
    Requirements 114
    Supplements 114, 116
Vitamin D3. *See* Vitamin D
Vitamin drops
    Collection difficulties 116
    Provided by NHS 66
Vitamin E 53
Vitamins
    Dietary sources 120
    Functions and sources 261
    How to obtain sufficient 122, 254

W

Waist circumference
    And fructose 249
    Recommended limits for children 248
Waist to hip ratio
    Recommended limits for adults 248
Walking
    Benefits 205
    Calories 5
Walnuts
    Omega-3 ratio 76
Warming up 222
Water 158
    Bottled 167
    Contaminants 169
    Daily requirements 159
    Home treatment methods 169
    Intoxication (hyponatremia) 159

    Jug filters 170
    Mineral 167
    NHS intake recommendations 158
    No evidence for NHS intake recommendations
        158
    Problems with chlorination 160
    Public drinking water supplies 160
    Purified 168
    Spring 168
    Summary of daily requirements 255
    Types 167
Water Act, 2003
    Promoted fluoridation 165
Waterson, S.
    Commando Workout 213
Weight gain
    Worst snacks 198
Weight loss 193
    And exercise 199
    And snacking 197
    Assisted by eating saturated fat 193
    Assisted by inclusion of dairy products 194
Weights
    Commercial sets 214
    Home made 215
    How heavy should they be? 215
Weight Watchers
    Pro Points plan 195
Wharram Percy excavation site 80
Wheaton, J.
    GM food labelling bill 16
Wheat sensitivity 144
Whey protein 251
Whitford, Dr. G.
    Tea in large quantities produces skeletal fluorosis
        166
Whitten, P. & Whiteside, P.J.
    Frequency of sexual intercourse among athletes
        204
Whorwell, Prof. P.
    Irritable bowel syndrome 148
WHR. *See* Waist to hip ratio
Wing, R.R. & Phelan, S.
    Study on maintaining weight loss 193
Wingspread Statement 161
Women
    And cholesterol 100
World Health Organization
    1990 report 46

    Coronary Prevention Study 24
    Dietary recommendations 45
    Glycaemic index... 97
World Wildlife Fund
    Endocrine disruption 161

X

Xenooestrogens.. 182

Y

Yerushalmy, J. & Hilleboe, H.
    Publication of Keys's full data 10
Yogurt making.. 149
Yudkin, Prof. J.
    Sugar and heart disease   89

Z

ZeroWater jug filters   170
Zinc   128
    Causes of deficiency   127
    Deficiency in children and adults   130
    Deficiency in infants   129
    Deficiency in older people   130
    Deficiency statistics   128
    Dietary sources   128, 187
    Effects of deficiency   129
    Functions   128
    Supplementation   131

ERRATA

Page v. Contents.
 Insert the following two lines:
 CHAPTER 16: WATER – A SPRING OF LIFE OR A LOW-LEVEL POISON?   158
 CHAPTER 17: ALCOHOL – THE SACRED COW   171

Page 10, paragraph 3, line 3.
 Insert 'even' before 'the association between deaths'.

Page 17, paragraph 2, line 1.
 Insert 'they' after 'the main reason'.

Page 24, paragraph 3, line 5.
 Change 'After 15 years' to '18 years after the trials began'

Page 40, Figure 10.
 Replace Figure 10 with the following figure.

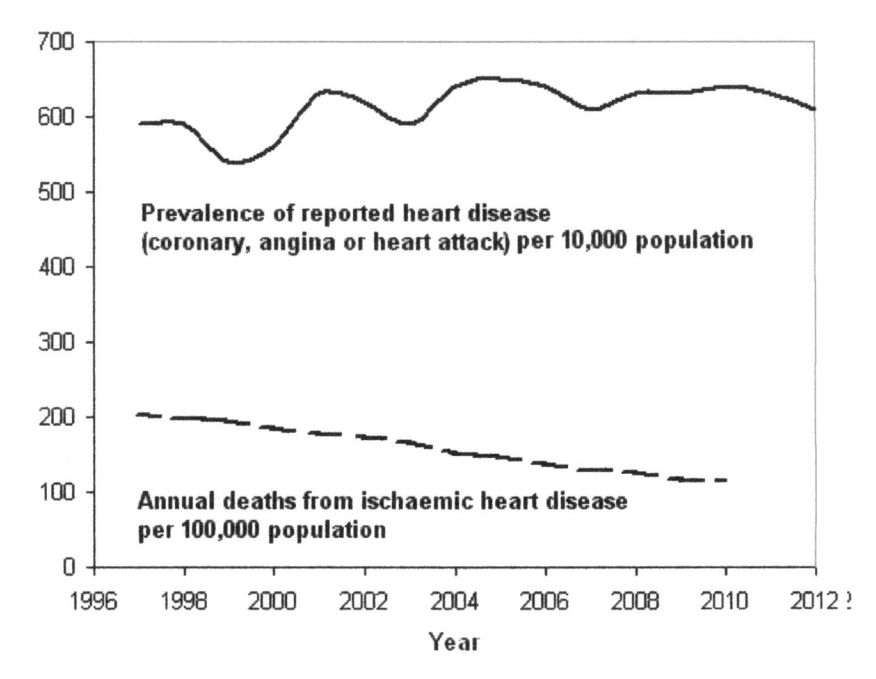

Page 70, Table 4. Insert three missing costs as follows:
 Krill oil capsules: £17.70
 Flaxseed oil capsules: £30.86
 Hemp oil: £21.64

Page 221, Table 14. The contents of this table have been printed in error on Page 222.